Supplement Field Guide
A CLINICAL PHARMACIST'S GUIDE TO YOUNG LIVING™ SUPPLEMENTS

DR. ASHLEY H. CRIBB

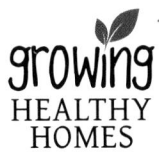

Copyright © 2022 Ashley Cribb. Photography copyright © 2022 Hannah Johnson. Book design copyright © 2022 Growing Healthy Homes. All rights reserved. No part of this publication shall be reproduced or transmitted in any form or by any electronic, mechanical, photocopying or recording means, or otherwise, without permission in writing from the copyright holder, except by a reviewer who may quote brief passages in a review.

No patent liability is assumed with respect to the use of the information contained herein. Although every precaution has been taken in the preparation of this publication, the author and publisher assumes no responsibility for errors or omissions. Neither is any liability assumed for damages resulting from the use of information contained herein.

ISBN: 978-1-7370846-4-8
Printed in the United States of America
First printing.

Growing Healthy Homes LLC
5701 SE Adams
Bartlesville, OK 74006

To obtain additional copies of this book, please visit
www.GrowingHealthyHomes.com.

Please note: I am not here to diagnose, treat, prevent or cure any diseases. Nor am I intending to take the place of your individual health practitioners. The information included in this book is for your own personal use and health empowerment. As always, I highly recommend finding a primary care provider that you love and trust to bring this information to and make decisions about your health.

For all supplements and regimens listed in this book, keep out of reach of children. If you are pregnant, nursing, taking medication, or have a medical condition, consult a health professional prior to use.

table of contents

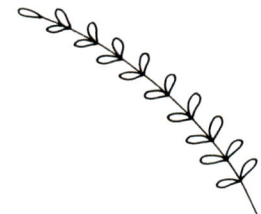

INTRODUCTION 7

CHAPTER 1 Why We Need To Supplement 9

CHAPTER 2 Conventional Supplements vs. Young Living Supplements 11
    Young Living Supplements at a Glance 13-19

CHAPTER 3 Foundational Supplements 21
    Protocols for Daily Health 59
        Overall Wellness (Male and Female)
        Options to Target Energy & Vitality
        Pre- and Post-natal

CHAPTER 4 Targeted Supplements 61

    PART 1: Supplements to Support the Endocrine System (Hormones, Thyroid, and Adrenals) 63
        Protocols For Thyroid, Adrenal, and Hormone Balance 87
            Mood & Emotions
            Stress Recovery (Adrenal Health)
            Thyroid Health
            Women's Health & Hormone Balance
            Men's Health & Hormone Balance

    PART 2: Supplements for the Immune System 91
        Protocols For Immune System Support 104
            Immune System (Daily Support)
            Immune System (Acute Needs)

    PART 3: Digestive Supplements 107
        Protocols For Digestive Health 126
            Overall Digestive Health (For Most Adults)
            Targeted Digestive Health

PART 4: Cleansing & Liver Support Supplements 129
    Protocols For Cleansing & Liver Health 145
        Cleansing
        Daily Liver Support

PART 5: Supplements For Bone & Muscle Support 147
    Protocols For Bone & Muscle Health 164
        Muscle & Bone Health
        Physical Fitness & Performance
        Aging Support

PART 6: Other Targeted Supplements (Heart, Bladder, Eyes, Brain) 167
    Protocols For Targeted Needs 179
        Cardiovascular Health
        Cognitive Support
        Diabetes Support
        Beauty & Skincare

PART 7: Children's Supplements 181
    Protocols For Children's Health 190
        Children's Health

PART 8: Nutritional Supplements 193

CHAPTER 5 Protocol Suggestions 205

Conventional Supplements & Young Living Alternatives 211

References 213

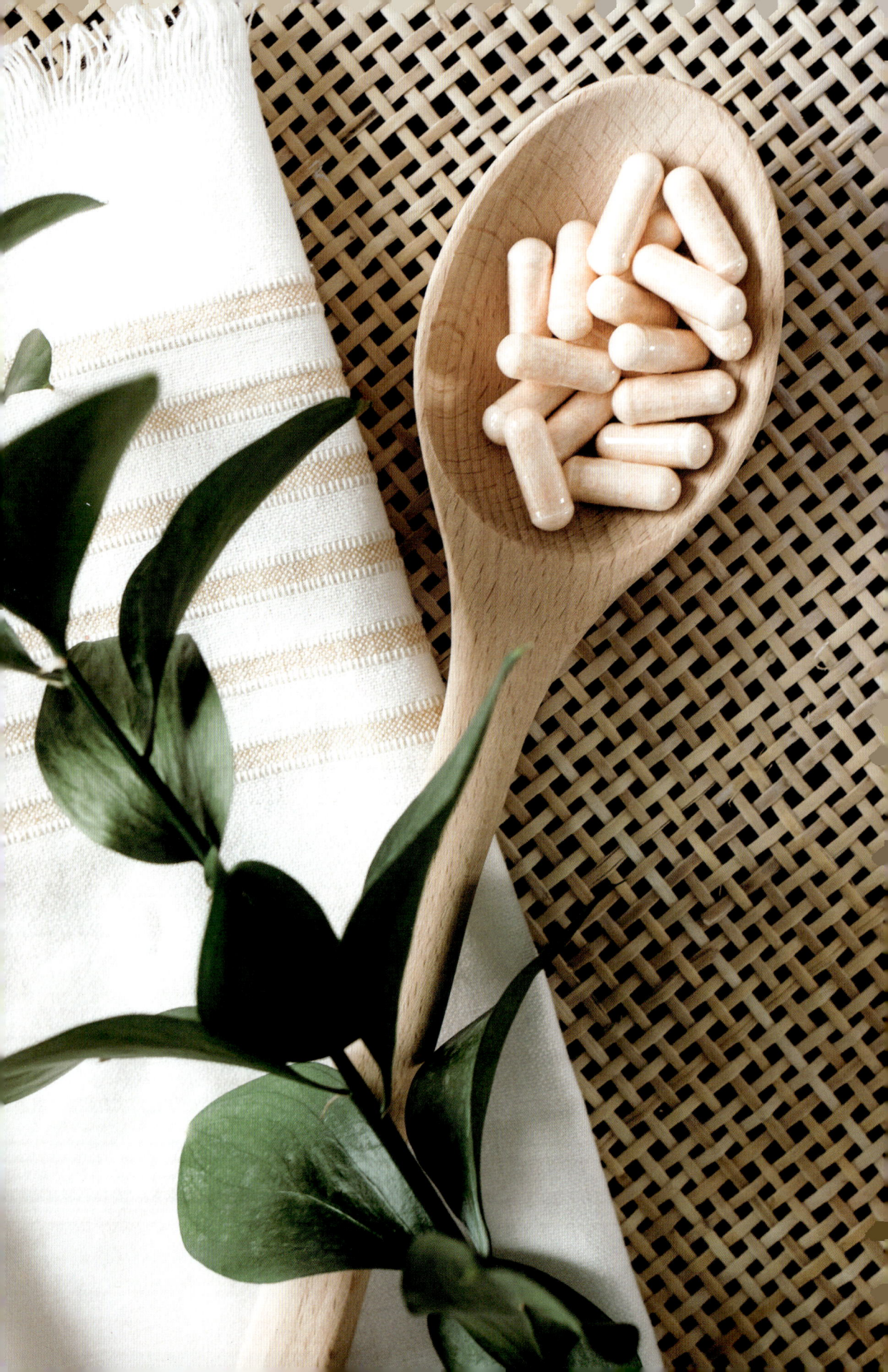

introduction

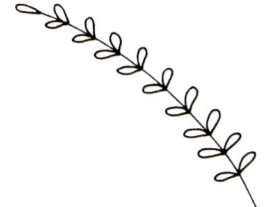

Hello! I am so glad that you are here and ready to jump in with powerful, essential oil-infused supplements that comprise such a huge part of health and vitality.

Like so many other people, I turned to Young Living after being continually let down and frustrated with the conventional options that were available to me for the health of both myself and my family. As a clinical pharmacist, I was frustrated with the lack of clean, sustainable, vitamins and supplements that were available over the counter. Why were all the vitamins filled with unnecessary colorants, pro-inflammatory diluents, such as corn starch or wheat, and chemically produced minerals? Why was it so hard to find a probiotic that was accessible and effective? These questions, alongside my own family's health needs, led me to Young Living, and for that I am forever grateful.

There are so many wonderful supplements available from Young Living, and I hope that this book gives you more insight into how, when, and why you should use each of them. As we don't know what we don't know, empowering ourselves with knowledge is the first step toward better health. Additionally, since health is such a nuanced part of our lives, we have to take our newfound knowledge and apply it to our individual bodies and lifestyles. That is the hope of this book—to empower you with the knowledge and tools that bring you closer to the health and vitality that you desire!

With love,
Dr. Ashley

I am not here to diagnose, treat, prevent, or cure any diseases, nor do I intend to replace your individual health practitioners. The information that is included in this book is for your own personal use and health empowerment. As always, I highly recommend finding a primary care provider that you trust to bring this information to and make decisions with regarding your health.

Keep all supplements that are listed in this book out of reach of children. If you are pregnant, nursing, taking medication, or have a medical condition, consult a health professional before use.

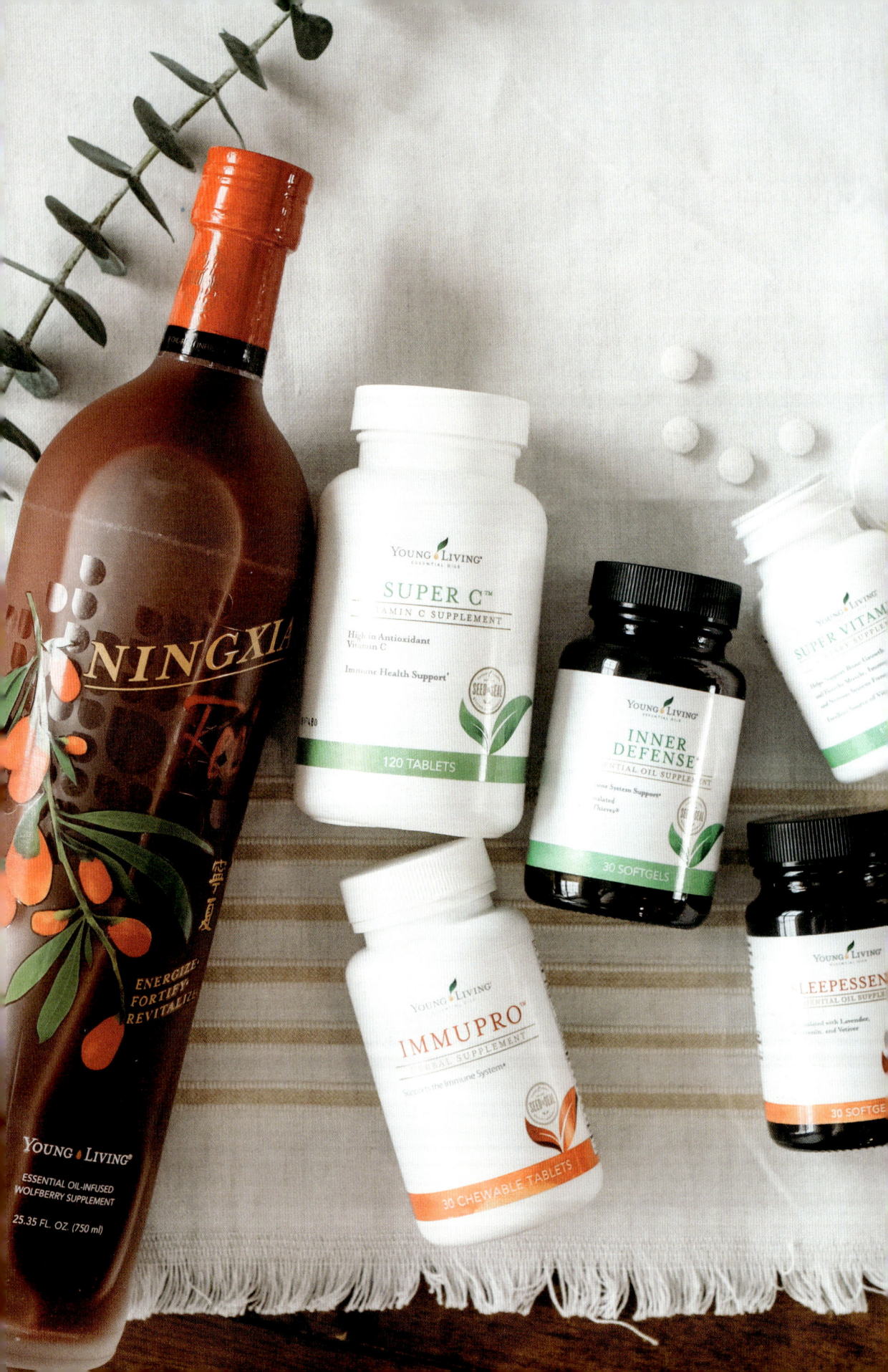

CHAPTER 1

WHY WE NEED TO *Supplement*

Have you ever heard someone say that taking vitamins is simply investing in expensive pee? (Side note—I hate that word!) It's an understandable sentiment among those who don't fully understand the role of vitamins and minerals in our diet and lifestyle. Let's debunk this myth before we jump into individual supplements.

Although we can do much for our bodies with a healthy diet and lifestyle, even on the best days, we still need a little extra help. The cleanest, most organic diet is still unable to provide every vitamin, trace mineral, and micronutrient that our bodies need, so supplementing is key. Supplemental vitamins, minerals, and herbs help to round out any missing nutrients in our diet, especially in a world where farming practices, soil conditions, and food transit times lead to foods that are less nutrient-dense than their ancestral counterparts. However, even if your produce is grown organically in your backyard, there are still gaps that need to be filled, which is where supplements come in.

HERE IS A GOOD EXAMPLE.

Some vitamins and minerals, such as B vitamins, cannot be made by the body and must be obtained through diet. While some plants contain B vitamins, those found in animal protein are much more readily absorbed by the body, making them a superior dietary source. This is why individuals who are vegetarian or vegan often suffer from pernicious anemia—a lack of both iron and B vitamins. However, even with high-quality animal protein in your diet, it is likely that you need more B vitamins. The body doesn't store B vitamins, making daily intake crucial.

Knowing which supplements are right for you can sometimes feel daunting. Which do you need? How do you choose? When do you take them? How do you know if the source is reliable? Unfortunately, the conventional options that are available at most health stores and pharmacies are lacking in many ways.

Young Living supplements contain only high-quality, sustainable ingredients that are a necessary part of the formulation. They are also infused with essential oils, which enhance absorption and add benefits of their own. This is what makes Young Living supplements far superior to anything you would find in a store, and this is why I recommend Young Living supplements in my practice and for my family.

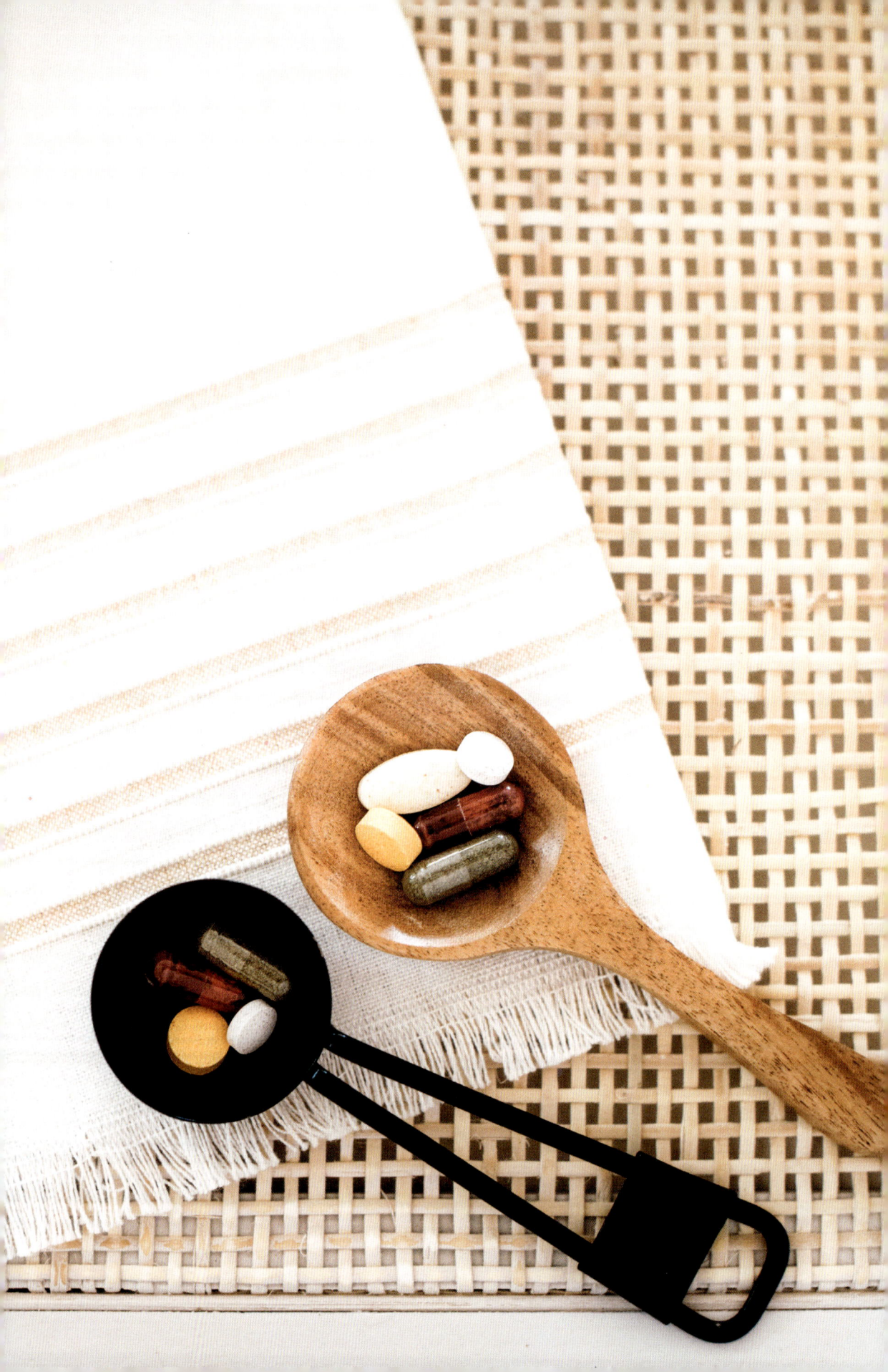

CHAPTER 2

CONVENTIONAL SUPPLEMENTS
vs. Young Living Supplements

Let's talk about bioavailability—a long word for a simple concept! Bioavailability refers to the amount of a substance that is recognized, absorbed, and utilized by the body. It's an important concept when it comes to supplements because no one wants to invest in things that aren't going to be used by the body. Even a supplement with the most impressive label and ingredient list will be useless if the vitamins and minerals aren't absorbed into the bloodstream and delivered in the appropriate form to the appropriate site in the body.

The source of the vitamin or mineral, how it is processed or prepared, and even what it is consumed with can all influence bioavailability. For example, in their natural forms, vitamin B12 and folic acid are poorly absorbed by most of the population, even though they are essential for the body (and a common component of multivitamins). Folic acid is essential but must be absorbed in the form of folate. It changes into folic acid once it is inside the body. Vitamin B12 is better absorbed as a liquid or in complex with the other B vitamins, which makes formulations and processes incredibly important.

THE ADDITION OF ESSENTIAL OILS TO THE FORMULA

All vitamins and minerals are more easily assimilated into the body in the presence of enzymes and essential oils. Supplements that are infused with essential oils are better absorbed and assimilated because the oils act as catalysts to improve nutrient absorption and assist in the removal of cellular waste. This is one significant reason why Young Living's supplements are far superior to anything you will find over the counter in a pharmacy.

Essential oils are small, lipophilic molecules, which means that they absorb most effectively in the presence of lipids. This allows essential oils to pass through the fatty layers of cell membranes in ways that vitamins and minerals cannot. Many essential oils are also rich in antioxidants, which makes them a fantastic addition to vitamins and supplements, as they can help to mitigate free radical damage at a cellular level. This in and of itself is beneficial for our health, and it also assists in nutrient absorption. A healthier cell can absorb and assimilate more effectively than a damaged one!

According to verbal heritage passed down from Young Living founder D. Gary Young, an experiment was conducted with MultiGreens™ to test the increased bioavailability of supplements containing essential oils. In this experiment, one formulation of MultiGreens™ contained essential oils, and one did not. Clinical data showed that the formula without essential oils had a 42% absorption rate in 24 hours. **The formula that contained Young Living essential oils had an absorption of 64% in 30 minutes and 86% in one hour**, which far surpassed the other formulation.

Even though we don't have documentation of these findings, we know that essential oils are powerful health tools, and having them infused into our supplements is a win!

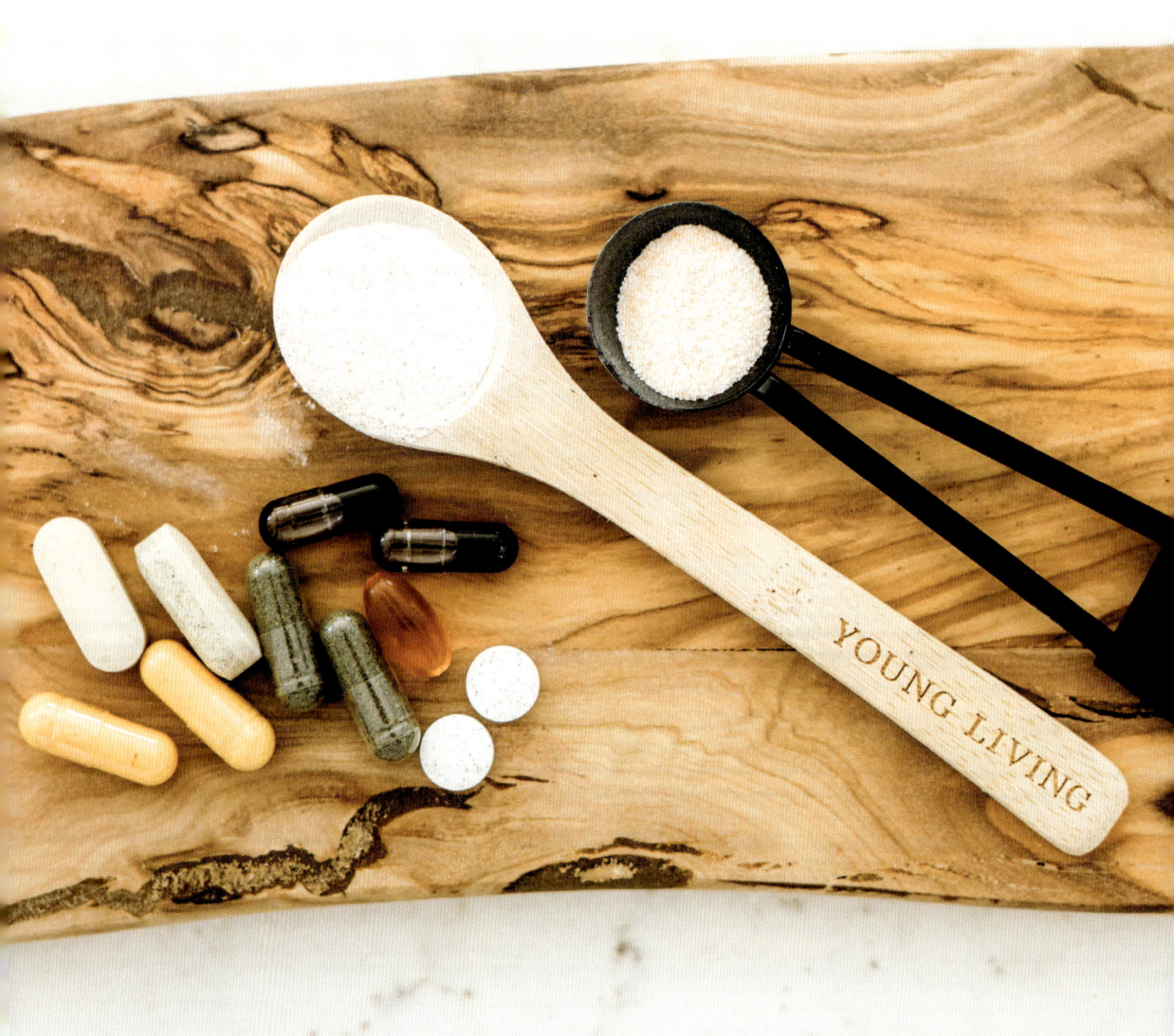

YOUNG LIVING SUPPLEMENTS *at a glance*

NAME	SOURCE OF	USED FOR	GOOD FOR
AGILEASE®	Collagen, glucosamine, hyaluronic acid, turmeric	Cartilage and joint health and maintenance	Athletes and individuals with an active lifestyle
ALKALIME®	Alkaline mineral salts	Occasional digestive upset and pH balance in the stomach	Individuals with dietary or environmental sensitivities and anyone needing pH balance
ALLERZYME™	Digestive enzymes (vegetarian formula)	Digestion and nutrient absorption and relief from digestive upset	Anyone wanting digestive support, vegetarians, and individuals with dietary or environmental sensitivities, such as seasonal allergies
AMINOWISE™	Antioxidants, branch chain amino acids, electrolytes	Muscle recovery and post-workout rehydration	Athletes and individuals with an active lifestyle
BALANCE COMPLETE™	Fiber, vitamins, minerals	Meal replacement and gentle cleansing	Healthy weight loss, gentle cleansing, and adding nutrients to the diet (*not* as a replacement)
BLM™ (BONES, LIGAMENTS, AND MUSCLES)	Collagen, glucosamine, methylsulfonylmethane (MSM), minerals	Bone, muscle, and ligament health and joint mobility	Athletes, aging individuals with arthritis or joint pain, and those with inflammatory bone, joint, or muscle conditions
CARDIOGIZE™	CoQ10, vitamin K2, selenium, garlic, astragalus root, dong quai, hawthorn berry	Heart and vascular health and circulation	Individuals wanting to lower cholesterol and/or blood pressure and/or reduce cardiac symptoms and those who need overall heart health support

NAME	SOURCE OF	USED FOR	GOOD FOR
COMFORTONE®	Cascara sagrada, fiber (psyllium seed), and tarragon and ginger essential oils	Cleansing and digestive support	Those with known digestive needs or dietary sensitivities that require gentle daily cleansing
CORTISTOP®	Pregnenolone, dehydroepiandrosterone (DHEA), phytoestrogens, black cohosh, clary sage	Reducing the effects of stress on women's bodies (weight gain, fatigue, decreased vitality)	Women with adrenal fatigue or elevated cortisol levels, individuals needing stress recovery, and men as needed for adrenal fatigue
DETOXZYME™	Digestive enzymes, cumin, and anise and fennel essential oils	Normal digestive function and cleansing, ideally used in conjunction with a cleansing or detoxifying program	Individuals needing to detox and cleanse the system or for occasional relief from digestive upset
DIGEST & CLEANSE™	Fennel, anise, ginger, peppermint, and caraway essential oils	Stimulating digestive health and maintaining overall balance	Anyone with dietary sensitivities, digestive needs or those wanting overall digestive support
ENDOGIZE™	Ashwagandha, DHEA, longjack root, clary sage, phytoestrogens	Balancing the overall female endocrine system, balancing estrogen, progesterone, and testosterone	Women wanting overall hormone support, or those with PMS symptoms or low libido
ESSENTIALZYME™	Digestive enzymes, pancreatic enzymes, bromelain, papain, and fennel, anise, tarragon and peppermint essential oils	Stimulates overall enzyme activity, digestive health, and pancreas health and activity	Anyone wanting digestive support, individuals with dietary or environmental sensitivities, and those needing pancreatic enzymes
ESSENTIALZYMES-4™	Digestive enzymes, bromelain, papain, and anise, ginger, fennel, tarragon, and rosemary essential oils	Nutrient absorption and proper digestion of fats, proteins, fiber, and carbohydrates	Anyone wanting digestive support, individuals with dietary or environmental sensitivities, and individuals whose diet includes animal proteins
FEMIGEN™	Phytoestrogens and phytoprogesterone, wild yam, black cohosh, dong quai, crampbark, and clary sage, fennel, ylang ylang, and sage essential oils	Balancing the female reproductive system and replenishing low estrogen and progesterone	Women wanting support for overall reproductive hormone balance, menstrual cycles, and menopause and women with low estrogen levels

NAME	SOURCE OF	USED FOR	GOOD FOR
GOLDEN TURMERIC™	Turmeric, antioxidants, boswellia extract, prebiotics	Inflammation and joint health, muscle recovery, immune and digestive health, mood and cognition, and overall vitality	Anyone looking to increase overall vitality, those with known inflammatory needs, athletes or those with an active lifestyle, and all adults
ICP™	Fiber (psyllium, oat bran, and flax) and fennel, anise, tarragon, ginger and rosemary essential oils	Intestinal cleansing, nutrient absorption, toxin removal, and heart health	Those looking for an intestinal cleanse (works best as part of the 'Cleansing Trio™')
ICP DAILY™	Prebiotics, fiber, prickly pear, and fennel, anise, tarragon, ginger, lemongrass, and rosemary essential oils	Gentle daily cleanse and a healthy gut flora balance	Anyone wanting digestive and immune support and those wanting to gently rid the body of toxic metabolites daily
ILLUMINEYES™	Lutein, zeaxanthin, vitamin A, vitamin E, antioxidants (wolfberry fruit)	Protection from age-related eye damage, blue light exposure, and eye strain and promotes skin and eye health	Those with age-related eye disorders, anyone wanting to support eye health, and individuals who are exposed to blue light/computer screens daily
IMMUPRO™	Antioxidants, reishi, maitake, and agaricus blazei mushrooms, melatonin	Immune system, sleep, and damage from oxidative stress	Anyone with immune system needs and anyone who needs restful sleep for recovery from stress (physical or emotional)
INNER DEFENSE®	Oregano, thyme, rosemary, cinnamon bark, and clove essential oils	Bolstering the immune and respiratory systems and supporting the removal of unwanted microbes	Anyone needing acute or chronic support for the immune system and those with known or suspected bacterial or viral infections
JUVAPOWER®	Antioxidants (spinach, broccoli, rice, and beet powders) and fennel and anise essential oils	Daily liver cleansing and support and binds acid and toxins	Anyone wanting daily liver support and elimination of toxins
JUVATONE®	Copper, choline, dl-methionine, Oregon grape root, bee propolis, echinacea, and lemon, German chamomile and rosemary essential oils	Advanced daily liver support, cleansing and toxin removal	Individuals needing more targeted liver support and individuals with a history of liver damage or disease

NAME	SOURCE OF	USED FOR	GOOD FOR
K&B™	Juniper berries, parsley, uva ursi, and clove, fennel, Roman chamomile, sage and juniper essential oils	Kidney and bladder cleansing and fighting against kidney and bladder infections	Anyone needing kidney and bladder support and individuals prone to or experiencing kidney or bladder infections
KIDSCENTS® MIGHTYPRO™	Prebiotics and probiotics (8 billion active, live cultures)	Gastrointestinal, digestive, and immune health and healthy gut flora balance	Children aged two and older (or at your discretion), children currently taking or with a history of antibiotic use (herbal or conventional), and adults wanting a powdered pre/probiotic
KIDSCENTS® MIGHTYVITES™	Full spectrum of vitamins, minerals, antioxidants, and phytonutrients, B vitamins, folate	Children's multivitamins, whole-food nutrients for overall health and wellness of children	Children aged four and older (use a lower dose for younger children, at your discretion) and adults wanting a chewable multivitamin
KIDSCENTS® MIGHTYZYME™	Digestive enzymes, broccoli, beet, barley grass, wolfberry powder	Digestive health and the absorption of nutrients, relief from symptoms of digestive upset, and overall health and vitality	Children aged two and older and adults wanting a chewable digestive enzyme
KIDSCENTS® UNWIND™	Magnesium, L-theanine, 5-HTP, and lavender and Roman chamomile essential oils	Restful sleep, irritability, and stress	Children aged four and older who need help winding down for sleep
LIFE 9®	Probiotics (17 billion live cultures)	Gastrointestinal, digestive, and immune health through balancing gut flora	All adults, anyone with known digestive needs, and anyone currently taking or with a history of antibiotic use (herbal or conventional)
LONGEVITY™	Antioxidants, and thyme, clove, frankincense and orange essential oils	Healthy docosahexaenoic acid (DHA) levels, brain function, cell integrity, liver and immune function, and protecting cells from oxidative damage	All adults, aging adults, individuals needing cognitive support, and those with a history of or concern for any type of cancer
MASTER FORMULA™	Full spectrum of vitamins and minerals, vitamins D, E, and K, turmeric, prebiotics	Adult multivitamins, whole-food nutrients for overall health and wellness, bone density, brain function, digestive and immune health, energy levels, and eye and heart health	All adults, anyone with a known nutrient deficiency, and women who are trying to conceive, pregnant, or postpartum

NAME	SOURCE OF	USED FOR	GOOD FOR
MEGACAL™	Magnesium, calcium, and lemon and lime essential oils	Heart, bone, and nerve health, muscle recovery, stress, and sleep	Those needing sleep or anxiety relief, athletes, and those looking to replace conventional magnesium powders or supplements
MINDWISE™	Vitamin D3, CoQ10, Omega-3 fatty acids, Acetyl-L-Carnitine (ALCAR), Glycerylphosphorylcholine (GPC)	Overall cognitive and cardiovascular health and helps with brain fog, concentration, and mood	Anyone under stress, those looking for a source of omega-3s, individuals who cannot take OmegaGize3*, women who are pregnant or nursing, anyone aged four or older needing help with brain fog or focus
MINERAL ESSENCE™	Antioxidants, magnesium, selenium, zinc, iodine and other trace minerals, royal jelly	Immune health, cognitive function, thyroid and cardiovascular health, hair, skin, bone, and teeth, and overall wellness and vitality	Anyone looking to improve overall health and wellness, those with known mineral or nutrient deficiencies, and those with a thyroid imbalance
MULTIGREENS™	Choline, spirulina, alfalfa sprouts, barley grass, bee pollen, Pacific kelp, and Melissa essential oil	Energy levels, heart health, and overall wellness and vitality	Anyone looking to improve overall health or energy levels and anyone with nutrient deficiencies
NINGXIA RED®	Antioxidants (wolfberry, blueberry, plum, pomegranate), and orange, tangerine, lemon, and yuzu essential oils	Protects against oxidative stress, supports healthy cell function, energy levels, hormones, immune system, and hair and skin health	Anyone looking to improve overall health, those needing energy or cognitive support, and anyone wanting immune, hormone, skin, hair, or antioxidant support
OLIVE ESSENTIALS™	Antioxidants from olives (Hydroxytyrosol), and parsley and rosemary essential oils	Heart and vascular health and healthy blood pressure and cholesterol levels	Individuals looking to lower blood pressure and cholesterol or promote overall heart health
OMEGAGIZE3®	Fish oil (omega-3 fatty acids), Eicosapentaenoic acid (EPA), Docosahexaenoic acid (DHA), vitamin D3, CoQ10, antioxidants, and clove essential oil	Heart, skeletal, and vascular health, mood and memory, and eye, skin, and joint health	Those needing a fish oil supplement, pregnant and postpartum women, and anyone wanting to lower triglycerides or promote heart health

NAME	SOURCE OF	USED FOR	GOOD FOR
PARAFREE™	Anise, fennel, vetiver, laurus nobilis, nutmeg, tea tree, thyme, clove, ocotea, tarragon, ginger and dorado azul essential oils	Cleansing of the entire digestive tract, specifically for unwanted pathogens and parasites	Anyone with known pathogens or parasites and those traveling to countries where exposure is possible
PD 80/20™ (PREGNENOLONE 80% AND DHEA 20%)	Pregnenolone and DHEA	Healthy hormone levels, memory, and cardiovascular and immune health	Individuals with known deficiencies of estrogen, progesterone, or testosterone
POWERGIZE™	Vitamin B6, zinc, ashwagandha, eurycoma longifolia, and blue spruce, goldenrod, and cassia essential oils	Stamina, muscle strength, tone, and performance, muscle recovery, hormone balance, energy levels and vitality, and testosterone levels for both men and women	Athletes or those with an active lifestyle, those wanting muscle support for physical stress and recovery, and those looking to support testosterone levels and athletic performance
PRENOLONE PLUS™ BODY CREAM	Progesterone, estrogen (plant-based), DHEA, St. John's wort, and ylang ylang and clary sage essential oils	Estrogen, progesterone, and testosterone balance in women	Women needing hormone balance or with known hormonal needs (acne, PMS, painful cycles)
PROGESSENCE PLUS™ SERUM	Bioidentical progesterone (plant-based)	Progesterone levels, hair and skin, mood, and menstrual cycles and fertility	Women needing balance, those with difficult periods, and those needing fertility support or with known menstrual cycle issues
PROSTATE HEALTH™	Saw palmetto, pumpkin seed oil, and geranium, fennel and myrtle essential oils	Prostate health and function	Men looking for prostate support (either acutely or proactively)
PURE PROTEIN COMPLETE™	Protein, branch chain amino acids, enzymes, probiotics	Nutrition, exercise recovery, and lean muscle mass, and energy levels and metabolism	Athletes or those with an active lifestyle and anyone looking for a nutrient-dense, high-quality protein powder
REGENOLONE™ MOISTURIZING CREAM	Progesterone, wild yam, phytoestrogens, black and blue cohosh, St. John's wort	Female hormone balance, PMS and painful periods, and skin health	Women with menstrual cycle needs and those looking for a plant-based hormone cream without DHEA
REHEMOGEN™	Cascara sagrada, red clover, prickly ash bar, burdock root, and rosemary, thyme and tea tree essential oils	Intestinal and blood cleansing and liver and lymphatic health	Adults looking for a digestive, liver, and blood cleansing supplement

NAME	SOURCE OF	USED FOR	GOOD FOR
SLEEP ESSENCE™	Melatonin and lavender, valerian, vetiver, and rue essential oils	Restful sleep and immune health and recovery	Adults needing support falling or staying asleep
SULFURZYME®	Antioxidants (wolfberry), Sulfur (MSM)	Bone, hair, joint, and skin health, circulation and muscle health, immune health, and thyroid and endocrine function	Athletes, those needing joint or muscle support, anyone with dull skin or hair or known thyroid issues, and anyone with skin needs (eczema, psoriasis, any inflammatory issues)
SUPER B™	All eight B vitamins, folate, minerals, nutmeg essential oil	Energy and muscle health, mood and cognition, heart health, stress response, and recovery	All adults, athletes or those with an active lifestyle, anyone under stress or needing energy support, and pregnant and postpartum mothers
SUPER C™ & SUPER C™ CHEWABLE	Antioxidants, vitamin C, citrus bioflavonoids, citrus essential oils	Immune, respiratory, and circulatory function, connective tissue, overall health, vitality, and longevity, and improves iron absorption	Anyone looking for a clean vitamin C supplement, those with acute or chronic immune system needs, individuals traveling or needing extra immune support, and those taking an iron supplement
SUPER CAL PLUS™	Calcium, magnesium, vitamins D and K, trace minerals, and spruce, copaiba, and vetiver essential oils	Bone density, structure, and integrity, muscles and teeth, and immune and cardiovascular health	Those with a risk or diagnosis of osteoporosis and anyone needing a calcium or bone health supplement
SUPER VITAMIN D	Vitamin D, lemon balm, Melissa essential oil	Respiratory, immune, and bone health, mood, and hormone production	Anyone looking for a vitamin D supplement, those with acute or chronic immune needs, those with or at risk for osteoporosis, and anyone with emotional needs or seasonal blues
THYROMIN™	Thyroid hormone, Iodine, vitamin E, and myrtle and myrrh essential oils	Metabolism and energy, body temperature, hair and skin, and mood	Anyone needing thyroid support

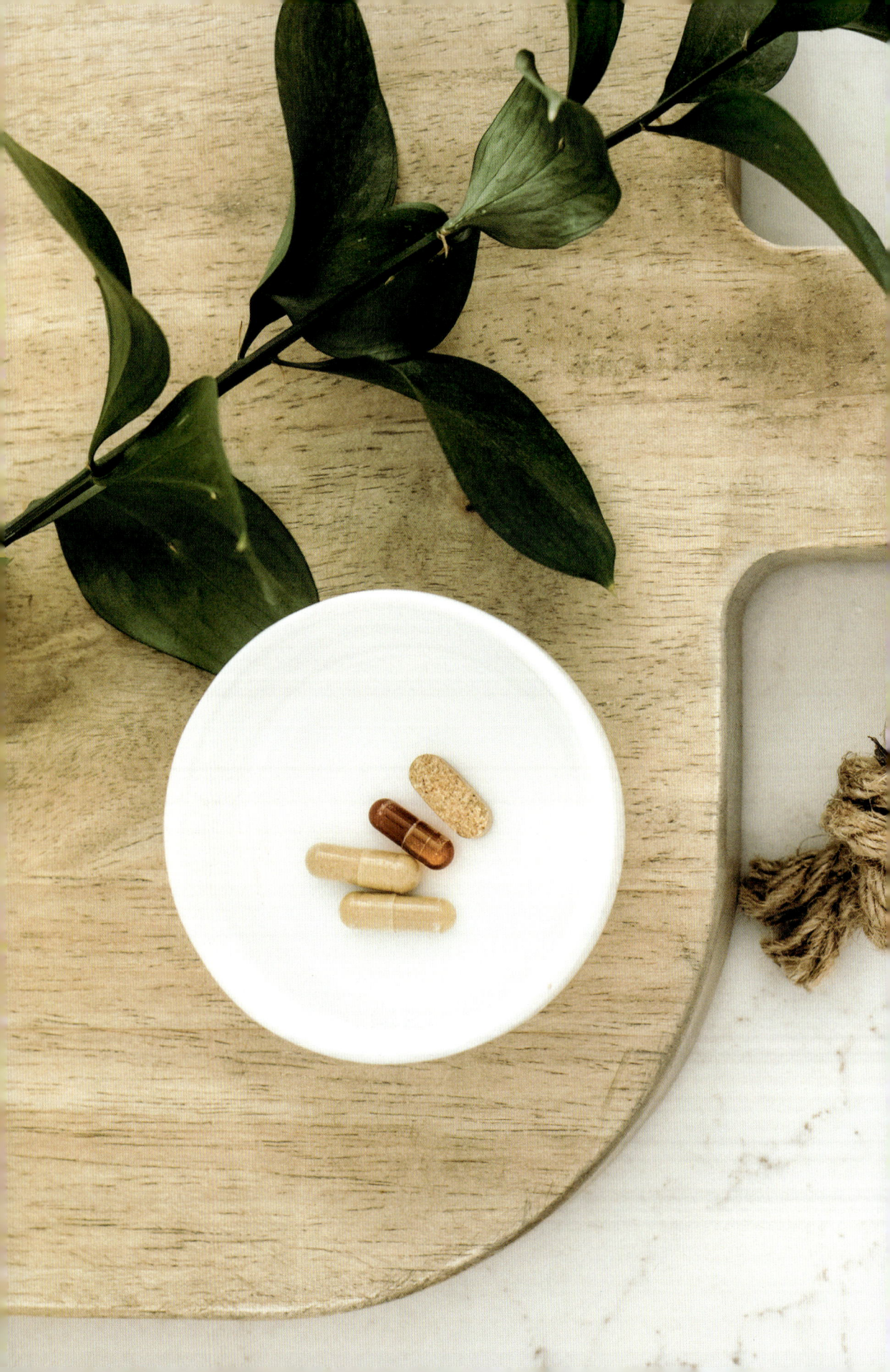

CHAPTER 3
FOUNDATIONAL *Supplements*

Although knowing where to get started with supplements can sometimes feel a bit overwhelming, there are a few great starting points for anyone. These supplements provide the core building blocks for the foundational functions of the body, including vitamins, probiotics, minerals, antioxidants, omega-3 fatty acids, and micronutrients, and are great choices for any adult.

A QUICK WORD ON ANTIOXIDANTS, OXIDATIVE STRESS, AND OXYGEN RADICAL ABSORBANCE CAPACITY (ORAC) VALUES...

Many of the Young Living supplements include antioxidant ingredients or essential oils that are powerful antioxidants, and while I cannot speak for the developers at Young Living, I would guess that this is deliberate. Antioxidants are a powerhouse when it comes to our health.

Antioxidants are substances or nutrients that are found in our plants and foods that can prevent or reduce oxidative damage to the body. When our body's cells use oxygen, they naturally produce free radicals as by-products, and these free radicals can cause damage. This happens at a cellular level, which is another reason why adding essential oils into a supplement routine is a great practice.

Free radicals are formed under natural circumstances, such as exercise, and are a result of environmental exposure to toxins from cigarette smoke, air pollution, and chemicals in food, drinking water, or household and personal care products. Oxidative stress is thought to play a role in a variety of diseases, including cancer, cardiovascular diseases, diabetes, Alzheimer's disease, Parkinson's disease, and eye diseases, such as cataracts and age-related macular degeneration.

Antioxidants act as "free radical scavengers" that neutralize the free radicals and help to prevent and repair the damage by the free radicals. Antioxidants work to keep our body systems functioning smoothly. They help prevent the onset of degenerative diseases, premature aging, cardiovascular disease, and mental decline. Examples of common antioxidants include vitamins C and E, selenium, and carotenoids, such as beta-carotene, lycopene, lutein, and zeaxanthin[1].

When it comes to measuring the antioxidant potential of a food, we typically speak in terms of the ORAC value. ORAC is a lab test that was developed by the National Institutes of Health that attempts to quantify the total antioxidant capacity (TAC) of a food. This is done by placing a food sample in a test tube, along with certain molecules that generate free radical activity and other molecules that are vulnerable to oxidation. After a while, scientists measure how well the food sample protected the vulnerable molecules from oxidation by the free radicals. The less free radical damage there is, the higher the antioxidant capacity of the test substance.

One benefit of using ORAC values as a standard is that it measures the antioxidant activity of a whole food rather than the levels of specific nutrients, such as vitamin C or E. There are thousands of unique antioxidant compounds in plants, and we have only scratched the surface identifying and understanding them. Measuring according to the ORAC value allows us to capture any synergy between the various components within a food substance or essential oil. However, it is important to note that the ORAC value of a given food/oil will vary slightly due to several factors, such as the growing and processing conditions and the specific variety that was tested. Therefore, the data is presented with the minimum, maximum, and mean values.

Bottom line? **Antioxidants are hugely important for overall health, as we age, and for the daily protection of our cells. Foods or essential oils with a higher ORAC value have more antioxidant potential and are definitely ones to include in your routine.**

Now let's dive in!

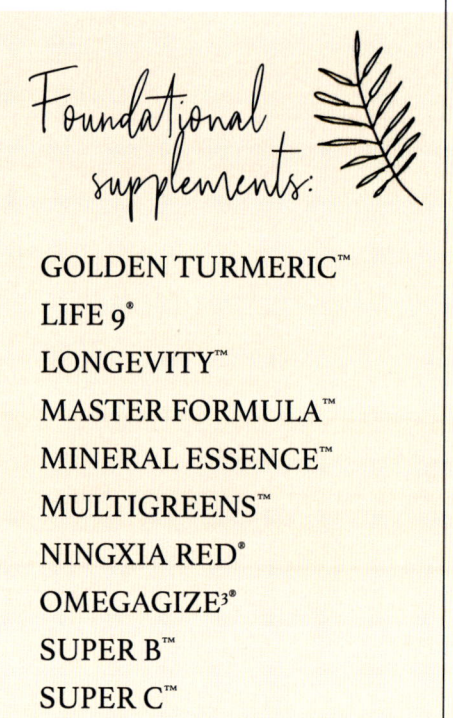

Foundational supplements:

GOLDEN TURMERIC™
LIFE 9®
LONGEVITY™
MASTER FORMULA™
MINERAL ESSENCE™
MULTIGREENS™
NINGXIA RED®
OMEGAGIZE$^{3®}$
SUPER B™
SUPER C™
SUPER VITAMIN D

GOLDEN TURMERIC™

Turmeric is no stranger to the health scene. This golden spice is well known for its ability to help the body during times of inflammation, both acute and chronic. Young Living's Golden Turmeric™ powder combines turmeric, Boswellia resin, and ginger, which work synergistically to support the body's natural response to inflammation, immune response, joint health, mobility, and physical recovery.

BENEFITS OF GOLDEN TURMERIC™
- Supports the body's natural response to inflammation
- Bolsters the immune response, joint health, mobility, and recovery after physical exertion
- 24 times more bioavailable than standard turmeric extract (your body absorbs the same amount of curcuminoids from just 300 mg of Golden Turmeric™ as it does from 1,926mg of standard turmeric)
- Contains prebiotics to support healthy digestion and the gut–brain axis
- Contains naturally occurring curcuminoids that support joint mobility
- Soy, milk, and gluten free, vegan friendly, no artificial flavors, colors, preservatives, or sweeteners

Golden Turmeric™ powder is an excellent source of curcuminoids, which help to support overall wellness in the body. Chronic, low-level inflammation plays a major role in almost every Western disease: from high cholesterol to heart disease, arthritis, and many others. Therefore, anything that can help fight chronic inflammation is important to prevent and treat these diseases and bolster overall health. Young Living's Golden Turmeric™ powder is a great choice for daily support.

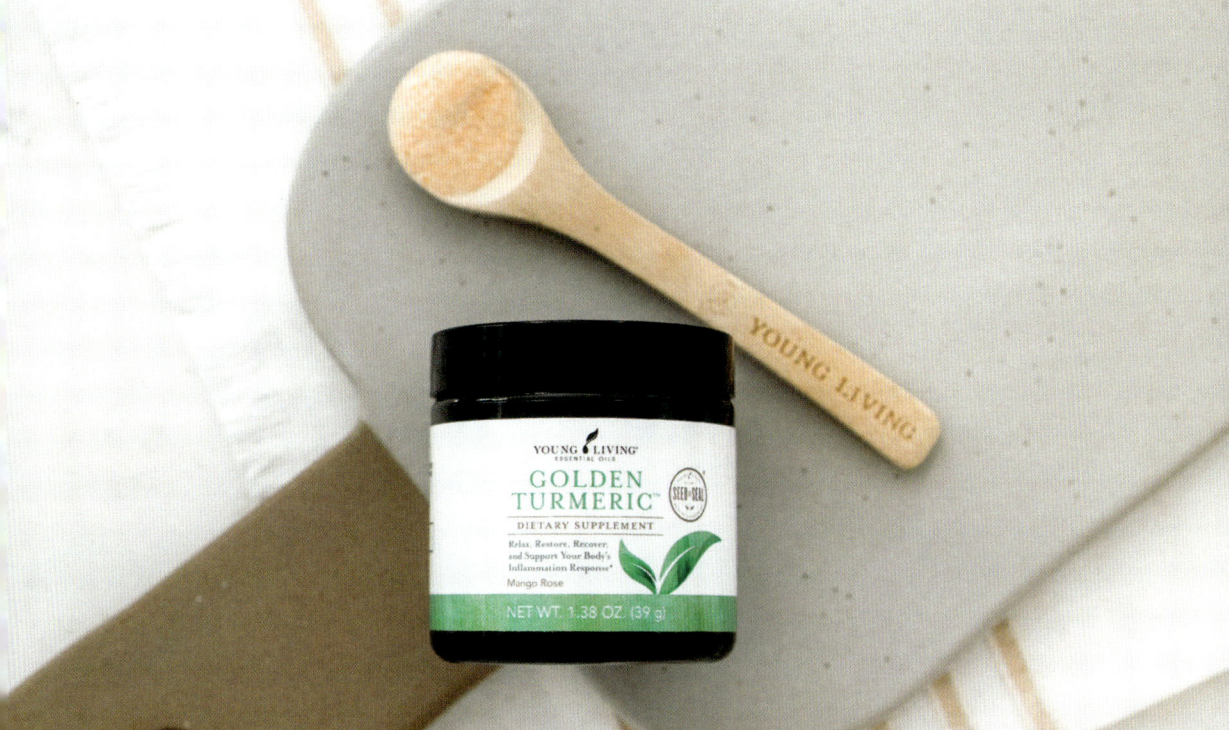

- **Turmeric extract (curcuma longa):** Turmeric has strong anti-inflammatory properties[2] that match the effectiveness of some anti-inflammatory drugs[3,4] and is a potent antioxidant that can neutralize free radicals[5] and boost the activity of the body's own antioxidant enzymes[6].
- **Boswellia resin extract:** Boswellia has both anti-inflammatory and antioxidant properties[7], strong immune-enhancing effects[8], and the ability to improve cognition and memory[9]. It may have anti-tumor effects[10], likely due to its antioxidant action.
- **Ginger essential oil:** Ginger has analgesic, anti-inflammatory, antibacterial, and antioxidant properties. It is great for soothing digestion[11], contains powerful antioxidants, which can protect against oxidative stress, helps to combat inflammation[12], and promotes liver health[13].
- **Lime essential oil:** Lime is high in limonene, a constituent known to strengthen the immune system and decongest the lymphatic system. Additionally, d-limonene alters the signaling pathways within cancer cells to stop cell multiplication and cause cell death[22].

INFLAMMATION & EMOTIONAL HEALTH

Chronic pain and inflammation are exhausting, both physically and emotionally. Chronic inflammation from injury, diet, or other illnesses are like tiny fires within our bodies, and our systems are constantly running to put out the fires. Our emotions follow suit—they run until we are at empty and feel extremely tired, run down, and depressed.

Because it is becoming such a widespread issue, modern science is researching the connection between inflammation and depression or anxiety. Studies show that chronic stress is associated with increased inflammation, depression, negative emotions, attention changes, and even dampened immune responses[14]. This proves that we need to take small, daily actions to give our bodies everything that they need to thrive!

Young Living's Golden Turmeric™ powder is a great choice for just about anyone, whether you have chronic health needs, are an athlete or avid exerciser who is prone to inflammation, or a health-conscious adult who wants to do everything you can to promote overall health, wellness, and vitality.

Safety notes: Keep out of reach of children. If you are pregnant, nursing, taking medication, or have a medical condition, consult a healthcare professional before use.

WHO SHOULD USE GOLDEN TURMERIC™?

- Anyone with known inflammation (acute or chronic)
- Athletes or those with an active lifestyle
- Anyone looking for overall health, vitality, and antioxidant support
- All adults, especially as we age

To use: Mix 1/2 tsp. in 6-8 oz. of water, juice, herbal tea, a smoothie, NingXia Red® or milk of choice once daily.

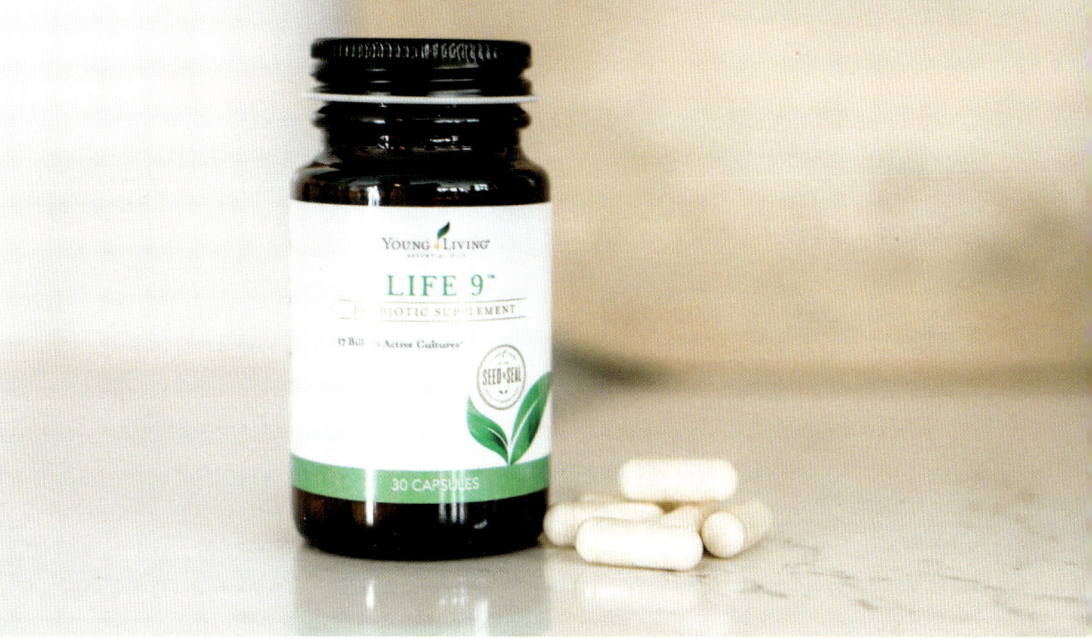

LIFE 9®

Life 9® is Young Living's high-potency probiotic and is one of Young Living's most popular supplements. Many health experts (myself included!) consider a high-quality, diverse probiotic to be a cornerstone of overall health. Research shows that a healthy gut is key to brain, immune, and skin health and emotional regulation.

Many components of our modern lifestyle, such as medications, chlorinated water, contaminated water supplies, sugar consumption, a lack of dietary fiber, and mental and emotional stress, increase our need to supplement with healthy bacteria. Although much of this is within our control, even with the best habits, we still need extra support.

GENERAL BENEFITS OF PROBIOTICS
- Replenish the body's good bacteria
- Assist the body with the production of B vitamins
- Improve nutrient absorption via healthy gut flora
- Support immune system function and recovery from infection
- Suppress unhealthy fungi and yeast, such as Candida
- Improve overall digestion

Your body contains approximately 100 trillion bacteria, which is more than ten times the number of cells you have in your entire body. Research has shown that the type and quantity of the microorganisms in your gut interact with your body in ways that can either prevent or encourage the development of many diseases. This means that maintaining an ideal bacterial balance is key. The ideal ratio between the bacteria in your gut is 85% "good" and 15% "bad," and it is attainable through simple, daily habits.

Not all probiotics are created equally, and unfortunately, the options at the pharmacy counter are less than desirable. We want a source of good bacteria that is diverse, can be easily absorbed, is potent enough to make a difference to our health, yet doesn't interact with each other or endogenous bacteria. That's why I love Young Living's Life 9®!

Life 9® includes nine probiotic strains for full-spectrum gut support throughout the entire digestive tract. There are Bifidobacterium that populate the entire gut, Lactobacillus that populate the small intestine, and Streptococcus thermophilus that populate the intestines.

- *Lactobacillus acidophilus*: This is the most common of the "friendly" bacteria that naturally lives in the body to protect against disease-causing bacteria.
- *Bifidobacterium lactis*: This probiotic is commonly used in fermented foods and supports the balance of healthy bacteria in the gut.
- *Lactobacillus plantarum*: This bacterium acts as an antioxidant, may support the body's response to inflammation, and may help maintain healthy blood sugar levels.
- *Lactobacillus rhamnosus*: This has beneficial properties for the digestive and immune systems, particularly against urinary and intestinal pathogens.
- *Lactobacillus salivarius*: This helps the body break down food, absorb nutrients, and fight off the overgrowth of organisms that might cause diseases.
- *Streptococcus thermophilus*: This strain helps stimulate disease-fighting cells, stunt the growth of tumors, and strengthen the immune system.
- *Bifidobacterium breve*: These bacteria live symbiotically in the intestines of humans, and have historically been used to treat constipation, diarrhea, irritable bowel syndrome, and even common colds and the flu.
- *Bifidobacterium bifidum*: This produces lactic acid and antibacterial substances, including acetic acid, to suppress harmful bacterial strains.
- *Bifidobacterium longum*: This bacterium is effective at supporting overall digestion, improving immune function, stabilizing gut microbiota, and improving the overall intestinal environment.

The blend of bacteria in Life 9® works synergistically to support normal gut health, promote healthy digestion, and maintain normal intestinal function. When the gut is healthy, the immune system can function well. When our guts are optimally populated with good bacteria, we are better able to digest food, and our liver is less burdened. Overall, our bodies win.

BENEFITS OF LIFE 9®
- Daily use supports overall health and wellness and a healthy, diverse gut microbiome
- Contains a diverse set of bacteria that work synergistically towards gut health
- Aids in healthy digestion and assists in digestive distress
- Helps to maintain immune health
- Helps with emotional health

A high-quality probiotic is always a cornerstone of health, but it is especially important to repopulate the gut with diverse, supportive bacteria after using antibiotics. I recommend taking Life 9® while on an antibiotic regimen (herbal, oil-based, or conventional) or you can start Life 9® after completing the regimen. If you choose to use Life 9® during the course of an antibiotic, separate the two by at least four hours.

PROBIOTICS

During the last several years, the connection between the gut and the brain has been a topic of extensive study, especially in the holistic health world, and studies show that a diverse microbiome has profound effects on emotional health—from easing social anxiety to decreasing depressive thoughts to enhancing memory and cognition[15,16,17].

The gut is often referred to as the "second brain," and for good reason! Gut bacteria produce and react to hundreds of the same neurochemicals that the brain uses for various processes, including mood regulation. In fact, almost 90% of the serotonin in our bodies is produced by the peripheral nervous system in the gut. Research has shown that probiotics have a positive influence on mood, especially when it comes to depression, stress, and anxiety[181].

Many things impact the gut's ability to produce and maintain adequate levels of serotonin, including food sensitivities and allergies, acute and chronic stress, gut flora imbalances, yeast overgrowth, acute and chronic illness, conventional medications, and antibiotic use. Some of these things are within our control to change, whereas with others, we have to simply support and rebuild the gut after experiencing them. Acute needs are going to require work, but the real ticket to health is in daily actions.

> **WHO SHOULD USE LIFE 9®?**
> - Anyone wanting to support overall health and wellness and immune health
> - Anyone with digestive needs or a known gut imbalance
> - Those taking antibiotics or using Young Living's Inner Defense® Capsules
> - Anyone struggling mentally and emotionally, as an imbalance or yeast overgrowth in the gut can be linked to anxious, dark feelings and thoughts and physical exhaustion
>
> **To use:** Take one capsule every night following a meal or as needed. For the best results, take one capsule eight hours after using Inner Defense®.

Safety notes: If you are pregnant, nursing, taking medication, or have a medical condition, consult a health professional before use.

LONGEVITY™

Longevity™ is a powerhouse antioxidant supplement—the name alone suggests that it should be in your daily rotation! This blend of essential oils includes clove, frankincense, thyme, and orange to help prevent and repair oxidative stress, protect DHA levels, maintain cellular integrity, and support brain, liver, and immune system function. This supplement is a powerful tool for overall health and well-being.

BENEFITS OF LONGEVITY™
- Helps prevent oxidative stress from free radicals
- Contains powerful antioxidant-rich essential oils to help maintain cell integrity
- Helps protect DHA levels, which is a nutrient that supports brain function
- Contains clove and frankincense oils, which are known for powerful health properties
- Contains the constituents eugenol, thymol, and d-limonene, which are known to have powerful effects
- Supports immune health and overall longevity and vitality

Although each essential oil in this blend plays a vital role in health and wellness, the addition of frankincense and clove makes it something that I want to have in my daily routine. Frankincense is mentioned in one of the oldest known medical records, the Eber's Papyrus, which dates back to the 16th century BC. This "holy anointing oil" has historically been used to treat "every conceivable illness known to man." Frankincense has been studied with respect to drug-resistant bacterial infections, hair growth, age-related diseases, and even cancer. There are too many incredible studies to list, so head over to www.pubmed.gov and search for "frankincense" or "boswellia."

Clove essential oil is high in the constituent eugenol, which boasts well-documented neuroprotective, antioxidant, anti-inflammatory, antipyretic, analgesic, antiparasitic, and antimicrobial properties. It protects our brains, hearts, lungs, immune systems, and the whole body. Additionally, eugenol helps to relieve pain, and at higher concentrations, it behaves as a prooxidant, meaning it shows strong anticancer activity[18].

One amazing benefit of this supplement is its ability to protect DHA levels. DHA is an omega-3 fatty acid that is found in abundance in the brain, eyes, and heart. It is essential for the function of these organs, and the body only manufactures a small amount. The vast majority of DHA comes from diet, and the turnover is quick because it is so heavily utilized. We want good dietary intake of DHA, and we want to protect it so that it can be utilized.

This blend of fat-soluble antioxidants should be taken daily to strengthen the body's systems to prevent the damaging effects of aging, diet, and the environment.

- **Clove essential oil**: Clove has a range of health benefits, most of which are due to its high antioxidant activity. It has an average ORAC value of over 290,000[19] and is effective at stopping the growth of some bacteria and fungi[20], including *Candida*[21], at higher doses.
- **Frankincense essential oil**: Frankincense has long been revered for its health properties, including strong immune-enhancing effects[8] and the ability to improve cognition and memory[9]. Additionally, it has promising anti-inflammatory and anti-tumor effects[10], which are likely due to its antioxidant activity.
- **Orange essential oil**: Orange is wonderful for supporting immune and digestive health and general well-being. It is high in d-limonene, a constituent that shows anti-inflammatory, wound-healing, and anticancer effects. D-limonene has been shown to alter the signaling pathways within cancer cells in a way that stops cancer cells from multiplying and causes their death[22].
- **Thyme essential oil**: Thyme is high in the constituent thymol, another potent antioxidant. It supports the immune, respiratory, cardiovascular, nervous, and digestive systems, protects DHA levels and brain function, has shown activity against antibiotic-resistant bacterial strains[23], and supports healthy hormone balance[24]. In addition, it acts as a circulatory stimulant and helps maintain healthy blood pressure and cholesterol levels[25].

LONGEVITY™ & EMOTIONAL HEALTH

The emotional health impact of Longevity™ is a result of the incredible antioxidant support that this supplement provides. Stress and anxiety are central to all mental health conditions: from everyday stress to more complex issues[26]. Antioxidants help repair physical stress on our cells, which in turn, affects our mood and emotions through an increase in neurotransmitters and "feel good" hormones. Relieving the physical oxidative stress on the body facilitates emotional healing at a cellular level. In addition, antioxidants help to promote the movement of grief through the body, which can further facilitate healing.

If Longevity™ softgels are out of stock, you can easily make your own. Longevity™ Vitality™ is the same combination of essential

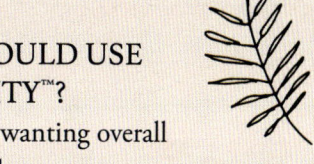

WHO SHOULD USE LONGEVITY™?

- Anyone wanting overall antioxidant support
- Individuals wanting health support as we age
- Anyone wanting healthy, glowing skin, especially as we age
- Individuals with the need for cardiovascular and cholesterol support
- Individuals who are struggling with mental and emotional needs or processing trauma
- In short, just about everyone!

To use: Take one softgel once daily with food or as needed.

oils and can be substituted for the Longevity™ Softgels with comparable results. Use Longevity™ Vitality™ Essential oil and add up to three drops into a clear, vegetarian capsule with olive oil and consume daily.

Safety notes: Keep out of reach of children. If you are pregnant, nursing, taking medication, or have a medical condition, consult a health professional before use.

MASTER FORMULA™

Master Formula™ is the Young Living equivalent of a multivitamin. However, it packs a much more powerful health punch than any multivitamin on the market.

This full-spectrum, multi-nutrient complex provides vitamins, minerals, and food-based nutrients that are great for anyone. This supplement has all the things that comprise a well-rounded multivitamin, is incredibly high quality, and is infused with powerful essential oils. Just like all Young Living supplements, Master Formula™ contains none of the fillers, coloring agents, or unnecessary ingredients that are common in conventional products.

BENEFITS OF MASTER FORMULA™
- Naturally supports health and well-being for the entire body
- Contains prebiotics that support gut flora
- Helps to neutralize free radicals in the body
- Includes antioxidants, vitamins, minerals, and other food-based nutrients
- Includes nutrition from 55 different natural botanical sources, including NingXia wolfberry powder
- Liquid Vitamin Capsule combines cardamom, clove, fennel, and ginger essential oils with fat-soluble vitamins
- Micronized Nutrient Capsule contains a blend of certified organic food extracts that provide vitamins B1, B2, B3, B5, B6, and B9
- Phyto-Caplet contains a powerful, nutrient-dense fruit, vegetable, and herb extract blend
- Pre-packaged sachets are convenient to take your vitamins on the go

Master Formula™ is a wonderful source of nutrients for general needs and has some incredible components that you won't find in any other multivitamin.
- **Turmeric root oil**: Turmeric has strong anti-inflammatory properties[2] that match the effectiveness of some anti-inflammatory drugs[3,4] and is a potent antioxidant that neutralizes free radicals[5], boosts the activity of the body's own antioxidant enzymes[6], and helps to improve mood and positive feelings[27,28].

- **Atlantic kelp**: This contains vitamins and minerals and is high in iodine, all of which are vital for a healthy thyroid and hormone balance and function. It is high in antioxidants, including carotenoids and flavonoids, which help fight against disease-causing free radicals, and contains antioxidant minerals, such as manganese and zinc, that combat oxidative stress and protect cardiovascular health.
- **Para-aminobenzoic acid (PABA)**: This is a structural component of endogenous folic acid, which is required to make DNA, and acts as an antioxidant to protect the body from free radical damage at a cellular level[29].
- **Cardamom essential oil**: Cardamom is a potent antioxidant with heart protective effects[30] that stimulates healthy digestion. It contains 1,8-cineole, a constituent that has shown antimicrobial activity in scientific studies.
- **Clove essential oil**: Clove has high antioxidant activity, with an average ORAC value of over 290,000[19]. It is effective at stopping the growth of some bacteria and fungi[20], including *Candida*[21] at higher doses, is high in the constituent eugenol, which boasts well-documented neuroprotective, antioxidant, anti-inflammatory, antipyretic, analgesic, antiparasitic, and antimicrobial properties, and protects the brain, heart, lungs, immune system, and the body as a whole[18].
- **Ginger essential oil**: Ginger has analgesic, anti-inflammatory, antibacterial, and antioxidant properties. It is great for soothing digestion[11], contains powerful antioxidants that protect against oxidative stress, helps combat inflammation[12], and supports liver health[13].
- **Fennel essential oil**: Fennel supports digestion, eases intestinal discomfort, supports the pancreas and liver, provides immune support, and promotes the excretion of toxins.

> **WHO SHOULD USE MASTER FORMULA™?**
> - Any adult looking for a general multivitamin for overall health and wellness
> - Anyone looking for a convenient supplement regimen
> - Any adult wanting to start adding supplements to a healthy lifestyle
> - Vegetarian adults needing a bioavailable source of nutrients, vitamins, and minerals
> - Anyone struggling mentally and emotionally, as a vitamin or mineral deficiency can be linked to anxious, exhausted, or dark feelings and thoughts
>
> **To use:** Take one packet (one liquid capsule, one caplet, two capsules) daily with water. May also be taken with 1-2 oz. of NingXia Red®.

If Master Formula™ is out of stock, here is a comparable regimen:
- Super B™
- MultiGreens™
- OmegaGize³⁺ (It's also fine to take OmegaGize³⁺ with Master Formula™)
- Super C™

Safety notes: Keep out of reach of children. If you are pregnant, nursing, taking medication, or have a medical condition, consult a health professional before use. An accidental overdose of iron-containing products is a leading cause of fatal poisoning in children under the age of six. In case of an accidental overdose, call a doctor or the poison control center immediately.

MINERAL ESSENCE™

Mineral Essence™ is a balanced, full-spectrum ionic mineral complex containing sixty ionic minerals, including iron, zinc, silicon, fluorine, boron, lithium, sodium, sulfur, magnesium, chloride, selenium, thallium, calcium, and potassium. Mineral Essence™ is also infused with peppermint, cinnamon bark, and lemon essential oils.

BENEFITS OF MINERAL ESSENCE™
- Balanced, full-spectrum ionic mineral complex that promotes overall health
- Enhanced with essential oils to improve mineral absorption
- Excellent source of magnesium, copper, and selenium
- Contains key minerals for a healthy thyroid

Trace minerals are incredibly important for our overall health. The body requires nearly two-thirds of all known elements to support optimal health, cognitive function, and overall performance, and keeping these minerals in balance is a complex yet incredibly vital task. Everyday life demands a continual ingestion of minerals, which ideally come from the diet. However, given current farming practices, diet alone isn't enough.

Traditionally, eating fresh, sprouted grains, fruits, and vegetables that are grown in nutrient-rich soil has been the primary source for a full spectrum of ionic minerals. Unfortunately, in today's world, naturally occurring, nutrient-rich soil is becoming increasingly rare. Decades and decades of vegetation growth and aggressive modern farming techniques have brought many of the earth's minerals to the surface, where they have been washed away. Although synthesized fertilizers are routinely applied to farms and fields where minerals have been depleted, man-made fertilizers only provide only enough mineral substance to support basic plant life. This has taken a huge toll on the amount of minerals that are present in our diets.

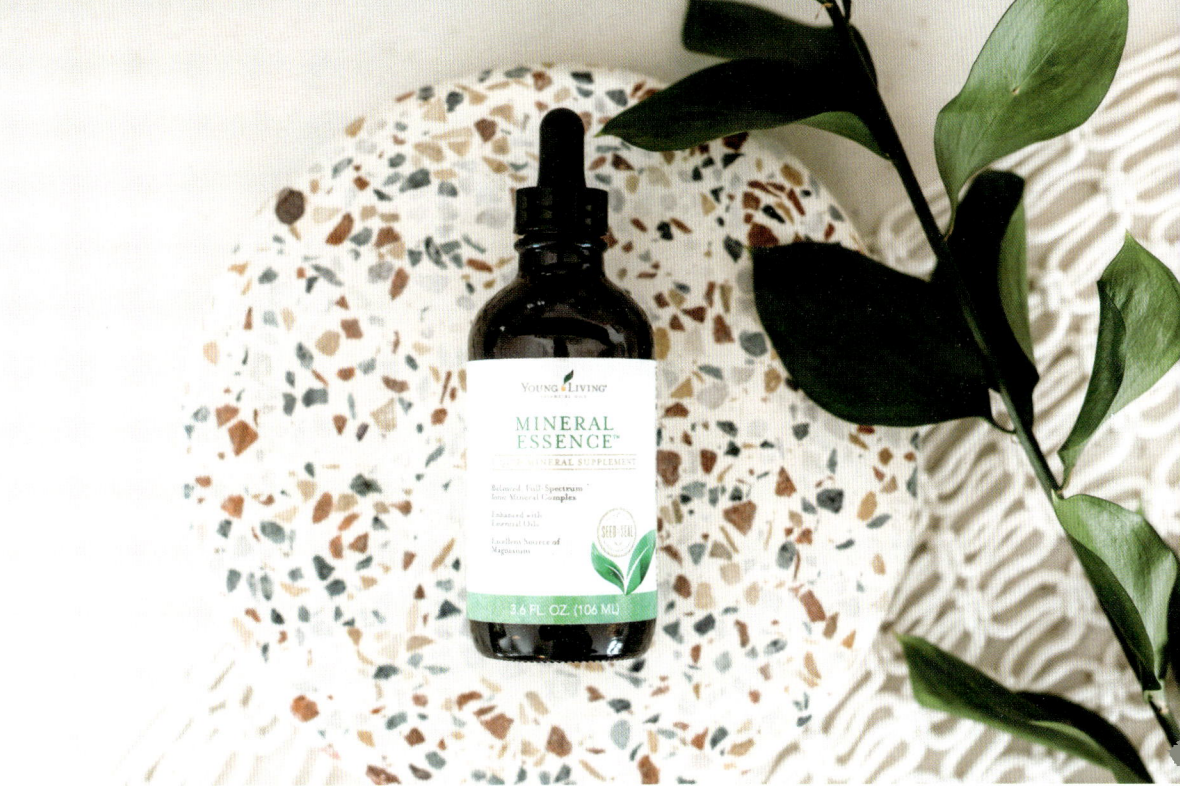

According to two-time Nobel Prize winner Linus Pauling, "You can trace every sickness, every disease, and every ailment to a mineral deficiency."

Deficiencies in iron, selenium, magnesium, and zinc are common in our society. Iron supports energy levels (among other things), selenium is key for thyroid health, magnesium is essential for muscle contraction, sleep, and emotional health, and zinc is used by more enzymes in the body than any other mineral and is essential for everything: from gut health to DNA repair. Minerals are critical to enzyme function, hormone production, bone building and breakdown, and long, luxurious hair and nails. They are used in every single cell in the body.

Each ingredient in Mineral Essence™ plays a specific role when it comes to supporting the body.
- **Calcium**: Calcium is the most abundant mineral in the body that assists in blood clotting, muscle contraction, cholesterol metabolism, healthy blood pressure levels, and nerve transmission. It enables normal bodily movement by keeping tissue rigid, strong, and flexible and is essential for healthy bones and teeth.
- **Chromium**: Chromium plays a role in carbohydrate, lipid, and protein metabolism, helps regulate blood sugar, and acts as an antioxidant to mitigate cellular damage.
- **Cobalt**: Cobalt is closely linked to vitamin B12, which is essential for energy and vitality. It promotes the formation of red blood cells, is involved in thyroid hormone production, and bolsters the immune system.
- **Copper**: Copper is essential for many processes in the body, including energy production, red blood cell formation, immune function, connective tissue formation, iron metabolism, brain development, and central nervous system function.

- **Iodine**: Iodine is essential for production of the thyroid hormones thyroxine (T4) and triiodothyronine (T3), which regulate numerous functions, including metabolism, energy levels, protein synthesis, and overall hormone balance. It may also play a role in immune system function.
- **Iron**: Iron is vital for oxygen delivery to the tissues through hemoglobin and is important for red blood cell formation, healthy energy levels, cognitive function, and emotional health.
- **Magnesium**: Magnesium is essential for more than 300 enzyme systems within the body to regulate everything from protein synthesis to muscle and nerve function, blood glucose levels, and blood pressure. It is required for energy production, contributes to the structural development of bone, is required for the synthesis of DNA, RNA, and glutathione, and plays a role in maintaining normal heart rhythm.
- **Molybdenum**: Molybdenum is a cofactor that is required for enzyme function that contributes to healthy growth and development.
- **Phosphorus**: Phosphorus is a component of DNA, RNA, cell membrane structure, and the body's key energy source, ATP. It works with calcium to contribute to healthy bones and teeth.
- **Potassium**: Potassium is the most abundant intracellular cation (a positively charged molecule) that is essential for normal cell function. It helps to regulate heartbeat, maintain fluid balance, and works closely with sodium to maintain proper nerve transmission, muscle contraction, and kidney function.
- **Selenium**: Selenium is an essential trace element that helps the body produce antioxidant enzymes and prevent cell damage, protects the body from the poisonous effects of heavy metals, plays a role in immune and reproductive health, and is necessary for normal growth and development[31].
- **Sulfur**: Sulfur provides structure and elasticity for our cells at a molecular level. It is important for skin health, wound healing, and soft, healthy hair, supports connective tissue, is key for muscle health, and is a significant component of glutathione, the most prevalent antioxidant in the body. Additionally, it is involved in detoxification and removes harmful substances from the body.
- **Zinc**: Zinc is involved in cellular metabolism, immune system function, wound healing, the ability to taste and smell, protein synthesis, reproduction, and more. It is essential during times of growth, and an inadequate intake can affect over 100 enzymes in the body. It is critical for eye health and has been shown to help with age-related macular degeneration[32] (and unless oysters are a part of your daily diet, achieving optimal zinc intake through food is incredibly difficult).
- **Cinnamon essential oil:** Cinnamon provides immune support through its antimicrobial activity and also acts as an antioxidant. It contains high levels of phenols, oxygenating compounds that function as catalysts for enzyme function within the body.

- **Lemon essential oil**: Lemon is high in limonene and promotes leukocyte production, which is an important factor in the immune system and for cleansing. D-limonene also alters the signaling pathways within cancer cells in a way that stops cancer cells from multiplying and causes their death[22].
- **Peppermint essential oil**: Peppermint soothes digestion, helps relax the digestive tract, acts as an antioxidant, and stimulates the immune system.

Like the other Young Living supplements, the addition of essential oils helps the body to absorb all the ionic minerals in this formula, which makes them more bioavailable (and useful) for our bodies.

Safety notes: Keep out of reach of children. If you are pregnant, nursing, taking medication, or have a medical condition, consult a healthcare professional before use. This product contains royal jelly, which may cause allergic reactions, especially in those with bee or honey allergies.

WHO SHOULD USE MINERAL ESSENCE™?
- Anyone looking to support overall health and vitality
- Anyone with a known nutrient or mineral deficiency
- Those suffering from emotional trauma, grief, anxiety, or depression, as a nutritional deficiency can worsen these needs
- Those with low or sluggish thyroid function
- Anyone looking to replace iron, selenium, or other trace minerals

To use:
- Take five half droppers (1 mL each) in the morning and evening or as needed as a mineral supplement. May be added to 4-8 oz. of distilled/purified water or juice before drinking. I recommend adding it to NingXia Red®, as this supplement has a spicy, mineral flavor. Shake well before using and refrigerate after opening.
- You can also apply this to the skin or use in an Epsom salt bath to enable absorption through the skin. Note, however, that this route of administration will provide less absorption than ingestion.

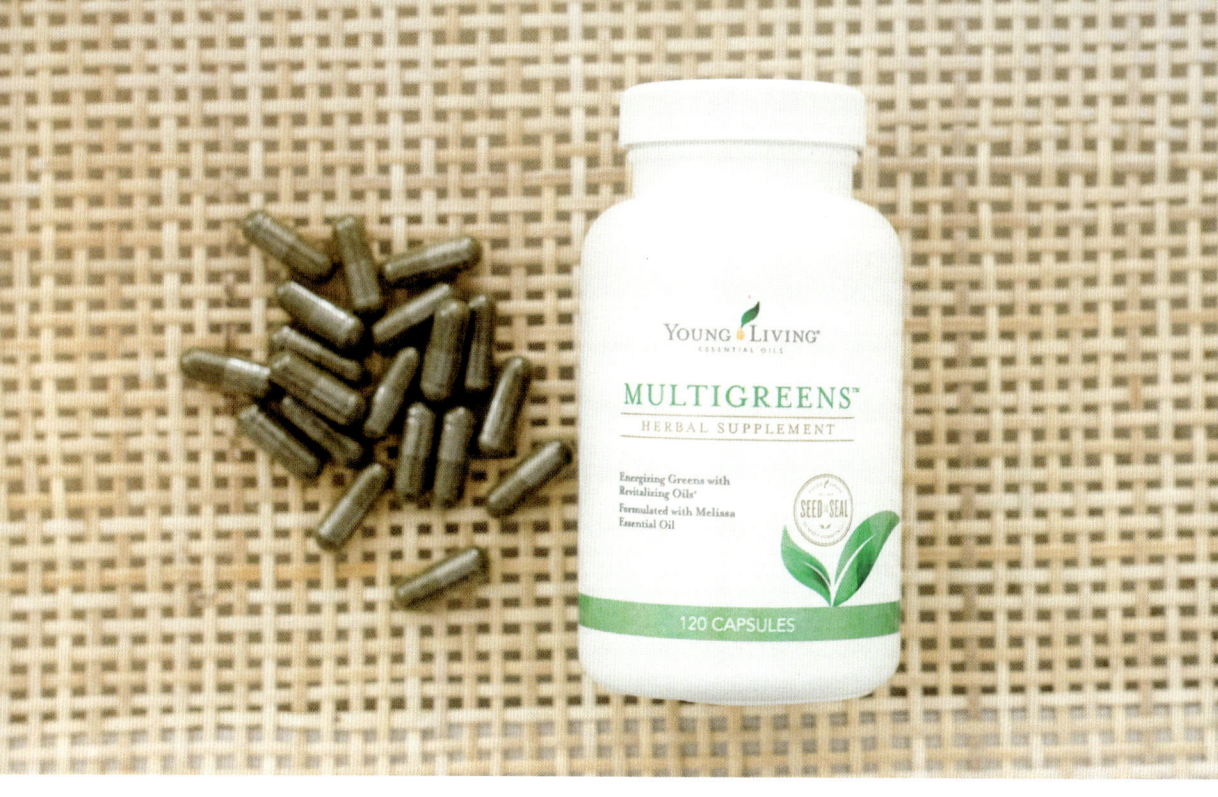

MULTIGREENS™

MultiGreens™ is your daily salad in a bottle. It fuels your system with lots of good things to help you feel amazing and increase vitality—much like eating a giant salad does!

MultiGreens™ is a blend of spirulina, alfalfa sprouts, barley grass, bee pollen, eleuthero root, Pacific kelp, and more. This nutrient-dense chlorophyll supplement combines invigorating greens and essential oils to support overall health, energy levels, and general well-being through supporting the glandular, nervous, and circulatory systems. MultiGreens™ provides a natural, sustainable energy source for the body and is an excellent source of choline, which is critical for energy production and mental clarity. MultiGreens™ also features a purifying essential oil blend that includes the powerhouse essential oil Melissa.

BENEFITS OF MULTIGREENS™
- Combines a powerhouse mix of greens, including spirulina and alfalfa
- Includes bee pollen and barley grass, which lower cholesterol and blood pressure
- Contains antioxidants that decrease inflammation
- Includes spirulina, which can relieve allergy symptoms
- Supports mental clarity, focus, and memory with choline and other ingredients
- Ingredients boast antimicrobial properties
- Promotes overall energy and vitality
- Purifies, mildly cleanses, and is a good source of fiber
- Formulated with Melissa essential oil, a cleansing antiviral oil

When we take Young Living's essential oil-infused vitamins supplements, the absorption rate increases dramatically compared to formulas without essential oils. This is because the essential oils help our bodies to take in and use the vitamins and minerals in our supplements. Essential oils work as little freight carriers to get the good things that we are taking into our bloodstream and cells. Additionally, they all have health benefits of their own, and MultiGreens™ contains several wonderful essential oils.

- **Bee Pollen**: Bee pollen is high in protein, vitamins, and minerals, including potassium, calcium, magnesium, zinc, and B vitamins. It has antifungal, antimicrobial, antiviral, anti-inflammatory, liver protective, and immune-stimulating properties that reduce chronic inflammation, aid in wound healing, and eliminate harmful bacteria[33,34]. It may have analgesic properties similar to some nonsteroidal anti-inflammatory drugs[34] and contains a wide variety of antioxidants, including flavonoids, carotenoids, quercetin, kaempferol, and glutathione[35], which boost the liver's antioxidant defense, remove waste products, safeguard the liver against damage from toxic substances, and promote liver healing. Moreover, it can lower the risk of heart disease[36] and assists with macronutrient assimilation.
- **Barley grass**: Barley grass is a nutrient-rich superfood that is loaded with vitamins A, B C, E, and K. It is full of antioxidants, which work to fight damage at a cellular level, works as a powerful cleansing agent, and can help relieve symptoms of ulcerative colitis[37,38]. It is an excellent source of both soluble and insoluble fiber. Insoluble fiber feeds the good bacteria in the gut, improving digestion and intestinal health. Soluble fiber helps the stomach to absorb sugar more slowly, which prevents blood sugar spikes and elevated cholesterol.
- **Spirulina**: Spirulina is a source of chlorophyll, antioxidants, and magnesium that protects against oxidative damage, supports the liver, intestines, immune and cardiovascular systems, energy levels, and improves allergy symptoms. It is a fantastic source of phycocyanin, the antioxidant that gives spirulina its unique blue-green color and has impressive anti-inflammatory effects[39,40]. It is effective at relieving allergy symptoms[41,42], can positively impact cholesterol[44] and blood sugar levels[46], and can lower blood pressure[45].
- **Choline**: Choline is an essential micronutrient that is necessary for numerous bodily processes, including nerve function, cholesterol processing, brain development, muscle mobility, and liver function. It ensures a healthy metabolism and works similarly to B vitamins, in that it supports energy, stimulates metabolism, and aids brain function. Additionally, it improves communication between nerves and muscles and boosts cardiovascular health, focus, and memory function. It helps maintain low levels of inflammation throughout the body and is necessary for mental and physical development in utero, which makes supplementation during pregnancy essential[47].
- **Eleuthero root**: Eleuthero root is an adaptogenic herb that soothes cortisol and boosts the body's resistance to stress by providing energy and strengthening immune cell and immune system function. It has been used to improve athletic performance, reduce fatigue[48], and ease the side effects of chemotherapy. Additionally, it acts as an antioxidant, lowers cholesterol[49], has analgesic and anti-inflammatory properties, and helps to prevent bone degeneration, especially when taken in combination with other joint- and muscle-supporting herbs[50].

- **Alfalfa leaf**: Alfalfa is high in chlorophyll, calcium, iron, potassium, phosphorus, and vitamins C and K. It has a positive effect on blood sugar, cholesterol, and blood pressure levels[51] and is beneficial in treating arthritis, urinary tract infections, menstrual problems, and an array of other disorders[52].
- **Pacific kelp**: Kelp contains iodine, vitamins, minerals, and antioxidants, all of which are vital for a healthy thyroid and hormone balance and function. It is high in antioxidants, including carotenoids and flavonoids, which help to fight against disease-causing free radicals, contains antioxidant minerals, such as manganese and zinc, that combat oxidative stress and protect cardiovascular health, and helps to reduce blood sugar levels, lower cholesterol, and increase antioxidant enzyme activities[53].
- **Amino acids L-arginine, L-cysteine, and L-tyrosine**: These amino acids help the body with proper circulation, cellular metabolism, liver function, and the production of dopamine and serotonin.
    - L-cysteine is broadly recognized as a precursor for glutathione, which is the body's main antioxidant that is involved in many necessary functions, including those that promote detoxification and longevity.
    - L-arginine is a precursor for nitrous oxide, a compound that plays a role in development, learning, and memory, protects against brain injury, and modulates stress-induced anxiety.
    - L-tyrosine acts as a precursor for the important neurotransmitters dopamine, norepinephrine, and epinephrine[54].
- **Rosemary essential oil**: Rosemary helps to balance the endocrine system and cleanse the liver. It cleanses, purifies, and provides immune support through direct bactericidal activity, even on certain drug-resistant bacteria and fungi[110].
- **Lemon essential oil**: Lemon is high in limonene, a constituent that is known to strengthen the immune system and help decongest the lymphatic system. D-limonene also alters the signaling pathways within cancer cells in a way that stops cancer cells from multiplying and causes their death[22].
- **Lemongrass essential oil**: Lemongrass is a highly cleansing oil. Some studies suggest that it has antimicrobial properties and is calming to the digestive system.
- **Melissa essential oil**: Melissa is helpful for diseases that are associated with inflammation, swelling, and pain[64]. It improves glycemic control and blood sugar levels[65], promotes healthy skin, and can improve acne and eczema[66]. It has antiviral properties and can stop bacterial infections, including those resistant to prescription medications[67].

MULTIGREENS™ AND EMOTIONAL HEALTH

When our physical bodies are tired and run down, our emotions are quick to follow. And sometimes it is our emotions alert us that our physical health is declining. The two are closely linked with one profoundly affecting the other.

Add in hormones. And stress. Thyroid, cortisol, and other essential hormones are always affected when we are tired, run down, and stressed. Our energy levels bottom out, and we have no "get up and go" left.

When we are feeling this way, it is especially important to supplement well. Ideally, we are already supporting both our physical bodies and our emotions daily with baseline supplements, such as MultiGreens™, NingXia Red®, and Super B™. Maintaining homeostasis (balance) within our hormones, and especially the thyroid, is essential for maintaining good energy levels. Pacific kelp is included in MultiGreens™ for just that purpose. Pacific kelp supports thyroid function and helps to keep our hormones balanced and in check. This is something that we need daily, especially when we are run down. Add in all the other powerful ingredients in this supplement, and it becomes something that can support us both physically and emotionally.

> **WHO SHOULD USE MULTIGREENS™?**
> - Anyone who needs to improve their iron levels
> - Anyone who needs minerals and nutrients
> - Individuals with environmental sensitivities or seasonal allergies
> - Anyone who wants to support the circulatory and nervous systems
> - Anyone who doesn't eat a strong, whole-food diet containing leafy greens
> - Anyone feeling weak and tired
> - Individuals with low or sluggish thyroid function
>
> **To use:** Take three capsules twice daily. Capsules may also be opened and sprinkled over food or in smoothies. This is a great option for children.

Safety notes: If you are pregnant, nursing, taking medication, or have a medical condition, consult a health practitioner before use. An accidental overdose of iron-containing products is a leading cause of fatal poisoning in children aged under six. Keep this product out of reach of children. In case of an accidental overdose, call a doctor or the poison control center immediately. Contains barley and bee pollen, so if you have a severe gluten sensitivity or are severely allergic to bee products, try using Mineral Essence™ instead for similar benefits.

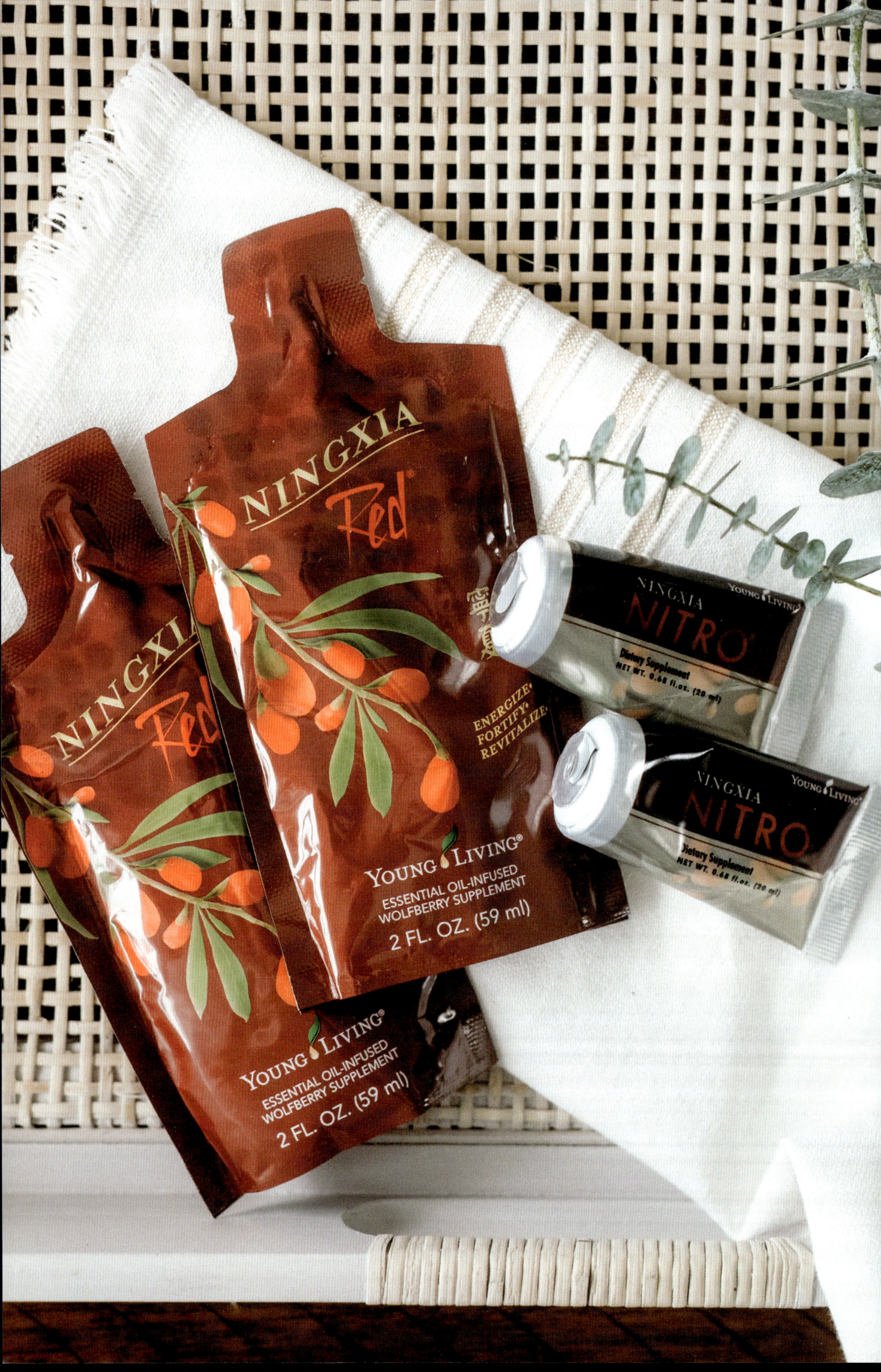
NINGXIA
Red
ENERGIZE•
FORTIFY•
REVITALIZE•
YOUNG LIVING
ESSENTIAL OIL-INFUSED
WOLFBERRY SUPPLEMENT
2 FL. OZ. (59 ml)
NINGXIA
Red
YOUNG LIVING
ESSENTIAL OIL-INFUSED
WOLFBERRY SUPPLEMENT
2 FL. OZ. (59 ml)
NINGXIA
NITRO
YOUNG LIVING
Dietary Supplement
NINGXIA
NITRO
YOUNG LIVING
Dietary Supplement

NINGXIA RED®

NingXia Red® is one of Young Living's most popular products, and for good reason. This wolfberry puree is so much more than a delicious addition to your day. NingXia Red® is a nutrient-dense fuel source for our bodies. Much like a car runs better with proper fuel, our bodies perform better when they are supplied with all the nutrients that they need.

BENEFITS OF NINGXIA RED®
- Supports a healthy immune system
- Provides energy and vitality
- A huge source of antioxidants
- Supports brain and joint health
- Supports healthy hormone levels
- Supports healthy blood sugar levels
- Can help curb sugar cravings
- Infused with citrus essential oils, which are high in limonene
- Whole-food, nutrient-dense supplement full of vitamins, minerals, amino acids, and polyphenols

NingXia Red® is a powerful antioxidant supplement drink made from wolfberry puree, blueberry, plum, cherry, Aronia, and pomegranate juices, grape seed extract, yuzu, tangerine, lemon, and orange essential oils, stevia and pure vanilla extract. The essential oils that are mixed in NingXia Red® act as catalysts to help deliver the antioxidants and nutrients through the cell membranes while assisting with the removal of cellular wastes.

In addition to its great taste, NingXia Red® has several amazing health benefits. It is the highest known protection against the dangerous superoxide free radicals, as documented in the S-ORAC test conducted by Brunswick Laboratories. One ounce of NingXia Red® has the same antioxidant power of:
- 4 pounds of carrots
- 2 quarts of carrot juice
- 8 oranges
- 1 pint of orange juice
- 2 pounds of beets
- 2 cups of beet juice
- 3 cups of raspberries
- 2 cups of blueberries
- ... **combined**!

NingXia Red® is rich in ellagic acid, polyphenols, flavonoids, vitamins, and minerals. In addition, it has 18 amino acids, 21 trace minerals, beta-carotene, and vitamins B1, B2, B6, and E. It is an excellent whole-food source of nutrients that provides energy and strength to the body without harmful stimulates. It also has an amazing low glycemic index of 11 that does not spike blood sugar levels.

- **Wolfberry puree:** The wolfberry powerful source of antioxidants that promote everything from eye and immune health to energy levels and hormone balance.
- **Blueberry, Aronia, cherry, pomegranate, and plum juices:** These antioxidant fruits repair DNA damage, provide energy and antioxidants to the cells, and support healthy blood sugar levels, cognitive function, and cardiovascular health.
- **Lemon, orange, yuzu, and tangerine essential oils:** These oils are high in limonene, which bolsters the immune system, provides antioxidant support to repair free radical damage, and has anti-inflammatory, wound-healing, and anticancer properties. D-limonene also alters the signaling pathways within cancer cells in a way that stops cancer cells from multiplying and causes their death[22].
- **Trace minerals:** Minerals are critical to enzyme function, hormone production, bone building, and all cellular functions within the body.
- **B vitamins:** B vitamins support normal cardiovascular and cognitive health, improve mood, and help to sustain healthy energy levels.
- **Vitamin E:** Vitamin E minimizes free radical damage within the body and promotes healthy cell function and overall health.

THE NINGXIA WOLFBERRY

The wolfberry (or goji berry) has been used in traditional Chinese medicine for centuries due to its ability to enhance immune function, improve eyesight, protect the liver, and improve circulation, among other effects. The wolfberry is rich in vitamin C, fiber, and B vitamins, as well as minerals, such as potassium, sodium, phosphorus, magnesium, iron, calcium, zinc, and selenium. Additionally, Chinese wolfberries have high levels of the antioxidant zeaxanthin, which is known to improve and prevent age-related declines in eye health[55]. To say that the NingXia wolfberry is a superfood is an understatement!

WHO SHOULD USE NINGXIA RED®?

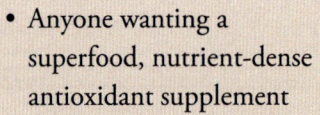

- Anyone wanting a superfood, nutrient-dense antioxidant supplement
- Anyone struggling with emotional health
- Individuals processing trauma or grief
- Anyone with known inflammatory conditions (acute or chronic)
- Women who are pregnant, nursing, or trying to conceive
- Children and adults, at your discretion
- In short: everyone aged two and older

To use: Take 2-4 oz. daily on its own or mixed with water, juice, or sparkling water. NingXia Red® can also be added to a smoothie.

NINGXIA RED® & EMOTIONAL HEALTH

Supporting our physical health is critical when it comes to emotional health, as they are so interconnected. Both NingXia Red® and NingXia wolfberries are full of antioxidants, which are essential when we are processing stress or trauma, and they are particularly helpful when feeling overwhelmed or experiencing grief or fear.

Relieving the physical oxidative stress on the body facilitates emotional healing at a cellular level. Furthermore, antioxidants help to promote the movement of grief through the body. To use the NingXia wolfberries, simply place them in a mug with some of your favorite herbal tea, add hot water, and steep. To use NingXia Red® for emotional health, simply drink it daily on its own or pair it with Mineral Essence™ and/or MindWise™ for additional support.

NINGXIA RED® FAQ:

Q: When can children begin drinking NingXia Red®?

A: This is your decision as the informed parent or caregiver. I choose to give it to my children when I am giving them other plant-based foods. It is usually best to begin with 1 oz. and then work up to the adult recommendation of 2 oz. My children who are above two years old, drink 2 or more oz. per day.

Q: Can I use NingXia Red® if I have diabetes?

A: You must answer that question based on your body's response to the product. Drink NingXia, wait 15 minutes, and then check your blood sugar. Add healthy fats and proteins whenever taking in sugars, even those naturally occurring in fruits. Although it falls well within the recommended guidelines for carbohydrate and sugar intake for those with diabetes, it is always wise to consult your trusted care provider.

Q: Can I use NingXia Red® if I need to avoid nightshades?

A: There is evidence to suggest that some nightshades can exaggerate inflammation in the body and should be avoided by those with autoimmune diseases. The NingXia wolfberry contains a balance between the polysaccharides and solanine, which suggests that a balance may be in place with this particular fruit.

Q: Can I use NingXia Red® if I'm on blood thinning medications?

A: Make sure that you research your specific medications and know your body. There have been people who have reported a thinning of blood with regular use of the wolfberry. If taking medications, be very sure that you consistently use the same amount of NingXia daily. This way, your doctor can help you adjust your dosage to work well with your NingXia intake in the same way that he or she would if you were to consume leafy greens on a regular basis.

OMEGAGIZE³®

We have all heard how wonderful fish oil can be for our health, and many people are supplementing with fish oil. Unfortunately, it is incredibly difficult to find a high-quality fish oil supplement that is free of mercury, sustainably sourced, and contains bioavailable vitamin D. Enter OmegaGize³®! Young Living's OmegaGize³® is an incredible, sustainably sourced fish oil supplement that is full of healthy omegas, vitamin D, and CoQ10, which supports heart, brain, eye, and joint health.

BENEFITS OF OMEGAGIZE³®
- Supports cardiovascular and skeletal health
- Supports normal, healthy brain function
- Supplies critical EPA and DHA nutrients
- Supports normal immune response and antioxidant levels
- Promotes normal eye, skin, and joint health
- Infused with clove, German chamomile, and spearmint essential oils that work as antioxidants to support health at a cellular level
- Trifecta of omega-3 fatty acids, vitamin D, and CoQ10

OmegaGize³® combines the power of three core daily supplements—omega-3 fatty acids, vitamin D3, and CoQ10 (ubiquinone)—in one capsule. CoQ10 is a great addition to this formula because it is required for ATP production. ATP is the energy currency of the body and is required for all cells to do what they do. Additionally, CoQ10 works synergistically with omega-3s and vitamin D. It can be difficult to get enough vitamin D each day through sun exposure and food alone, so supplementation can help. Moreover, since vitamin D is fat-soluble, it needs to be taken in the presence of fatty acids for proper absorption. OmegaGize³® has all that covered! When used daily, these ingredients work synergistically to support normal brain, heart, eye, and joint health and overall health and wellness.

IMPORTANCE OF OMEGA-3 FATTY ACIDS
Although the human body can make most of the fats that it needs from other fats or raw materials, that isn't the case for omega-3 fatty acids. These are essential fats, which means that the body can't make them from scratch and must get them from outside sources. Even if your diet is high in wild-caught fish, you still need supplementation.

Omega-3s are an integral part of cell membranes throughout the body and affect the function of the cell receptors in these membranes. This means that they are vital for all of our cellular functioning and are especially important during pregnancy. Omega-3s provide the starting point for making hormones that regulate blood clotting, the contraction and relaxation of artery walls, and inflammation. Research has shown that omega-3s can…
- Help prevent heart disease and stroke
- Support a healthy heart and blood pressure

- Support healthy hormone levels by aiding the body in keeping the cellular receptor sites (where hormones bind) repaired and in optimal condition
- Support autoimmune needs and conditions
- Support the body's natural response to inflammation and joint pain
- Assist the body in hormone productions associated with mood disorders
- Support those with ADHD and focus needs
- Support normal brain and nerve function which is important for older individuals

In addition to the health benefits of omega-3s, OmegaGize³® contains other ingredients that work together to promote overall health and well-being.

- **Vitamin D**: Vitamin D is an essential supplement that supports optimal brain health, hormone levels, immune function, bone and joint health, and overall well-being. Research shows that vitamin D:
    - Supports immunity
    - Helps regulate mood and fight depression
    - Supports the body's natural response to inflammation
    - Supports normal growth and the development of bones and teeth
- **CoQ10:** CoQ10 is a powerful antioxidant that supports every cell in the body. It acts as a battery for our cells, helps with the production and exchange of energy, and helps to facilitate the production of ATP. As CoQ10 levels naturally decline with age, supplementation is a great health habit. Several studies show that CoQ10:
    - Is required in every cell in the body
    - Helps protect the body from free radical damage
    - Produces the energy that your body needs for daily functions
    - Boosts the immune system

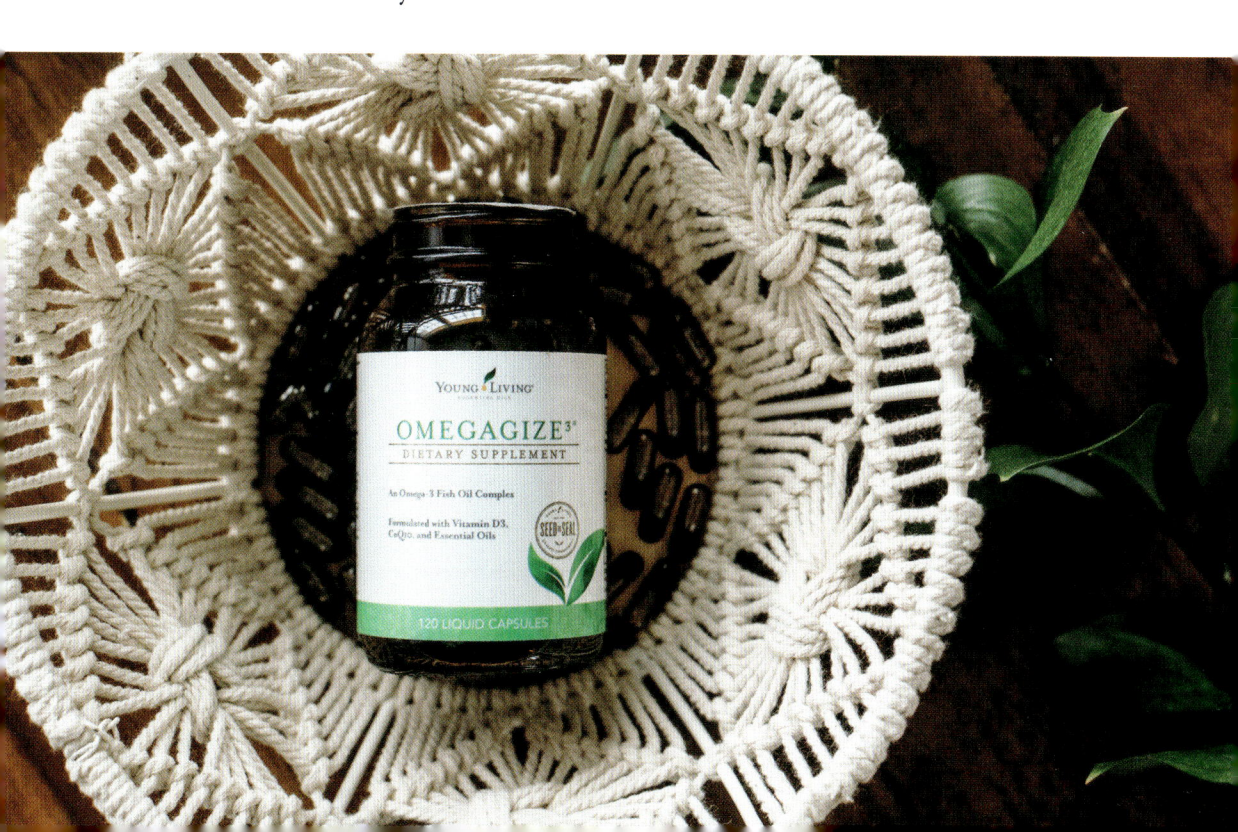

- **Clove essential oil**: Clove has long been used in eastern medicine for a range of health benefits due to its high antioxidant activity. It has an average ORAC value of over 290,000[19], is high in the constituent eugenol, which boasts well-documented neuroprotective, antioxidant, anti-inflammatory, antipyretic, analgesic, antiparasitic, and antimicrobial properties, and protects the brain, heart, lungs, immune system, and the whole body[18].
- **Spearmint essential oil**: Spearmint is high in the constituents carvone and limonene. It is wonderful for digestive health, soothes intestinal discomfort, and decreases inflammation.
- **German chamomile essential oil**: German chamomile is a powerful antioxidant that supports healthy cholesterol levels, liver and gallbladder health, and the body's natural response to inflammation.
- **Vitamin E** (as rice bran oil): Vitamin E minimizes free radical damage within the body, promoting healthy cell function and overall health.

OMEGAGIZE3® & CARDIOVASCULAR HEALTH

Because we're usually thinking about cholesterol in the diet, most people don't realize that cholesterol in the body comes from two places: the diet and your internal production of cholesterol. Cholesterol is important to your body because it is one of the major components of cell membranes. It's also the precursor for all of the sex hormones. It's not all bad. Cholesterol becomes an issue when there is an overt excess of it and when the types of cholesterol are way out of balance.

Omega-3 fatty acids primarily support heart health through their ability to reduce triglyceride levels. Triglycerides are a type of storage cholesterol in the body. When we eat, our bodies convert any unused calories into triglycerides and store them in fat cells. Later, hormones release the triglycerides for energy between meals. When triglyceride levels become too high, this can cause health problems. Therefore, most clinicians will monitor triglyceride levels along with other cholesterol levels. Omega-3 fatty acids are a simple way to support healthy triglyceride levels. Omega-3 fatty acids modestly raise HDL ("good" or "protective" cholesterol) levels.

Most Americans who need support for healthy cholesterol levels take a "statin" prescription drug to lower cholesterol. Statins work by inhibiting the enzyme HMG-CoA reductase, which is one of the facilitators of the body's production of cholesterol. However, statins also impair the production of CoQ10 and inhibit the conversion of vitamin K1 to vitamin K2. Both CoQ10 and vitamin K conversion are essential for body processes, including a healthy heart. The depletion of CoQ10 and vitamin K reduces ubiquinol levels and can have very severe consequences, such as low energy, fatigue, and muscle pains.

I don't preach mutual exclusivity when it comes to health tools. I believe that you can use both Eastern and Western medicine to reach your health goals. However, no matter how you look at it, it is obvious that we need better options for maintaining healthy cholesterol levels than what conventional Western medicine has to offer.

OMEGAGIZE3® & EMOTIONAL HEALTH

Several studies have shown the importance of omega-3 fatty acids when it comes to emotional health, especially in females and during pregnancy and the surrounding time frame. Omega-3 fatty acids are essential for cell growth and development, and they assist with mental clarity—these functions are often "off" during times of increased emotional need or stress[56,57].

Studies have found that a reduced omega-3 status may predispose individuals toward anxiety and depression, as well as other conditions[58]. As always, we want to do all we can to stay above the health line and support our bodies daily. Therefore, supplementing with OmegaGize3® is a great starting point. If you need extra support, I always recommend finding a healthcare provider, such as a naturopath or functional medicine physician, who you trust.

WHO SHOULD USE OMEGAGIZE3®?

- Anyone wanting to achieve or maintain healthy cholesterol levels
- Women who are pregnant, nursing, or trying to conceive
- Individuals with emotional health needs, stress, anxiety, or depression
- Anyone with a history of nutrient depletion through chronic or acute illness, childbearing and breastfeeding, or mycotoxin exposure
- Anyone wanting to support overall health and wellness

To use: Take two to four capsules twice daily. Do not exceed eight capsules per day. Store in a cool, dark place.

OMEGAGIZE3®

Sadly, conventional fish oil supplements are full of synthetic fillers, artificial colorants, and flavors and are irresponsibly sourced. Some even contain high levels of mercury, which we don't want to consume. The fish oil complex in OmegaGize3® is derived from some of the cleanest waters on the planet. OmegaGize3® capsules are rigorously tested to ensure a lack of these pollutants. Even the capsule of OmegaGize3® is ocean-derived, which ensures the best quality and no fishy taste.

"The oil in OmegaGize3® is produced from carefully selected, wild-caught Peruvian and Chilean coastal marine fish oil, one of the cleanest ocean areas in the world. Consisting mainly of anchovy, sardine, mackerel, skipjack, yellowfin, albacore, and bigeye fish species. The fish oil used in OmegaGize3® is in triglyceride form (research shows this is the best form).—Young Living.

Safety notes: Keep out of reach of children. If you are pregnant, nursing, taking medication, or have a medical condition, consult a healthcare professional before use. Contains fish (Basa).

SUPER B™

B vitamins are essential to our health and well-being, and each B vitamin performs a unique and separate function, which is why a B complex vitamin is necessary. Unfortunately, B vitamins must be replenished daily, as they are water soluble and are therefore not stored in the body. It is difficult to gain all the B vitamins we need from our food, even in the best-case scenario, which is why it's a good idea to supplement. This is also a great addition to your routine if you are currently expecting or are wanting to grow your family in the near future.

BENEFITS OF SUPER B™
- Known for supporting normal cardiovascular and cognitive health
- Improves mood
- Helps sustain healthy energy levels
- Contains all eight essential, energy-boosting B vitamins
- Contains nutmeg essential oil and bioavailable chelated minerals, such as magnesium, manganese, selenium, and zinc
- Contains Orgen-FA, which is a natural folate source that is derived from lemon peels
- Contains methylcobalamin, which is a more bioavailable source of B12

Many commonly used medications can wreak havoc on the body's B-vitamin levels. Some of these include hormonal birth control of all types, acid suppressing drugs, such as Prilosec (omeprazole) or Zantac (ranitidine), diabetes medications (metformin), and even some antibiotics (minocycline, azithromycin, ciprofloxacin, and others). And while conventional medications are a tool in the toolbox, having an awareness of their side effects allows us to support our bodies well and take preventative measures when possible.

Young Living's Super B™ is a B complex. It contains all eight essential, energy-boosting B vitamins, nutmeg essential oil, and bioavailable chelated minerals, and folate. Our bodies struggle to absorb and utilize folic acid. We need it in the form of folate for adequate absorption, and many individuals require a methylated version, which is why Orgen-FA is a great addition to this supplement.

Here is a closer look at each ingredient in Super B™ and how it supports our system.
- **Thiamin** (Vitamin B1): Thiamin is essential for energy production, carbohydrate metabolism, and nerve function at the cellular level.
- **Riboflavin** (Vitamin B2): Riboflavin assists with the production of cellular energy and helps to regenerate the liver while supporting normal cellular health.
- **Niacin** (Vitamin B3): Niacin is important for the metabolism of carbohydrates into an energy source and can lower cholesterol and regulate blood sugar.
  - *Note: Niacin may cause a phenomenon known as "niacin flush." This is a normal reaction where the hands, face, and elbows may turn red and feel warm to the touch. It will go away on its own.*

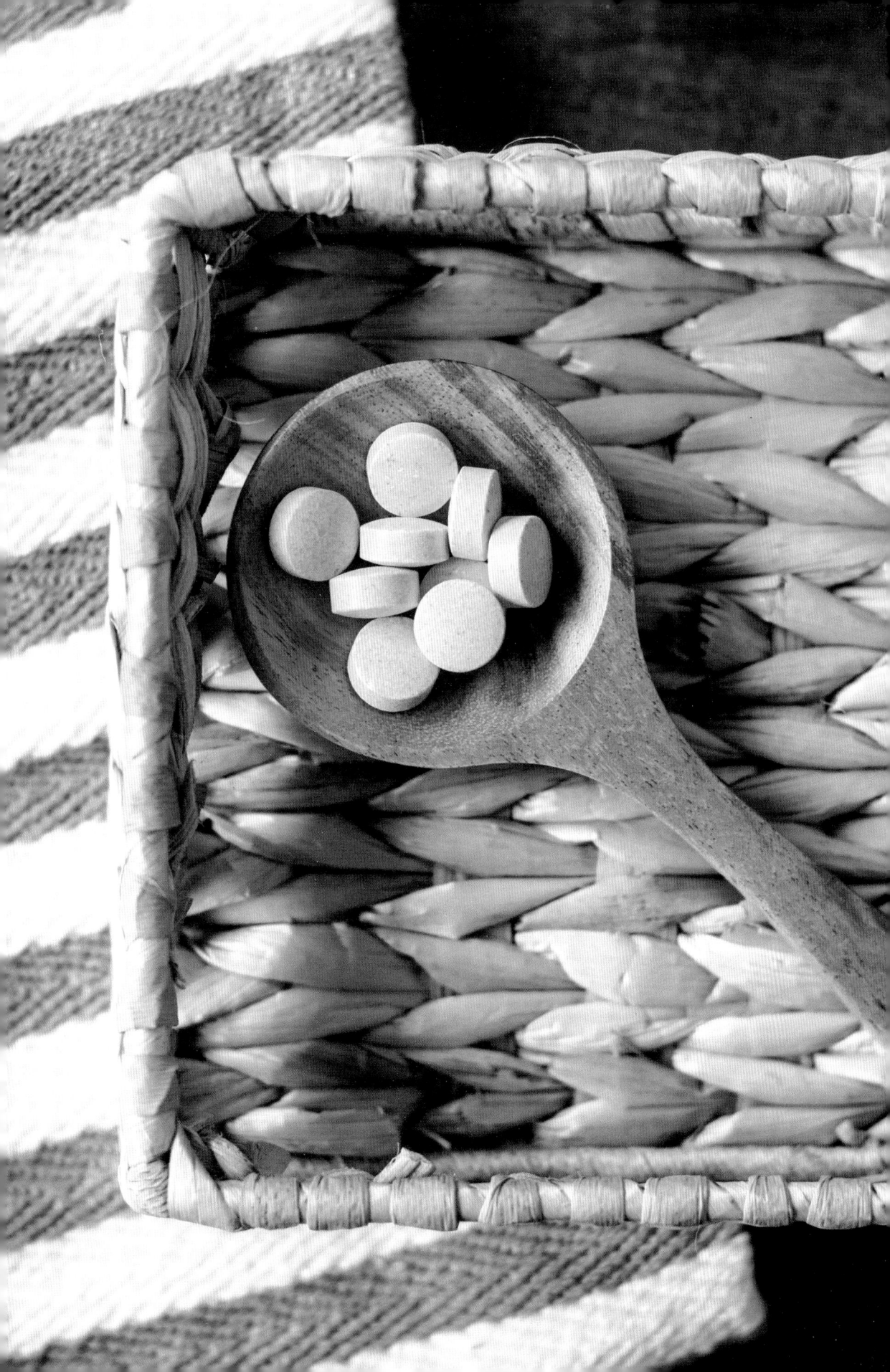

- **Pyridoxine** (Vitamin B6): B6 supports the cardiovascular system, specifically the blood vessels.
- **Orgen-FA**: This is a natural folate source derived from lemon peels. Folate is essential for vitamins B6 and B12 to be assimilated into the body, and folate is superior to folic acid, as the body cannot easily convert folic acid into folate.
- **Methylcobalamin** (Vitamin B12): B12 is essential for red blood cell production, immune function, and nervous system function. It works with vitamin B6 to support the cardiovascular system. The specific methylcobalamin included is a more bioavailable source of B12, so our bodies absorb it more readily.
- **Biotin** (Vitamin B7): B7 helps to convert fats and amino acids into energy, supports healthy hair and nail growth, and can combat yeast and fungus overgrowth.
- **Pantothenic acid** (Vitamin B5): B5 assists with the secretion of hormones and supports the adrenal glands.
- **Magnesium** (Magnesium oxide): Magnesium is essential for the proper function of enzymes, muscle contractions, and heart rhythm, supports the cardiovascular system, and helps to maintain blood pressure and healthy insulin levels.
- **Zinc** (Zinc gluconate): Zinc is necessary for immune support, cell regeneration, and the proper function of hormones, such as insulin and the growth hormones.
- **Selenium** (Selenium yeast): Selenium supports the immune system and is an essential trace element that helps the body produce antioxidant enzymes and prevents cell damage. It also helps protect the body from the poisonous effects of heavy metals, plays a role in immune and reproductive health, and is necessary for normal growth and development[31].
- **PABA** (Para Amino Benzoic Acid): PABA works with the "good" bacteria of the gut to produce folic acid, helps to produce red blood cells, and acts as an antioxidant to protect the body from free radical damage[29].

WHO SHOULD USE SUPER B™?

- Anyone under stress, as stress depletes B vitamins in our bodies
- Anyone who battles *Candida*. Some believe that a lack of it causes overgrowthAnyone struggling with energy levels
- Anyone struggling mentally and emotionally, as a deficiency can be linked to anxious, exhausted, and dark feelings and thoughts
- Anyone who struggles with anemia, is pregnant, or doesn't eat a strong whole-food diet
- All adults, unless otherwise contraindicated

To use: Take two tablets daily with a meal, ideally with your first meal of the day. Alternatively, you can take one tablet with your first meal and one tablet midday.

B VITAMINS & EMOTIONAL HEALTH

Vitamin deficiencies, such as zinc, B vitamins, and vitamin D, among others, are gaining the spotlight when it comes to emotional health. B vitamins are essential for proper brain function and energy levels. Vitamin B12 and folate are both needed to produce norepinephrine, serotonin, and dopamine and play important roles in regulating and maintaining a healthy central nervous system. Low folate and vitamin B12 levels have been associated with depression, although the mechanisms are somewhat unclear.

The bottom line is that when you are feeling low, sad, anxious, or just "off" emotionally, it is often a signal that your body is deficient in a necessary vitamin or mineral. Don't discount the power of nutrition! Super B™ is a great choice if you are feeling fatigued, low, or lethargic. Lab testing with a trusted care provider may give you additional insight.

Safety notes: Keep out of reach of children. If you are pregnant, nursing, taking medication, or have a medical condition, consult a health professional before use. If taken on an empty stomach, you may experience a temporary niacin flush/warming sensation.

SUPER C™ (AND SUPER C™ CHEWABLE)

We all know that vitamin C is good for us and can help boost immunity, and Young Living's Super C™ and Super C™ Chewable don't disappoint! Super C™ contains 2,166% of the recommended dietary intake of vitamin C per serving and is fortified with rutin, citrus bioflavonoids, and minerals to balance electrolytes and enhance the effectiveness and absorption of vitamin C. This is a *much* better option than the sugary packets that you find in health food stores.

BENEFITS OF SUPER C™
- Supports immune health, respiratory function, and overall wellness
- Provides the body with powerful antioxidants that promote vitality and longevity
- Supports eye health and vision
- Promotes the formation of collagen
- Infused with citrus essential oils that are high in limonene, which is a powerful antioxidant
- Vitamin C is essential for bone, ligament, tendon, and blood vessel health
- Vitamin C aids with iron absorption (add to a protein-rich meal or iron supplement)

Super C™ tablets contain orange, tangerine, grapefruit, lemon, and lemongrass essential oils. When combined with the other ingredients, these play a role in normal immune and circulatory functions, help to strengthen connective tissues, and promote overall health, vitality, and longevity[59]. As our bodies cannot manufacture vitamin C, it must be consumed daily.

In addition to being a potent antioxidant, vitamin C is one of the most important vitamins required by our bodies. Vitamin C is essential for the growth and repair of tissues in all parts of the body. It is necessary to form collagen, which is an important protein used for scar tissue, tendons, ligaments, and blood vessels. It is essential for healing wounds and the repair and maintenance of cartilage, bones, and teeth.

Super C™ tablets include:
- **Orange, tangerine, and grapefruit essential oils**: These citrus oils are high in d-limonene, a constituent that shows anti-inflammatory, wound-healing, and anticancer effects. D-limonene alters the signaling pathways within cancer cells in a way that stops cancer cells from multiplying and causes their death[22].
- **Citrus bioflavonoids**: These help to maximize the benefits of vitamin C by inhibiting its breakdown in the body. Additionally, they protect against oxidative stress, inflammation, elevated blood sugar and cholesterol, damage to the lining of cells, and plaque buildup in the arteries[60].
- **Cayenne powder:** Cayenne aids digestion and helps to decrease inflammation and maintain healthy arteries[61].
- **Rutin powder**: Rutin is a bioflavonoid with antioxidant properties that promotes heart and brain health.

Super C™ Chewable tablets include vitamin C from whole-food plant sources.
- **Acerola cherry powder**: Acerola cherries are very high in vitamin C,

WHO SHOULD USE SUPER C™ OR SUPER C™ CHEWABLE?
- Anyone wanting to bolster the immune system daily (everyone!)
- Those needing support for bones, joints, and inflammation
- Those with acute infections (note, higher doses are needed)
- Anyone wanting daily antioxidant support
- Those entering circumstances of increased bacterial and viral exposure (note, higher doses are needed for acute exposures)

To use Super C™: For reinforcing immune strength, take up to three tablets daily, making sure to separate the doses by a few hours. For other needs or daily maintenance, take one tablet once or twice daily. It works best when taken before meals.

To use Super C™ Chewable: Take one chewable tablet three times daily or as needed. Take daily or when additional vitamin C is desired.

The Super C™ Chewable tablets are perfect for a chewable option and for little ones. We love these for keeping us healthy all year round, when our defenses go down, or while traveling, and always take them when getting on a plane or when we are around extra germs.

contains vitamin A, which acts as an antioxidant, and supports immune and cognitive function.
- **Camu camu fruit powder**: This food source is high in vitamin C, which boosts immunity and supports liver detoxification, as well as manganese and other antioxidants.
- **Rose hip fruit powder**: Rose hips are naturally high in vitamin C, plant phenols, flavonoids, ellagic acid, lycopene, and vitamin E and boosts immunity.
- **Orange essential oil**: Orange is high in d-limonene, a constituent that shows anti-inflammatory, wound-healing, and anticancer effects. D-limonene alters the signaling pathways within cancer cells in a way that stops cancer cells from multiplying and causes their death[22].
- **Citrus bioflavonoids**: These help to maximize the benefits of vitamin C by inhibiting its breakdown in the body and protect against oxidative stress, inflammation, elevated blood sugar and cholesterol, damage to the lining of cells and plaque buildup in the arteries[60].

Vitamin C and immune health are almost synonymous. Vitamin C bolsters immunity by supporting various functions of both the innate and adaptive immune system, prevents pathogens from entering cells, and acts as a free radical scavenger to reduce cellular damage[62].

Note: Vitamin C absorption is saturable, so you can only absorb a limited amount at one time. It is better to take smaller doses (up to 2,000 mg for adults) multiple times throughout the day instead of all at once.

WHAT IS THE DIFFERENCE BETWEEN SUPER C™ AND SUPER C™ CHEWABLE?

- Super C™ tablets provide 1,300 mg of vitamin C as ascorbic acid in one serving (two tablets). It contains calcium, zinc, and manganese, as well as citrus bioflavonoids, rutin flower bud powder, cayenne fruit powder, and orange, tangerine, grapefruit, lemon, and lemongrass essential oils.
- Super C™ Chewable tablets provide 150 mg of plant-based vitamin C in one serving (one tablet). The vitamin C in these tablets is from Arerola cherry powder, camu camu fruit powder, and rose hip fruit powder. Super C™ Chewable tablets also contain organic stevia, citrus bioflavonoids, and orange essential oil.

	SUPER C™	SUPER C™ CHEWABLE
VITAMIN C SOURCE	Ascorbic acid	Acerola cherry, camu camu, and rose hip powder
AMOUNT OF VITAMIN C PER TABLET	650 mg	150 mg
ESSENTIAL OILS	Orange, tangerine, grapefruit, lemon, lemongrass	Orange
NOTES	Enhanced with rutin, citrus bioflavonoids, and minerals to balance electrolytes and enhance vitamin C absorption	Chewable tablets

Safety notes: Keep out of reach of children. If you are pregnant, nursing, taking medication, or have a medical condition, consult a healthcare professional before use. Super C™ Chewable contains milk.

SUPER VITAMIN D

Vitamin D is one of those supplements that gets a lot of hype, and for good reason. It's estimated that between 40%-70% of the United States population is deficient in vitamin D[63], and this vitamin is a powerhouse when it comes to our health. Immune, respiratory, bone, and joint health, emotions, and autoimmune needs are all supported with healthy vitamin D levels.

Vitamin D is important for…
- Supporting healthy bones and helping to prevent osteoporosis
- Regulating the absorption of calcium and phosphorus (essential for health)
- Facilitating normal immune function
- Regulating mood and emotions and warding off depression
- Reducing seasonal depression and seasonal affective disorder
- Reducing the risk of other diseases

"The Vitamin D Council—a scientist-led group promoting vitamin D deficiency awareness—suggests vitamin D treatment might be found helpful in treating or preventing autoimmune disease, chronic pain, depression, diabetes, heart disease, high blood pressure, flu, and osteoporosis."—WebMD

"Vitamin D" is a term that refers to several different compounds, all of which are various states of the same thing. The difference is in the chemical structure. Whether from sun, food, or a supplement, the liver converts most vitamin D3 into 25(OH)D (calcidiol). This is the form that we measure in the blood because it is present in the highest quantities and lasts for the longest time (for two to three months). The conversion of 25(OH)D calcidiol into 1,25(OH)2D calcitriol occurs in the kidneys. This is the hormonal form of vitamin D that circulates in the blood to the cells.

VITAMIN D3 FROM SUPPLEMENTS → CALCIDIOL (LIVER) → CALCITRIOL (KIDNEYS) → CIRCULATES IN THE BLOOD TO THE CELLS

As only a limited number of foods contain vitamin D, exposing the skin to UV-B rays in sunlight is how we get 70%-80% of the vitamin D that our body needs. Unfortunately, sunlight is not always a reliable source of vitamin D. The current season, geographic latitude, use of sunscreen, city smog, skin pigmentation, and a person's age are just some of the factors that affect how much vitamin D is produced in the skin through sunlight. This makes supplementation essential!

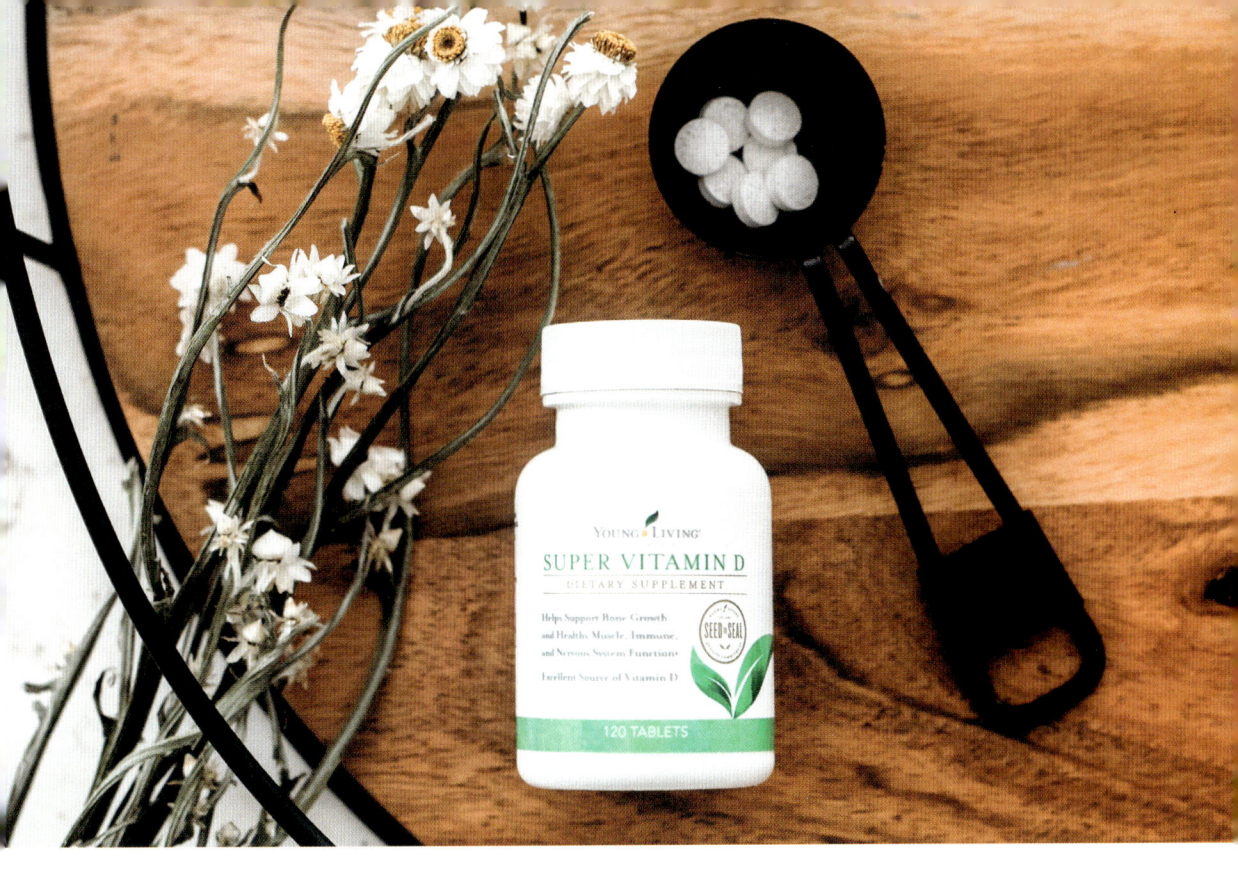

BENEFITS OF SUPER VITAMIN D
- Contains vitamin D3, which is derived from lichen that is sustainably grown and harvested in the United States
- Plays a key role in respiratory health
- Supports the body's respiratory immune system through its innate, adaptive defense mechanisms
- Helps to boost healthy immune systems
- Supports mood and hormone regulation with vitamin D and lemon balm
- Supports bone growth and healthy muscle
- Supports calcium balance and bone growth
- Infused with lemon balm (Melissa) essential oil

Young Living's Super Vitamin D is a highly absorbable, vegan-friendly tablet made with lemon balm extract and lime and Melissa premium essential oils. Melissa essential oil is a wonderful addition to this supplement. These essential oils help to increase the bioavailability of vitamin D and support mood and hormone regulation. Furthermore, vitamin D is supplied as D3, which is an important designation. This active metabolite is responsible for all the wonderful health benefits of vitamin D.

- **Vitamin D3**: Vitamin D3 is a fat-soluble vitamin that is required for mood and hormone regulation, healthy bones and teeth, immune function, and reproduction.
- **Melissa essential oil:** This oil is beneficial for diseases that are associated with inflammation, swelling, and pain[64]. It improves glycemic control and blood sugar levels[65], promotes

healthy skin, and can improve acne and eczema[66]. It has antiviral properties and can stop bacterial infections, including those resistant to prescription medications[67].
- **Lime essential oil:** Lime is high in limonene, a constituent that is known to strengthen the immune system, and helps to decongest the lymphatic system. D-limonene alters the signaling pathways within cancer cells in a way that stops cancer cells from multiplying and causes their death[22].

VITAMIN D AND BONE HEALTH

Regarding healthy bones, calcium is likely to be the nutrient that you think of first. However, vitamin D is just as important for keeping bones strong and preventing the bone disease osteoporosis. Vitamin D helps your intestines to absorb calcium from the food that you eat, so getting enough of both nutrients is an important part of ensuring that your bones are dense and strong.

VITAMIN D AND EMOTIONS

Healthy vitamin D levels are crucial for emotional health. Having adequate levels of vitamin D allows your brain to perform executive functions, such as reasoning, attention, critical thinking, and flexibility[68]. It is also helpful for women who suffer from premenstrual symptoms of cramping and fatigue[69].

Healthy vitamin D levels lower the risk of seasonal blues, can improve depressive mental health states[70], and can improve memory. As we naturally have higher vitamin D levels from sun exposure during the warmer months, most people are happier and more at ease during this time. Since we can't always be out in the sun, and since we need higher vitamin D levels than previously thought, supplementation is key.

WHO SHOULD USE SUPER VITAMIN D?
- Individuals with a risk of or known osteoporosis
- Individuals needing emotional support
- Anyone suffering from seasonal blues, depression, or seasonal affective disorder
- Anyone wanting to bolster their immune system
- Anyone with a known vitamin D deficiency
- Those looking to support overall health and vitality

To use: Take one to two tablets daily with food. Place in mouth and allow to dissolve for 5-10 seconds, then chew for optimal results. Note: Each sublingual tablet contains 1,000 IU vitamin D.

ACHIEVING OPTIMUM VITAMIN D LEVELS

Depending on who you ask, blood levels above 20 ng/mL or 30 ng/mL are considered "sufficient." However, there are multiple factors that affect how much vitamin D an individual may need. A generally recognized dosage for an otherwise healthy individual would be 1,000 IU-4,000 IU (25-100 micrograms) daily. This dose should be enough to ensure optimal blood levels in most people. However, individuals who are deficient in vitamin D may need 5,000 IU daily to reach optimum levels[71].

Safety notes: Keep out of reach of children. If you are pregnant, nursing, taking medication, or have a medical condition, consult a healthcare professional before use.

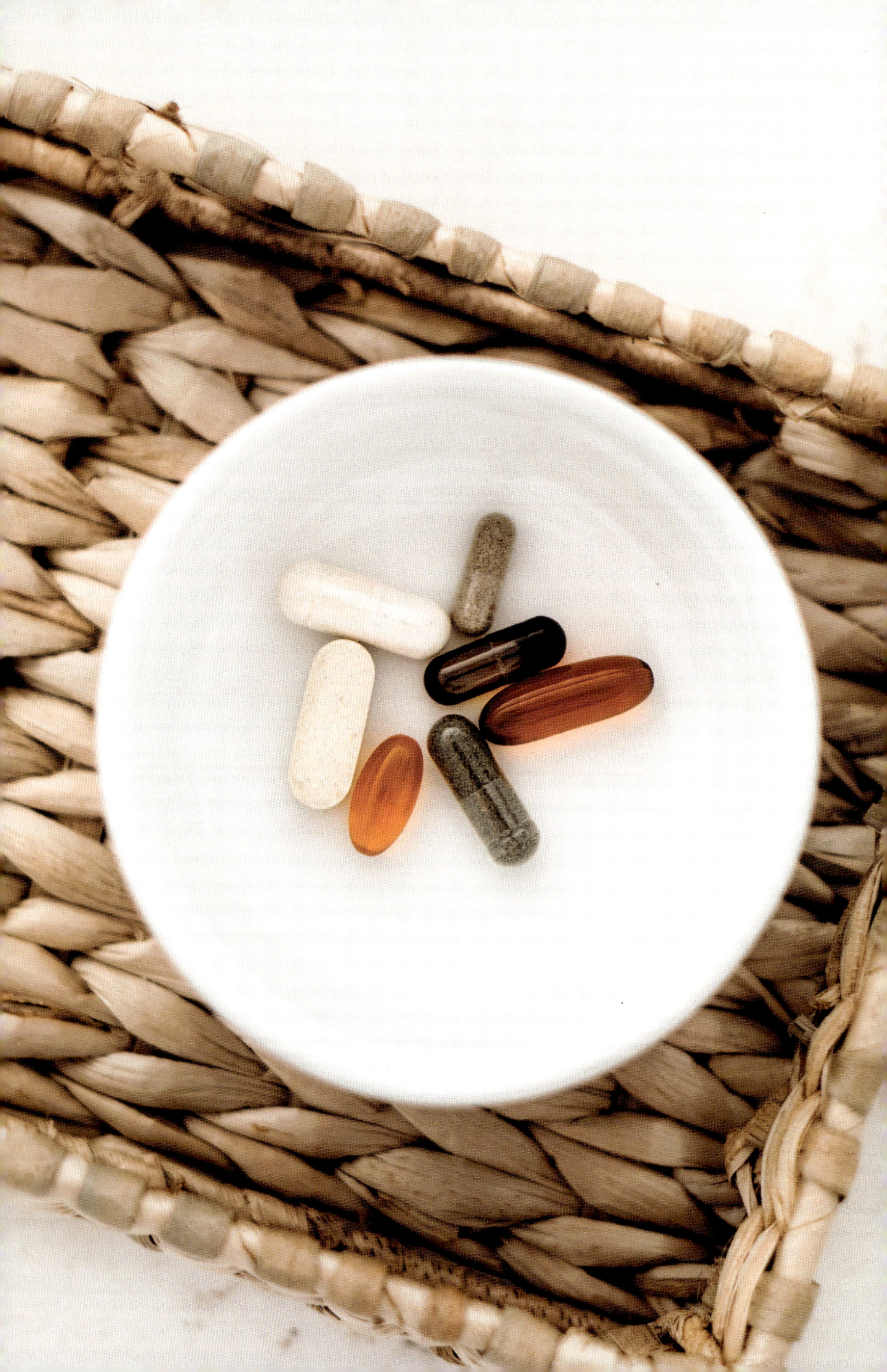

Protocols for Daily Health

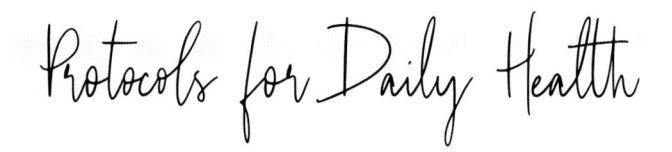

Here are a few ideas to get you started with a supplement routine for overall health and wellness. Start with these basics and add any other targeted support you may need.

OVERALL WELLNESS (MALE AND FEMALE)
- Golden Turmeric™
- Life 9®
- Longevity™
- Master Formula™
- Mineral Essence™
- MultiGreens™
- NingXia Red®
- OmegaGize³®
- Super B™
- Super C™/Super C™ Chewable
- Super Vitamin D

OPTIONS TO TARGET ENERGY & VITALITY™
- Golden Turmeric™
- Longevity™
- MindWise™
- Mineral Essence™
- NingXia Red®
- Super B™

PRE- AND POST-NATAL
- Life 9®
- Master Formula™
- MultiGreens™
- NingXia Red®
- OmegaGize³®
- Super B™
- Super C™ Chewable
- Super Vitamin D

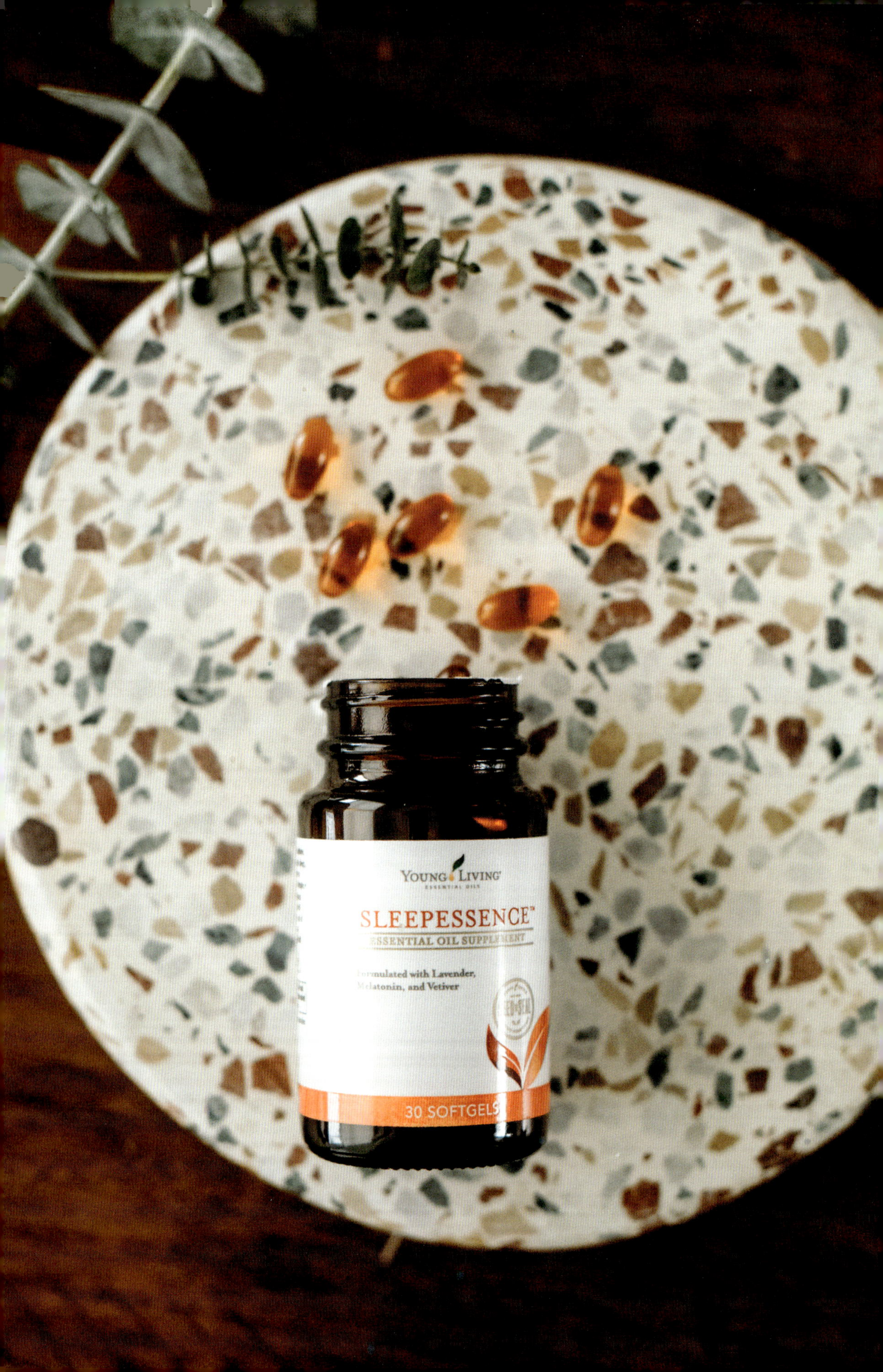
YOUNG LIVING
SLEEPESSENCE™
Formulated with Lavender, Melatonin, and Vetiver
30 SOFTGELS

CHAPTER 4
TARGETED *Supplements*

One of the best things about Young Living's supplement line is the vast array of targeted supplements. These formulations contain multiple herbs and essential oils to suit every need, which means that you don't have to search the health food store for subpar options and end up taking ten capsules for one need.

Some of these supplements are great options for just about anyone, whereas others are targeted at specific needs or areas of support. Some supplements, such as CortiStop®, should be used intermittently to help mitigate high levels of cortisol during times of stress. Specific and acute needs, I highly recommend finding a healthcare provider who you trust to help you monitor lab values and make decisions regarding treatment changes and therapies. A good provider will be open to your questions and to using the brand of supplements that you prefer.

FEELS
GOOD
TO BE
HOME

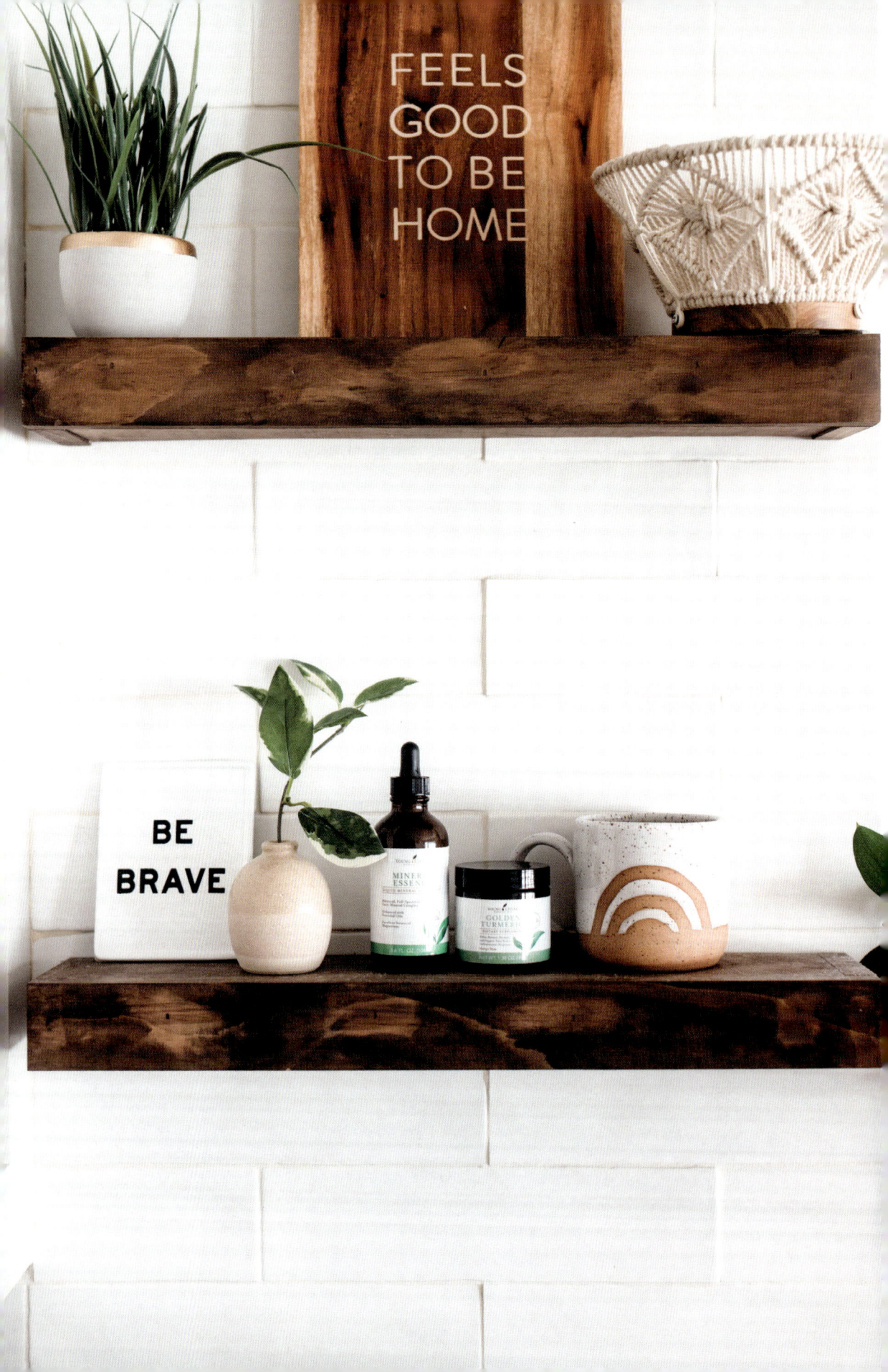

BE
BRAVE

Part 1: SUPPLEMENTS TO SUPPORT THE ENDOCRINE SYSTEM (HORMONES, THYROID, AND ADRENALS)

The endocrine system is a network of glands throughout the body that make hormones, including insulin, thyroid hormones, cortisol, and sex hormones. The hormones that are made in the endocrine system are responsible for almost every cell, organ, and function in the body.

The hypothalamus, pituitary gland, and pineal gland are in your brain. The thyroid and parathyroid glands are in your neck. The thymus is between your lungs, the adrenals are on top of your kidneys, and the pancreas is behind your stomach.

While all of these glands are important, the thyroid and adrenals are often the target of support because they are often out of balance. Energy levels, heart and breathing rates, body temperature, weight, mood and emotions, and even menstrual cycles are affected by these systems. Another important component of the endocrine system is the sex hormones—estrogen, progesterone, and testosterone.

The adrenal, thyroid, and sex hormones work together in a cycle. The thyroid hormones affect sex hormones, adrenal hormones affect thyroid hormones, and sex hormones affect adrenal hormones. Therefore, when one part of the cycle is out of balance, there are consequences for the entire endocrine system.

Unfortunately, conventional treatments for hormone imbalances are lacking. These typically include birth control pills, injections, synthetic hormone replacements, and prescription drugs that simply mask the symptoms of the imbalance without solving the underlying problem. A more ideal treatment would include a combination of lifestyle changes (including removing potential mycotoxins, such as mold), imbalance-specific dietary modifications, and natural, high-quality supplements.

THE ADRENALS

The adrenal glands are located just above the kidneys and are known for the "fight-or-flight" response. This response is natural and necessary. Although it protects us in high stress situations (such as running from a lion), the constant stress of daily life often keeps our adrenals on overdrive.

When we are stressed, our bodies activate the hypothalamic-pituitary-adrenal (HPA) axis, which is the loop of neurotransmitters and hormones that includes cortisol. When we're being chased by a lion or experience a car accident, this loop is a good thing. It keeps us focused, alert, moving, and safe. The harm comes when the loop doesn't turn off. Consistent psychological stress causes the overproduction of cortisol and keeps this loop going… and going… and going. This means that our systems are literally flooded with stress, which starts to suppress immunity, slow digestion, tank energy levels, and disrupt emotions and can have long-lasting effects.

THE THYROID

The thyroid gland performs a myriad of tasks in the body. It regulates metabolism, energy, body temperature, and hormone production, which impacts just about every other body system in some way. Although thyroid support is always important, it is especially so for women aged 25-45 and before/during/after pregnancy. The hormonal changes during these times place a load on the thyroid that often goes unsupported or unnoticed.

SEX HORMONES

Estrogen, progesterone, and testosterone play a huge role in our overall health—they affect everything from reproduction to muscle tone, mood, and energy levels. Chronic stress, improper nutrition, low vitamin D levels, prescription drugs, an unhealthy gut balance, and yeast overgrowth can all negatively affect estrogen, progesterone, and testosterone. These reproductive cells are the most delicate cells in the body and are most sensitive to oxidative damage, especially when out of balance.

Bottom line? **The endocrine system is involved in every single body process and is essential to overall well-being. Many common issues are linked to the endocrine system, which means that support for this area is vital.**

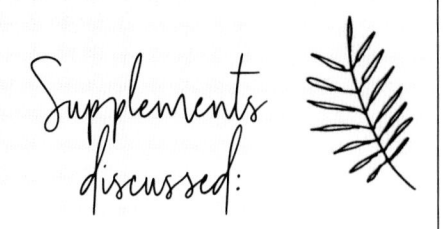

Supplements discussed:

CORTISTOP®
ENDOGIZE™
FEMIGEN™
PD 80/20™
POWERGIZE™
PRENOLONE PLUS™ BODY CREAM
PROGESSENCE PLUS™ SERUM
PROSTATE HEALTH™
REGENOLONE™ CREAM
SUPER B™
THYROMIN™

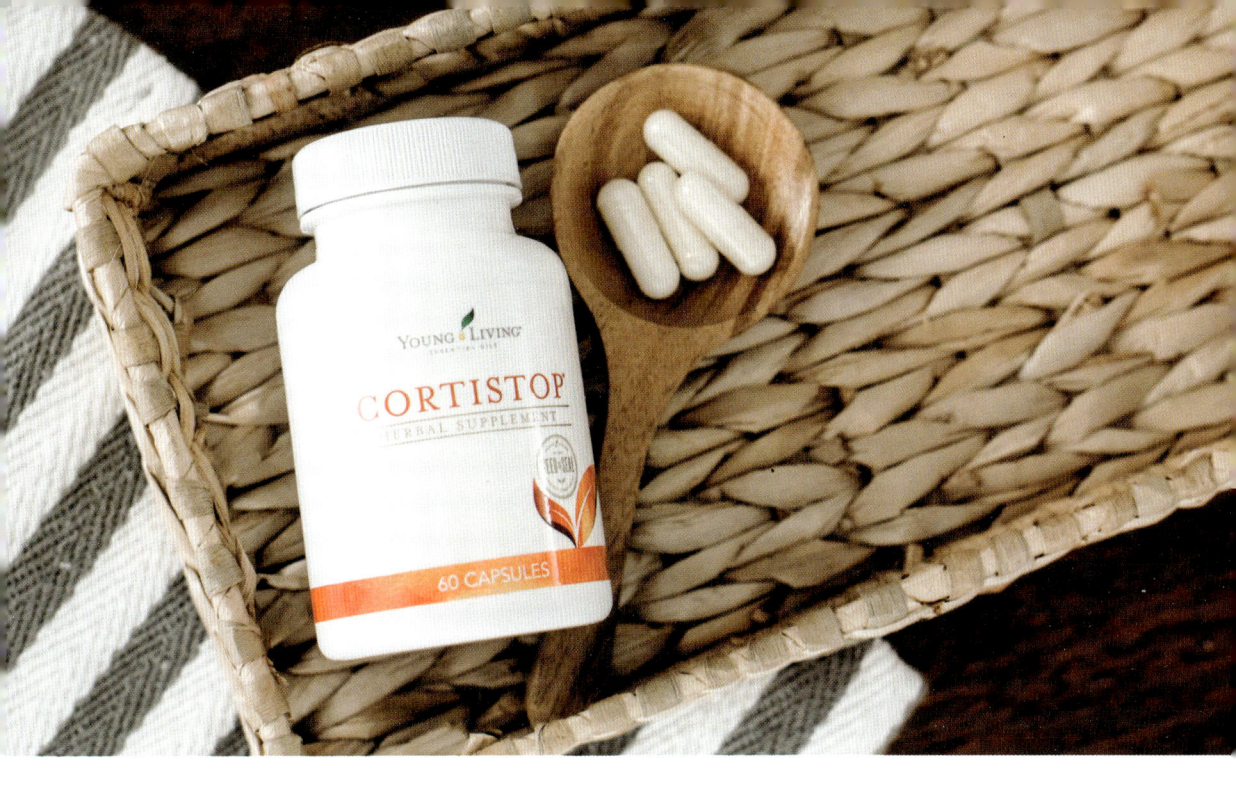

CORTISTOP®

Stress that is experienced and stored by the body is a huge danger to our well-being, especially in our modern world. Making sure that we have the tools to help our bodies both physically and emotionally deal with stress is one of the biggest changes toward better health, and CortiStop® is the perfect supplement for that.

BENEFITS OF CORTISTOP®
- Works with the body's natural balancing systems
- Supports women's hormones through a combination of pregnenolone, herbs, and essential oils
- Contains DHEA, a precursor for hormone development
- Supports emotional and physical health through stress mediation
- Supports healthy restfulness and wakefulness patterns

When you're stressed, either physically or psychologically, the adrenal glands go into overdrive and raise cortisol levels. High levels of cortisol cause the body to scavenge for protein to convert into glucose to send to the brain so that it has enough energy to deal with the perceived stress. Because of high cortisol and protein scavenging, adrenaline levels rise. Adrenaline is the fight-or-flight hormone that is responsible for short-term increases in energy and strength (i.e., a mother lifting a car off her child). Although this is fine in the very short-term, it has serious consequences when it happens too frequently.

When cortisol is produced too frequently, it can cause fatigue, difficulty maintaining a healthy weight, suppressed immunity (which manifests as frequent infections or *Candida* overgrowth), anxiety and depression, and difficulty maintaining optimal heart health. Chronically elevated cortisol affects the HPA axis, which affects all the body's hormones and disrupts the natural feedback loop. This causes the body to be less sensitive to the cortisol "Stop Signal" and creates a vicious cycle of elevated stress hormones and messengers. This is the root cause of adrenal fatigue.

When the adrenals release cortisol spikes, it creates a short burst of energy, followed by a crash with extreme fatigue. In the case of chronic stress, this looks like feeling fine in the morning, but as the day progresses, you become extremely tired or feel overwhelmed, even when contemplating work. Any type of stress will cause the adrenal glands to either overreact or fail to respond. You either become extremely anxious, nervous, or hyperactive or you feel extremely tired and unmotivated to do anything. This is adrenal fatigue.

Triggers for elevated cortisol levels include:
- Excess heat/cold
- Alcohol abuse
- Caffeine
- Depression
- Anxiety
- Malnutrition
- Personal relationships
- Physical and emotional trauma
- Surgery
- Diseases
- Major life events, such as job changes, family changes, or moving house

CortiStop® is designed to address how women's bodies react to the cortisol that is produced when under stress, both acute and chronic. CortiStop® combines herbs and essential oils to help to balance the stress response by calming the body and lowering cortisol levels. As cortisol declines, strength and energy return, and the body returns to a state of equilibrium.

Each ingredient in CortiStop® is included for a specific reason and system support.
- **Pregnenolone**: Pregnenolone reduces the corticotropin-releasing hormone (CRH) in experimental models (CRH is the first step in the production of the stress hormone cortisol). Additionally, it is a precursor hormone from which all other hormones are created and is important for the body's production of progesterone, which blocks cortisol receptors.
- **DHEA**: DHEA is a hormone precursor for estrogen, progesterone, and testosterone. It helps to prevent bone loss, improves estrogen production, lowers inflammation, and improves heart health. (Note: DHEA is not recommended during pregnancy or breastfeeding or for those being treated for prostate or breast cancer, unless directed by a physician.)

- **Phosphatidylcholine**: Phosphatidylcholine helps to protect the brain, liver, and stomach during times of stress and is a key component for every cell in the body.
- **Phosphatidylserine**: Phosphatidylserine helps to balance the hypothalamus–pituitary axis, benefits cognitive function, and may blunt cortisol production. The effects may be more pronounced in people under chronic stress.
- **Black cohosh**: Black cohosh is a phytoestrogen that helps to counteract the effects of cortisol, stop stress responses, and may elevate the mood.
- **Clary sage**: Clary sage is a phytoestrogen that supports hormone balance, reduces cortisol levels[80], lowers elevated blood pressure and cholesterol[81], and helps to uplift the mood.
- **Frankincense essential oil**: Frankincense is a grounding and uplifting oil that also works as a powerful antioxidant within the body. It also helps to balance endocrine hormones.
- **Fennel essential oil**: Fennel supports digestion, eases intestinal discomfort, supports the pancreas and liver, promotes the excretion of toxins, and provides immune support.
- **Peppermint essential oil**: Peppermint helps to soothe the stomach, aids digestion, and has natural anti-inflammatory properties to soothe physical stress on the body.

CortiStop® is a wonderful choice for women who need support for physical or emotional stress or who feel the effects of adrenal fatigue. Men can also take this supplement when needed. Dr. Purser, the doctor who formulated Progessence Plus™, taught that men can take CortiStop® in times of high stress and anxiety. Use at your discretion, and as always, speak with your healthcare provider if you have any concerns.

See page 76 for a comparison chart of CortiStop®, EndoGize™, FemiGen™, PD 80/20™, and PowerGize™.

> **CORTISTOP®**
>
> **To use:** Take two capsules in the morning before breakfast. If desired, for extra benefits, take another two capsules before bed. Use daily for eight weeks. Discontinue use for two to four weeks before resuming.

Safety notes: This is not recommended during pregnancy. Use while breastfeeding at your discretion and need. Contains soy. Keep out of reach of children. For adult use only.

ENDOGIZE™

EndoGize™ is a women's daily hormone support supplement that is powered by a blend of minerals and essential oils, as well as ashwagandha root, which is a well-known herb for hormone balance. These ingredients work synergistically to create a formula that supports a healthy endocrine system for women.

BENEFITS OF ENDOGIZE™
- Specially formulated to support a balanced endocrine system in women
- Includes ashwagandha, a well-known adaptogen that helps to mitigate stress in the body
- Provides overall hormone support
- Helps to balance estrogen, progesterone, and testosterone levels
- Contains DHEA, a hormone precursor
- Supports healthy menstrual cycles and libido
- Enhanced with essential oils

Increased cortisol levels reduce estrogen and testosterone levels, which creates an unhealthy scenario when it comes to endocrine balance. Impaired metabolism, low libido, painful menstruation, and low energy levels are just some of the symptoms of this imbalance. Each ingredient in EndoGize™ works synergistically to create a 1+1=3 scenario to balance female hormones.

- **Ashwagandha root extract**: Ashwagandha is an ancient herb that works as an adaptogen, helping your body to manage stress. It can boost brain function, lower blood sugar and cortisol levels, and fight symptoms of anxiety and depression. Moreover, it helps to improve thyroid-stimulating hormone (TSH) and thyroxine (T4) levels in individuals with low thyroid function[84].
- **Muira puama bark**: This herb is commonly used to help with cramps, PMS, and other menstrual issues.
- **L-arginine:** This amino acid is required to produce nitric oxide, which supports blood vessel tone and encourages healthy blood flow within the body.
- **Epimedium leaf:** Epimedium is commonly used in Chinese herbal medicine to support libido and hormone balance. It is a phytoestrogen that is high in flavonoids, which help to relax the nervous system. Additionally, it balances estrogen and estradiol levels and improves menopause symptoms.
- **Tribulus terrestris extract**: This herb supports muscle tone, libido, and overall hormone balance without raising hormone levels above the normal range.
- **DHEA**: DHEA is a hormone precursor for estrogen, progesterone, and testosterone. It helps to prevent bone loss, improves estrogen production, lowers inflammation, and improves heart health. (Note: DHEA is not recommended during pregnancy or breastfeeding or for those being treated for prostate or breast cancer, unless directed by a physician.)

- **Black pepper extract:** Black pepper improves the absorption and assimilation of nutrients.
- **Longjack root extract:** Longjack root enhances the body's production of hormones, improves muscle tone and strength, and contains antioxidants that support overall health and longevity.
- **Glucoamylase, acid-stable protease, amylase, and cellulase**: These enzymes help to break down starches, proteins, sugars, and cellulose, respectively, to aid digestion and ease digestive inflammation.
- **Ginger essential oil**: Ginger has analgesic, anti-inflammatory, antibacterial, and antioxidant properties, is great for soothing digestion[11], contains powerful antioxidants that can protect against oxidative stress, helps to combat inflammation[12], and promotes liver health[13].
- **Myrrh essential oil**: Myrrh is a powerful essential oil for overall health. Myrrh contains terpenoids and sesquiterpenes, constituents that have both anti-inflammatory and antioxidant effects.
- **Clary sage essential oil**: Clary sage is a phytoestrogen supports hormone balance, reduces cortisol levels[80], lowers elevated blood pressure and cholesterol[81], helps to uplift the mood, and supports healthy sleep patterns.
- **Cassia essential oil**: Cassia supports the body's response to inflammation. It is one of the oldest known medicinal herbs (in the cinnamon family, though it has a distinctly different chemical profile) and promotes healthy blood sugar levels.
- **Canadian Fleabane essential oil**: Canadian fleabane contains the powerful constituents limonene, cis-matricaria ester, and trans-alpha-bergamotene, which have incredible health benefits—they bolster immunity, balance hormones, and help the body to manage stress signals.
- **Zinc**: Zinc is an essential trace element that helps to strengthen the immune system and is essential for reproductive health.
- **Vitamin B6**: B6 is an essential B vitamin that must be obtained through the diet. It plays a critical role in the function of essential chemical reactions in the body.

> **ENDOGIZE™**
>
> **To use:** Take one capsule twice daily. Use daily for two weeks. Discontinue for two weeks before resuming.

See page 76 for a comparison chart of CortiStop®, EndoGize™, FemiGen™, PD 80/20™, and PowerGize™.

Safety notes: Contains soy. Not recommended during pregnancy or when breastfeeding. Intended for adult use only.

WHAT IS THE DIFFERENCE BETWEEN ENDOGIZE™ AND CORTISTOP®?

EndoGize™ and CortiStop® are similar in that they both work to dampen stress signals and balance overall hormone levels. However, CortiStop® is more geared toward cortisol and stress, while EndoGize™ is more geared toward balancing estrogen, progesterone, and testosterone. When cortisol is balanced, levels of estrogen, progesterone, and testosterone also become balanced, and vice versa. When choosing which of these two supplements to begin, look at whether you primarily need support for elevated cortisol or for estrogen, progesterone, and testosterone imbalance.

FEMIGEN™

FemiGen™ is a women's supplement that supports the overall reproductive system through estrogen balance and helps to balance hormones during menopause. FemiGen™ combines whole-food herbs, amino acids, and essential oils that are known for nourishing the body from development through menopause.

BENEFITS OF FEMIGEN™
- Supports the female reproductive system with herbs and essential oils
- Helps to maintain hormone balance during menopause
- Provides relief from common menstrual cycle and menopause symptoms
- Formulated with whole-food herbs that nourish the body

FemiGen™ is a twice-daily supplement that combines wild yam, damiana, and dong quai with synergistic amino acids and clary sage, fennel, ylang ylang, and sage essential oils. FemiGen™ specifically supports the female reproductive system through estrogen balance and helps to maintain the reproductive system from development through menopause.

- **Damiana leaf powder**: Damiana leaf is used in herbal medicine to both relax the body and improve energy levels. It fights symptoms of PMS and works as a diuretic to remove excess fluid.
- **Epimedium leaf powder**: Epimedium leaf is a phytoestrogen high in flavonoids that help to relax the nervous system. It balances estrogen and estradiol levels and supports menopause relief.
- **Dong quai leaf powder:** Dong quai is an ancient Chinese medicinal herb that improves bone density[72], reduces symptoms of menopause, and regulates hormone balance[73]. Additionally, it may decrease depression[74], lower blood sugar levels, ease inflammation, and improve heart health.
- **Wild yam root powder**: Wild yam helps to regulate blood sugar, raises HDL ("good" cholesterol) levels, lowers LDL ("bad" cholesterol") levels[75], supports estrogen and progesterone levels, and has anti-inflammatory properties that soothe muscle spasms.

- **Muira Puama bark powder**: This herb is commonly used to help with cramps, PMS, and other menstrual issues.
- **Licorice root**: Licorice root helps to mitigate an unhealthy stress response, has anti-inflammatory properties that soothe the body overall, helps to improve digestion, and acts as a mild cleansing agent to the digestive system.
- **Ginseng root and leaf powder:** Ginseng helps to relieve inflammation, improves immune function, acts as an adaptogen to help reduce the effects of stress, and reduces menopause symptoms[76].
- **Black cohosh powder**: Black cohosh is a phytoestrogen that helps to counteract the effects of cortisol, stops stress responses, and may elevate the mood. It helps with symptoms of menopause, anxiety, and Polycystic Ovarian Syndrome (PCOS)[77].
- **L-Carnitine L-Tartrate:** This is an amino acid complex that plays a role in energy metabolism and production. It reduces muscle soreness, boosts physical performance, and regulates blood sugar levels.
- **L-Phenylalanine:** This is an essential amino acid that improves mental clarity, energy levels, and mood and helps to alleviate symptoms of PMS and depression.
- **L-Cystine, L-Cystine HCl:** These amino acids are required for thyroid health, glutathione production, and the utilization of B vitamins. They are involved in insulin production in the pancreas.
- **Crampbark powder:** Crampbark naturally contains methyl salicylate, which is known to have pain-relieving and anti-inflammatory properties. It is helpful for relieving PMS cramps, afterbirth pains, and symptoms of endometriosis[78,79].
- **Squaw vine powder:** Squaw vine helps to treat infections, water retention, and menstrual pain.
- **Fennel essential oil**: Fennel supports digestion, eases intestinal discomfort, supports the pancreas and liver, provides immune support, and promotes the excretion of toxins.

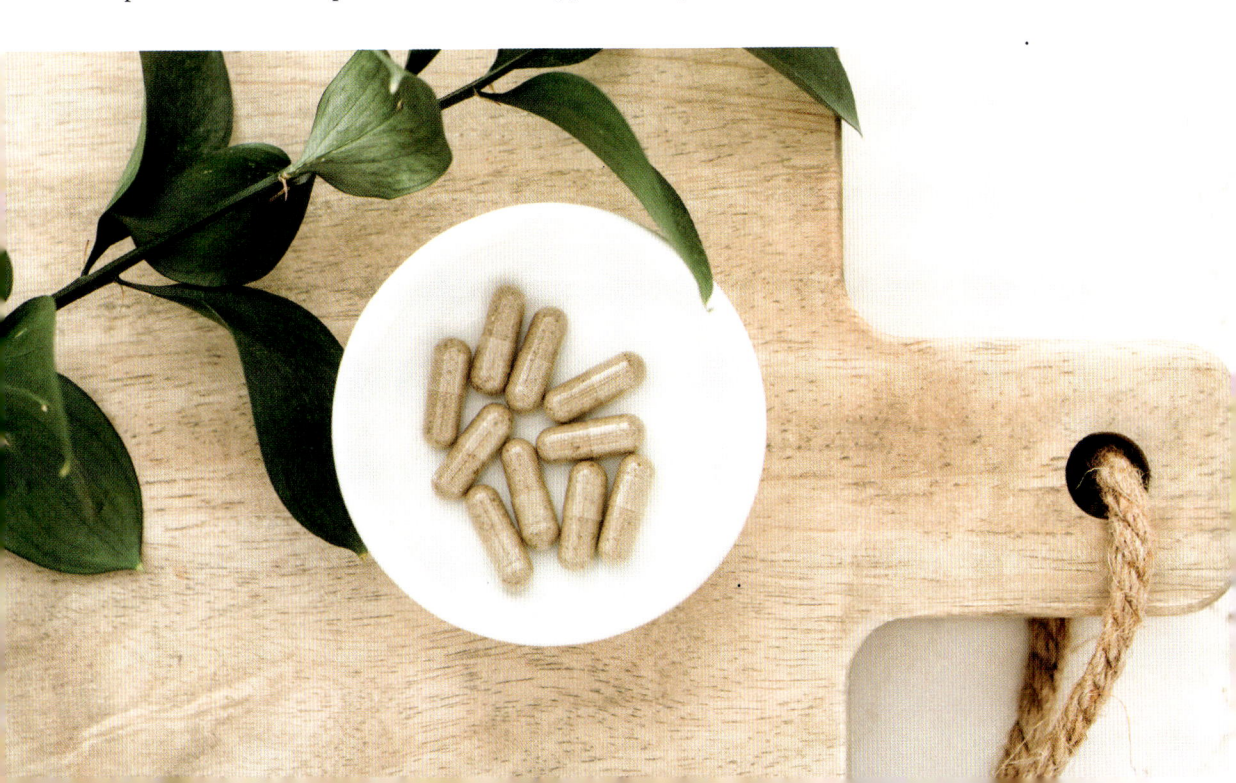

- **Clary sage essential oil**: Clary sage is a phytoestrogen that supports hormone balance, reduces cortisol levels[80], lowers elevated blood pressure and cholesterol[81], and helps to uplift the mood.
- **Ylang ylang essential oil:** Ylang ylang promotes healthy blood flow, balances hormones, relieves inflammation, and uplifts the mood.
- **Sage essential oil**: Sage helps to regulate hormones, promotes healthy digestion, has antioxidant, antiseptic, antiviral, and antifungal properties, stimulates the gallbladder, and supports healthy cholesterol levels[82].

See page 76 for a comparison chart of CortiStop®, EndoGize™, FemiGen™, PD 80/20™, and PowerGize™.

Safety notes: Keep out of reach of children. If you are pregnant, nursing, taking medication, or have a medical condition, consult a healthcare professional before use. An accidental overdose of iron-containing products is a leading cause of fatal poisoning in children under the age of six. Keep this product out of reach of children. In case of an accidental overdose, call a doctor or the poison control center immediately.

> **FEMIGEN™**
>
> **To use:** Take two capsules with breakfast and two capsules with lunch.

PD 80/20™

PD 80/20™ is a daily supplement that contains pregnenolone and DHEA in an 80%/20% ratio. These two substances are produced naturally by the body and are essential for hormone production, though levels decline with age.

BENEFITS OF PD 80/20™
- Contains DHEA, a precursor for hormones in the body
- Contains pregnenolone, a precursor for estrogen and progesterone
- Supports overall hormone health
- Supports internal health

We've already mentioned the importance of hormone balance, especially when it comes to estrogen, progesterone, and testosterone. PD 80/20™ is a very targeted supplement for supporting sex hormones.

Pregnenolone is a prohormone that serves as a precursor for numerous steroid hormones, including cortisol, progesterone, and DHEA. It has an impact on mental acuity, energy levels, and memory, as well as many other body processes, such as sleep/wake cycles and reproduction. Pregnenolone may also play a role in regulating anxiety and depression[83].

DHEA is often used by athletes to promote muscle growth and strength. However, this pro-hormone is also involved in maintaining the health of the cardiovascular and immune systems, improving bone density and cholesterol levels, and producing sex hormones. DHEA is one of the most abundant hormones in the human body and is required for more than 150 metabolic functions. The adrenal glands naturally produce DHEA for the body to convert into other hormones. DHEA levels naturally start to decline after the age of 30, which can lead to weight gain, low energy, low libido, and higher levels of inflammation.

This combination of pregnenolone and DHA is a powerful tool for supporting the endocrine system and maximizing internal health.

- **Pregnenolone**: Pregnenolone is a precursor hormone that is important for the body's production of progesterone. Progesterone blocks cortisol receptors. Pregnenolone also reduces corticotropin-releasing hormone (CRH). CRH is the first step in the production of the stress hormone cortisol.
- **DHEA**: DHEA is a hormone precursor for estrogen, progesterone, and testosterone. It helps to prevent bone loss, improves estrogen production, lowers inflammation, and improves heart health. (Note: DHEA is not recommended during pregnancy or breastfeeding or for those being treated for prostate or breast cancer, unless directed by a physician.)

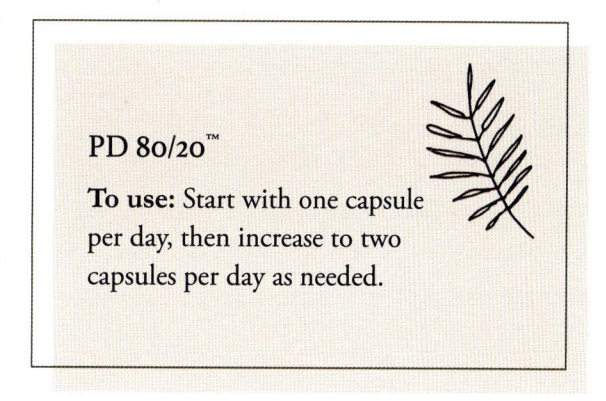

PD 80/20™

To use: Start with one capsule per day, then increase to two capsules per day as needed.

See page 76 for a comparison chart of CortiStop®, EndoGize™, FemiGen™, PD 80/20™, and PowerGize™.

Safety notes: Not for use by individuals under the age of 18. Keep out of reach of children. Do not use if pregnant or nursing. Consult a physician or licensed, qualified health professional before using this product if you have or have a family history of breast cancer, prostate cancer, prostate enlargement, heart disease, low "good" cholesterol (HDL), have a medical condition, or if you are using any other dietary supplement, prescription drug, or over-the-counter drug. Do not exceed the recommended serving. Exceeding the recommended serving may cause serious adverse health effects. Possible side effects include acne, hair loss, hair growth on the face (in women), aggressiveness, irritability, and increased levels of estrogen. Discontinue use and call a physician or licensed, qualified health professional immediately if you experience rapid heartbeat, dizziness, blurred vision, or other similar symptoms.

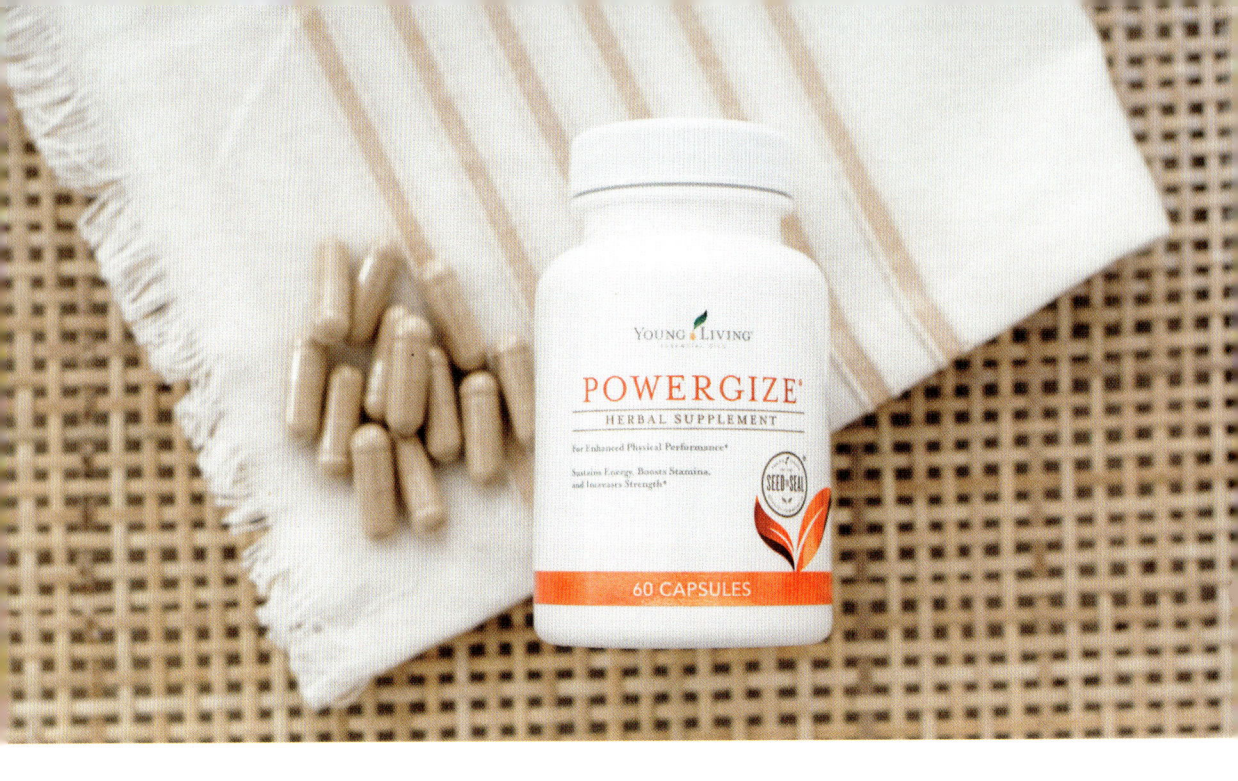

POWERGIZE™

PowerGize™ is an endocrine and muscle support supplement that helps to sustain energy levels, strength, mental and physical vibrancy, and vitality when used in addition to physical activity. PowerGize™ is a great option for men and women of all ages who want to improve their physical performance, increase muscle size and strength, and enhance their muscle tone and rate of muscle recovery.

BENEFITS OF POWERGIZE™
- Improves energy levels for physical performance and endurance
- Boosts stamina and enhances sports performance
- Sustains energy levels, strength, and vitality when paired with physical activity
- Supports healthy muscles, increases muscle size and strength, and enhances muscle tone and the rate of muscle recovery
- Formulated with ashwagandha root, a powerful adaptogen for managing stress
- Promotes mental clarity, concentration, alertness, and a sense of energy and calm
- Promotes overall well-being and hormonal balance
- Contains Eurycoma longifolia to support healthy testosterone levels in both men and women

PowerGize™ is infused with blue spruce, goldenrod, and cassia essential oils and is formulated to boost the stamina and performance of individuals of all ages. It's great for athletes, maintaining performance as we age, for parents or anyone needing extra support. Additionally,

PowerGize™ contains ashwagandha root extract, which is touted for its properties that support stress management and antioxidant levels. The formula also includes KSM-66, which supports immunity, mental clarity, concentration, and alertness.

- **Ashwagandha root extract**: Ashwagandha is an ancient herb that works as an adaptogen, which helps your body to manage stress. It can boost brain function, lower blood sugar and cortisol levels, and fight symptoms of anxiety and depression. Additionally, it improves thyroid stimulating hormone and thyroxine (T4) levels in individuals with low thyroid function[84].
- **Eurycoma longifolia**: This is a well-studied herb that supports healthy testosterone levels in both men and women. It supports male reproductive health and reproductive disorders[85].
- **Tribulus terrestris extract**: This herb supports muscle tone, libido, and overall hormone balance without raising hormone levels above the normal range. It improves inflammation and swelling in muscle tissue[86].
- **Idaho Blue Spruce essential oil**: Idaho blue spruce is high in alpha-pinene, a constituent that reduces inflammation and oxidative stress, supports hormone balance, testosterone levels, and immunity, and helps the body to reduce pain signals[87].
- **Cassia essential oil**: Cassia supports the body's response to inflammation. It is one of the oldest known medicinal herbs (in the cinnamon family, though distinctly different chemical profile) and promotes healthy blood sugar levels.
- **Goldenrod essential oil**: Goldenrod supports the cardiovascular and vascular systems, enables healthy blood flow and circulation, and balances testosterone levels.
- It also includes vitamin B6, magnesium, zinc, and fenugreek, all of which support muscle and immune health and energy levels.

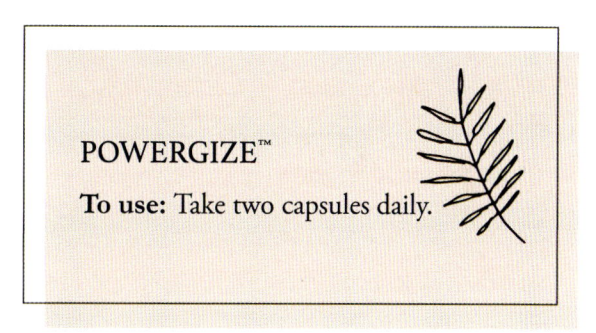

POWERGIZE™

To use: Take two capsules daily.

Safety notes: Keep out of reach of children. If you are pregnant, nursing, taking medication, or have a medical condition, consult a health professional before use. Contains milk.

COMPARISON OF CORTISTOP®, ENDOGIZE™, FEMIGEN™, PD 80/20™, AND POWERGIZE™

	DAILY OR INTERMITTENT USE	ADAPTOGENIC?	IMPROVES ESTROGEN, PROGESTERONE, AND TESTOSTERONE?	CONTAINS DHEA?	FORMULATED FOR MEN OR WOMEN?	ADDITIONAL NOTES
CORTISTOP®	Use daily for eight weeks, then take 2-4 weeks off	Yes, through herbs and essential oils	Contains pregnenolone, DHEA, and phytoestrogens	Yes	Women, though men can use if needed	Specifically formulated to dampen the stress response
ENDOGIZE™	Use daily for two weeks, then take two weeks off	Contains ashwagandha	Contains DHEA, phytoestrogens	Yes	Women	Has more phytoestrogens than CortiStop®. Formulated for overall endocrine support for women
FEMIGEN™	Use daily (no break required)	No	Contains phytoestrogens and progesterone	No	Women	Formulated for women's reproductive health
PD 80/20™	Use daily (no break required)	No	Very targeted sex hormone support	Yes	Both	Pregnenolone and DHEA
POWERGIZE™	Use daily (no break required)	Contains ashwagandha	Supports healthy testosterone levels	No	Both, though great for men	Supports healthy testosterone levels

PRENOLONE PLUS™

Prenolone Plus™ Body Cream is a topical cream that contains pregnenolone, DHEA, blue and black cohosh, and essential oils to nourish the skin and help to maintain healthy hormone levels in women.

BENEFITS OF PRENOLONE PLUS™
- Specifically designed for women's hormonal health
- Moisture-rich cream nourishes and hydrates dry skin
- Absorbs easily without a greasy feel
- Made from plant-based, moisturizing ingredients and premium essential oils

This body cream smells incredible and provides many wonderful hormone-supporting herbs, such as St. John's wort, wild yam extract, ginkgo biloba leaf extract, and green tea leaf extract. These herbs and essential oils work synergistically to promote a healthy balance of hormones while also nourishing the skin.
- **DHEA**: DHEA is a hormone precursor for estrogen, progesterone, and testosterone. It helps to prevent bone loss, improves estrogen production, lowers inflammation, and improves heart health. (Note: DHEA is not recommended during pregnancy or breastfeeding or for those being treated for prostate or breast cancer, unless directed by a physician.)
- **Blue and black cohosh**: These are phytoestrogens that helps to counteract the effects of cortisol, stop stress responses, and may elevate the mood. These herbs help improve symptoms of menopause, anxiety, and PCOS[77], support the body through painful menstrual cycles, and promote healthy estrogen levels.
- **Pregnenolone**: Pregnenolone is a precursor hormone that is important for the body's production of progesterone. Progesterone blocks cortisol receptors. Pregnenolone also reduces corticotropin-releasing hormone (CRH). CRH is the first step in the production of the stress hormone cortisol.
- **St. John's wort:** St. John's wort is often used to improve low mood. It may also improve symptoms of PMS[88] and menopause[89].
- **Ylang ylang essential oil:** Ylang ylang promotes healthy blood flow, balances hormones, relieves inflammation, and uplifts the spirits.
- **Clary sage essential oil**: Clary sage a phytoestrogen that supports hormone balance,

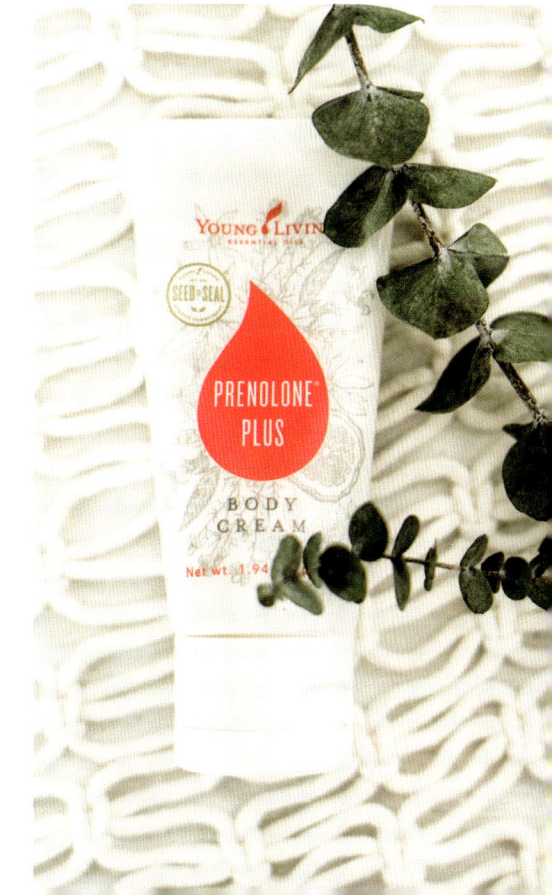

reduces cortisol levels[80], lowers elevated blood pressure and cholesterol[81], and uplifts the mood.
- **Geranium essential oil:** Geranium promotes healthy hormone balance and aids circulation. It is a natural diuretic with anti-inflammatory and antimicrobial properties.
- **Bergamot essential oil:** Bergamot supports hormonal balance and helps to relieve feelings of depression and anxiety[90,91]. It contains limonene, a constituent with wonderful health boosting properties.
- **Fennel essential oil**: Fennel supports digestion, eases intestinal discomfort, supports the pancreas and liver, provides immune support, and promotes the excretion of toxins.
- **Yarrow essential oil:** Yarrow has anti-inflammatory properties, promotes healthy digestion, and may help to ease feelings of anxiety.
- **Sage essential oil**: Sage helps to regulate hormones and promotes healthy digestion. It has antioxidant, antiseptic, antiviral, and antifungal properties, stimulates the gallbladder, and supports healthy cholesterol levels[82].

> **PRENOLONE PLUS™**
>
> **To use:** Begin using one day after the menstrual cycle ends or as desired. Apply 1/4-1/2 tsp. one to two times daily for 21 consecutive days. Discontinue use for seven days, then repeat. Massage cream thoroughly into soft-tissue areas of the body until it is absorbed (inner thigh or inside of the forearm). Individual needs may vary.

See page 83 for a comparison chart with Prenolone Plus™.

Safety notes: Contains gluten and soy.

PROGESSENCE PLUS™

Progessence Plus™ contains USP-grade, super-micronized progesterone from wild yam blended with essential oils and vitamin E to balance hormones naturally. The unique formulation maximizes the effects of natural progesterone and allows enhanced absorption through the skin.

BENEFITS OF PROGESSENCE PLUS™
- Designed especially for women and made with natural, bioidentical progesterone from wild yam
- Promotes well-being and feelings of relaxation, harmony, and balance

- Absorbs easily and contains skin-nourishing premium essential oils and vitamin E
- 100% plant-based and naturally derived vegan formula
- Promotes healthy progesterone levels

Wild yams help to normalize blood sugar levels, combat weight gain and hair loss, and reduce the occurrence of hormonal headaches. Progessence Plus™ promotes restfulness and sleep through the natural effects of progesterone and essential oils. Each of the ingredients and essential oils in this blend plays an important role for the body:

- **USP-grade progesterone from wild yam extract:** This helps to regulate blood sugar, raises HDL levels, lowers LDL levels[75], supports estrogen and progesterone levels, and has anti-inflammatory properties that soothe muscle spasms.
- **Sacred frankincense essential oil**: Frankincense is a potent antioxidant that supports healthy-looking skin, promotes feelings of grounding, and has anti-inflammatory properties.
- **Bergamot essential oil**: Bergamot supports healthy circulation and the immune system, helps to relieve feelings of overwhelm, depression and anxiety[90,91], and contains the constituents limonene, linalyl acetate, and linalool, which are known for their anti-inflammatory, antioxidant, and anti-stress benefits.
- **Cedarwood essential oil**: Cedarwood has a calming and soothing aroma. It promotes the appearance of healthy skin and hair and is high in sesquiterpenes, which help to calm the body and mind.
- **Peppermint essential oil**: Peppermint contains the constituents menthol and menthone, which have anti-inflammatory properties and enhance the absorption of other ingredients.
- **Clove essential oil**: Clove is an antioxidant and anti-inflammatory agent with an average ORAC value of over 290,000[19]. It is high in the constituent eugenol, which boasts well-documented neuroprotective, antioxidant, anti-inflammatory, antipyretic, analgesic, antiparasitic, and antimicrobial properties, and protects the brain, heart, lungs, immune system, and entire body[18].

See page 83 for a comparison chart with Progessence Plus™

> **PROGESSENCE PLUS™**
>
> **To use:** Apply two to four drops to the stomach, feet, or inner thighs each day. Rotate the application sites to avoid applying to the same area two days in a row. For added effect, one to two extra drops may be applied.

Safety notes: Keep out of reach of children. If you are pregnant, nursing, taking medication, or have a medical condition, consult a health professional before use. Avoid direct sunlight or UV rays for up to 12 hours after applying this product.

PROSTATE HEALTH™

As the name suggests, Prostate Health™ supports the male glandular system and is specifically formulated for men, as it focuses on maintaining healthy, normal prostate function. This supplement combines herbs and essential oils that support prostate health and can be used proactively or acutely as desired.

BENEFITS OF PROSTATE HEALTH™
- Promotes healthy prostate function in men
- Includes saw palmetto, which is an herb that is known for prostate health
- Formulated with an essential oil blend that is specific for male needs
- Can be used proactively or acutely for prostate needs

The prostate is a gland in the male reproductive system that serves many important roles, including hormone metabolism, fluid production, and effective reproduction. Not only is this gland essential for male health, but when problems arise, they can cause painful and aggravating symptoms that affect daily life. Furthermore, the incidence of prostate enlargement or prostate cancer increases with a family history. While we can't completely prevent the occurrence of every single possible disease, there is much we can do every day to support our bodies.

Prostate Health™ features saw palmetto and pumpkin seed oil, both of which have documented benefits for prostate health and function. The formula includes an essential oil blend that further improves the function and absorption of these botanicals.
- **Saw palmetto fruit extract:** Saw palmetto is a well-known herb for men that is often used to treat an enlarged prostate and improve symptoms of prostate disfunction[92]. It may help to prevent prostate cancer from developing[93] and supports urinary and sexual health.
- **Pumpkin seed oil:** Pumpkin seed oil supports overall prostate health and function and urinary health. It reduces inflammation and prevents the growth of prostate cancer cells[94].
- **Geranium essential oil:** Geranium promotes healthy hormone balance and aids circulation. It is a natural diuretic with anti-inflammatory and antimicrobial properties.
- **Fennel essential oil**: Fennel supports digestion, eases intestinal discomfort, supports the pancreas and liver, provides immune support, and promotes the excretion of toxins.
- **Lavender essential oil:** Lavender is well known for its ability to support physical and emotional relaxation and decrease the stress response within the body[115]. Additionally, it has also shown antidepressant activity in clinical studies[116] and balances the hormones.

PROSTATE HEALTH™

To use: Take one capsule twice daily.

For maximum benefit, Prostate Health™ should be taken consistently.

- **Myrtle essential oil**: Myrtle balances thyroid hormones, has positive effects on glandular imbalances, and aids detoxification in the liver.
- **Peppermint essential oil:** Peppermint contains menthol, a natural anti-inflammatory that helps to decongest the prostate and promotes a healthy urinary flow.

Safety notes: Keep out of reach of children. If you are pregnant, nursing, taking medication, or have a medical condition, consult a health professional before use.

REGENOLONE™ MOISTURIZING CREAM

Regenolone™ Moisturizing Cream contains nourishing plant extracts, such as wild yam and black and blue cohosh, that support female hormone health and estrogen levels. The formulation is rounded out with a special blend of premium essential oils that help to balance hormones and promote healthier, more youthful-looking skin.

BENEFITS OF REGENOLONE™ MOISTURIZING CREAM
- Helps to balance female estrogen levels with plant extracts, such as wild yam, blue cohosh, and black cohosh
- Moisturizes dry skin to create skin that feels soft, smooth, and comfortable
- Contains antioxidant-rich essential oils
- Formulated with skin-supporting minerals and vitamins
- Contains pregnenolone and adaptogens

Regenolone™ is a natural estrogen support cream with plant-based phytoestrogens that soothe the skin and can provide an alternative to conventional estrogen creams.
- **Pregnenolone**: Pregnenolone is a precursor hormone that is important for the body's production of progesterone. Progesterone blocks cortisol receptors. Pregnenolone also reduces corticotropin-releasing hormone (CRH). CRH is the first step in the production of the stress hormone cortisol.
- **Wolfberry seed oil, shea butter, and aloe vera leaf:** These are sources of antioxidants that are soothing and moisturizing to the skin and act as carriers for the herbs and essential oils in this formula.
- **Calendula flower extract:** Calendula is a powerful source of antioxidants that soothes the skin, promotes healing, and may help with menstrual pain[95].
- **Roman chamomile flower extract:** Roman chamomile contains natural antioxidants and anti-inflammatory properties that may be beneficial for overall health and calms the mind and body.
- **Rosebud flower extract:** This is a rich source of vitamin C. It is a powerful antioxidant that soothes and moisturizes the skin.

- **Green tea leaf extract:** Green tea high in polyphenols, antioxidants that promote skin health, reduce inflammation, and support cellular health.
- **St. John's wort:** St. John's wort is often used to improve low mood. It may help to improve symptoms of PMS[88] and help with symptoms of menopause[89].
- **Ginkgo biloba leaf extract:** Ginkgo biloba may help to improve PMS symptoms[96], mitigate migraines, and improve sleep quality.
- **Wintergreen essential oil:** Wintergreen is extremely high in methyl salicylate, an anti-inflammatory constituent that supports healthy blood pressure and blood vessels. It also has anticoagulant properties.
- **Peppermint essential oil**: Peppermint contains the constituents menthol and menthone, which have anti-inflammatory properties and enhance the absorption of other ingredients.
- **Douglas fir essential oil:** Douglas fir contains antioxidants and has anti-inflammatory properties which support the prostate and the body overall.
- **Oregano essential oil:** Oregano has powerful antioxidant and antimicrobial properties. It boosts immunity, eases inflammation, and promotes feelings of security.
- **Vitamin E:** This is a natural antioxidant that minimizes free radical damage within the body, promoting healthy cell function and overall health.
- **Wild yam root extract:** Wild yam is a natural source of plant-based progesterone that helps to regulate blood sugar, raises HDL levels, lowers LDL levels, supports estrogen and progesterone levels, and has anti-inflammatory properties that soothe muscle spasms.
- **Eleuthero root extract**: Eleuthero root is a wonderful adaptogen that boosts the body's resistance to stress, provides energy, and strengthens the immune system function. It acts as an antioxidant, lowers cholesterol[49] and may have analgesic, anti-inflammatory, and anti-osteolytic effects, especially when taken in combination with other joint- and muscle-supporting herbs.
- **Kelp extract:** Kelp soothes and moisturizes the skin and is high in antioxidants, including minerals, carotenoids and flavonoids, which help to fight against disease-causing free radicals.
- **Retinyl palmitate (vitamin A):** Vitamin A is a powerful antioxidant that increases collagen production, treats mild acne, and moisturizes the skin.

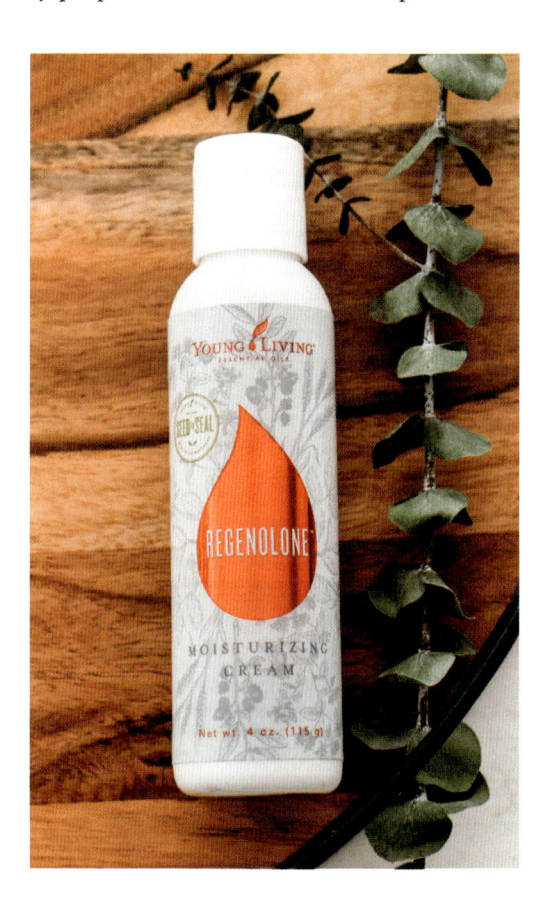

- **Black cohosh root extract**: This is a phytoestrogen that helps to counteract the effects of cortisol, stops stress responses, improves bone density, and may elevate the mood. It helps with symptoms of menopause, anxiety, and PCOS[77].
- **Blue cohosh extract:** This is a phytoestrogen that promotes healthy blood flow in the female reproductive system, relieves cramping, and balances estrogen levels.

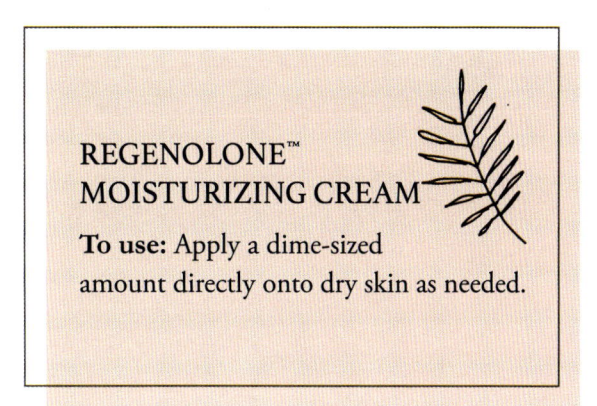

> REGENOLONE™ MOISTURIZING CREAM
>
> **To use:** Apply a dime-sized amount directly onto dry skin as needed.

See below for a comparison chart with Regenolone™.

PRENOLONE PLUS™ CREAM, PROGESSENCE PLUS™, AND REGENOLONE™ MOISTURE CREAM COMPARISON

	ESTROGEN	PROGESTERONE	DHEA	MOOD SUPPORT	NOTES
PRENOLONE PLUS™	Contains the phytoestrogensblue and black cohosh	Yes	Yes	Contains St. John's wort	Contains pregnenolone
PROGESSENCE PLUS™	No	Contains wild yam extract	No	Contains sacred frankincense and bergamot essential oils	
REGENOLONE™	Contains the phytoestrogensblue and black cohosh	Contains wild yam extract	No	Contains St. John's wort and adaptogenic herbs	Contains pregnenolone

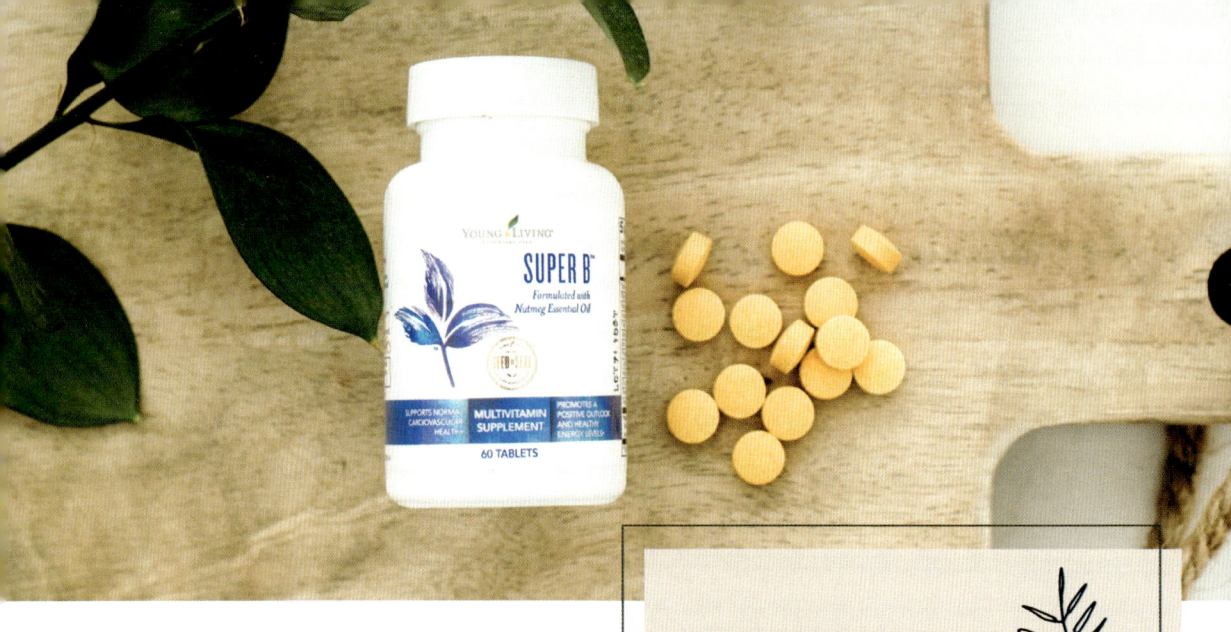

SUPER B™

See page 48 for more information on Super B™.

Young Living's Super B™ is a B complex. It contains all eight essential, energy-boosting B vitamins, nutmeg essential oil, and bioavailable chelated minerals, and folate. Our bodies struggle to absorb and utilize folic acid. We need it in the form of folate for adequate absorption, and many individuals require a methylated version, which is why Orgen-FA is a great addition to this supplement.

SUPER B™

To use: Take two tablets daily with a meal, ideally with your first meal of the day. Alternatively, you can take one tablet with your first meal and one tablet at midday.

SUPER B™ & HORMONES

The B vitamins are critical for a healthy endocrine system. They are involved in the production and metabolism of hormones and neurotransmitters, are required for liver detoxification of heavy metals, histamines, and bacterial toxins, and have dramatic energy and mood-elevating effects. Super B™ is a great choice for:

- Anyone under stress, as stress depletes B vitamins in our bodies
- Anyone who battles candida. Some believe that a lack of B vitamins causes overgrowth.
- Anyone who needs energy. Super B™ nourishes the adrenals and combats fatigue.
- Anyone struggling mentally and emotionally, as a vitamin deficiency can be linked to many anxious, exhausted, or low feelings and thoughts

Safety notes: Keep out of reach of children. If you are pregnant, nursing, taking medication, or have a medical condition, consult a health professional before use. If taken on an empty stomach, you may experience a temporary niacin flush/warming sensation.

THYROMIN™

Thyromin™ is a blend of porcine glandular extracts, herbs, amino acids, minerals, and essential oils that maximizes nutritional support for healthy thyroid function. The thyroid gland regulates body metabolism, energy, and body temperature and is connected to all the body's functions. Being proactive and supporting the thyroid with proper amino acids and minerals is important to support an overall healthy lifestyle.

BENEFITS OF THYROMIN™
- Nutritionally supports a healthy thyroid function
- Helps to balance thyroid hormones naturally
- Provides the body with iodine, herbs, and essentials oils to support a healthy thyroid
- Nourishes the thyroid to regulate energy levels, body temperature, and a healthy weight

Most women have or will have a thyroid imbalance at some point in their lives, and it often goes undiagnosed due to widely ranging lab values. Subclinical hypothyroidism is incredibly common. Sadly, many individuals are suffering from symptoms of low thyroid function but have "normal" values on a lab test. Find a care provider who will take a closer look, especially in the presence of symptoms, such as fatigue, brain fog, cold or heat intolerance, constipation, or fluid retention. When it comes to support, Thyromin™ contains a wonderful blend of herbs, minerals, and oils that can give the thyroid gland the daily support that it needs.
- **Bovine thyroid powder:** This improves energy levels, metabolism, and weight management and supplements the thyroid hormone that is made in the body.
- **Porcine pituitary powder:** This helps to regulate overall endocrine function, cortisol and sex hormone production, secretion of hormones, and bone resorption.
- **Porcine adrenal powder:** This helps to regulate the body's natural response to stress and improve symptoms of fatigue and muscle weakness.
- **CoQ10**: CoQ10 is an enzyme used by every cell in the body to convert food into energy. It is a powerful antioxidant that supports every cell in the body. It acts as a battery for our cells, helping with the production and exchange of energy, and facilitates the production of ATP *(see page 45-46 for more information on CoQ10).*
- **Vitamin E**: Vitamin E is a natural antioxidant that minimizes free radical damage within the body, promotes healthy cell function, overall health, and healthy hair, skin, and nails.
- **Kelp:** Kelp contains vitamins, minerals, antioxidants and iodine, all of which are vital for a healthy thyroid and hormone balance and function.
- **Parsley leaf powder:** Parsley is commonly used in herbal medicine to cleanse and purify the urinary tract. It is high in antioxidants, which support liver health.
- **L-cystine:** This is an amino acid that is required for the utilization of B vitamins and helps to supply insulin to the pancreas.
- **L-cysteine HCL**: This amino acid is essential for thyroid health and promotes glutathione production and liver health.

- **Spearmint essential oil**: Spearmint is high in carvone and limonene, which promote thyroid function. It is wonderful for digestive health, as it soothes intestinal discomfort and decreases inflammation.
- **Peppermint essential oil**: Peppermint is highly regarded for supporting normal digestion and promoting healthy intestinal and pancreatic function.
- **Myrtle essential oil**: Myrtle is an adaptogen that can increase or decrease thyroid activity, depending on the body's needs. It supports the respiratory system, skin, and hair and helps to restore glandular balance to the thyroid and ovaries.
- **Myrrh essential oil**: Myrrh is a powerful antioxidant that supports healthy hormones and overall longevity.

> ### THYROMIN™
>
> **To use:** Take one or two capsules daily before bed or rotate one in the morning and one in the evening. If you are currently taking a thyroid medication, consult your doctor before starting this supplement.

Safety notes: Keep out of reach of children. If you are pregnant or nursing, taking medication, or have a medical condition, consult a health professional before use.

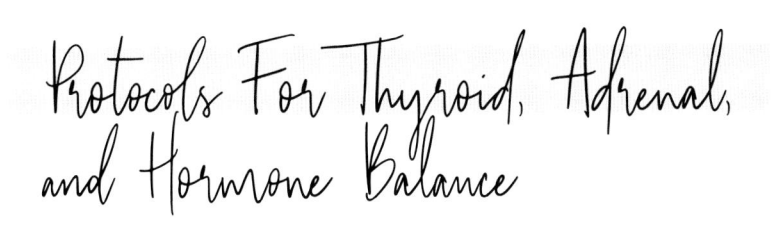

Protocols For Thyroid, Adrenal, and Hormone Balance

Here are a few suggestions for getting started in this area of health. Remember—you are your own health advocate. Your body will intuitively give you clues regarding what it needs, so it's our job to pay attention and pull in providers who we trust and who align with our values. It is often helpful to keep a journal of your symptoms, the date, and any seemingly significant factors. Our bodies are grand designs that are constantly telling us what they need!

MOOD & EMOTIONS

Although this is a complex area of support, our emotions and physical health are closely linked. Supporting your body in these areas is a powerful tool for emotional health.

- Life 9®
- MindWise™
- NingXia Red®
- OmegaGize³®
- Super B™
- Super Vitamin D
- Options for more support: Inner Defense®, Cleansing Trio™, CortiStop®, Progessence Plus™ (women), FemiGen™ (women), EndoFlex™ Vitality™

STRESS RECOVERY (ADRENAL HEALTH)

Signs that you may need support in this area include dizziness, emotional instability, feeling easily triggered, anxiety, feeling overwhelmed, and feeling tired but having difficulty falling asleep ("tired but wired"). These supplements are great support tools for times when you know that you have/are experiencing a lot of psychological and emotional stress.

- CortiStop® (intermittently)
- Golden Turmeric™
- Mineral Essence™
- NingXia Red®
- Super B™
- Super Vitamin D
- Options for more support: EndoFlex™ Vitality™ Essential Oil, Nutmeg Essential Oil

THYROID HEALTH

Signs that you may need support in this area include fatigue, dizziness, feeling cold all the time, feeling hungry all the time, lethargy, and exercise intolerance. Thyroid imbalance is incredibly common in women aged 30-50 and women who are pregnant and postpartum.

- Golden Turmeric™
- MultiGreens™
- Mineral Essence™
- NingXia Red®
- Sulfurzyme®
- Thyromin™
- Options for more support: Myrtle Essential Oil, EndoFlex™ Vitality™ Essential Oil

WOMEN'S HEALTH & HORMONE BALANCE

Signs that you may need support in this area include painful periods, symptoms of PMS (physical and emotional), irregular cycles, low libido, and any known issues, such as PCOS or endometriosis. Adding more estrogen support with Prenolone or Regenolone™ is a great option for these symptoms. These supplements are a good place to start when creating an overall wellness plan for women.

- FemiGen™
- Mineral Essence™
- Progessence Plus™
- NingXia Red®
- Sulfurzyme®
- Super B™
- Super Cal Plus™
- Optional for more targeted support: Thyromin™, Prenolone Plus™, Regenolone™ Moisture Cream

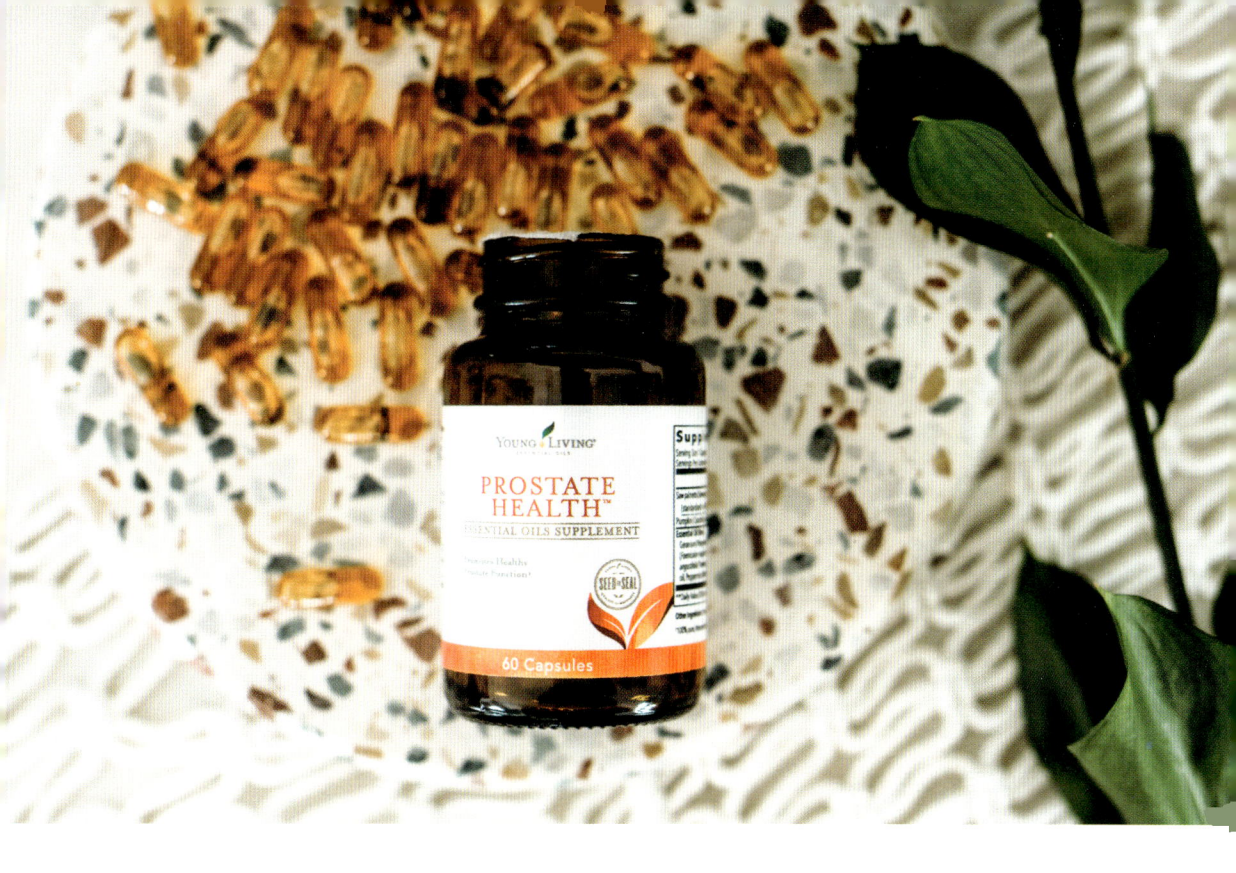

MEN'S HEALTH & HORMONE BALANCE

Signs that you may need support in this area include fatigue, stress, anxiety, feeling low, loss of interest in things that used to interest you, difficulty gaining lean muscle mass, and low libido.

- Golden Turmeric™
- Life 9®
- Longevity™
- MultiGreens™
- Mineral Essence™
- NingXia Red®
- PowerGize™
- Super B™
- Super Vitamin D
- Options for more targeted support: Prostate Health™, CortiStop® as needed for stress recovery, Shutran™ Essential Oil Blend, Idaho Blue Spruce Essential Oil, Mister™ Essential Oil Blend

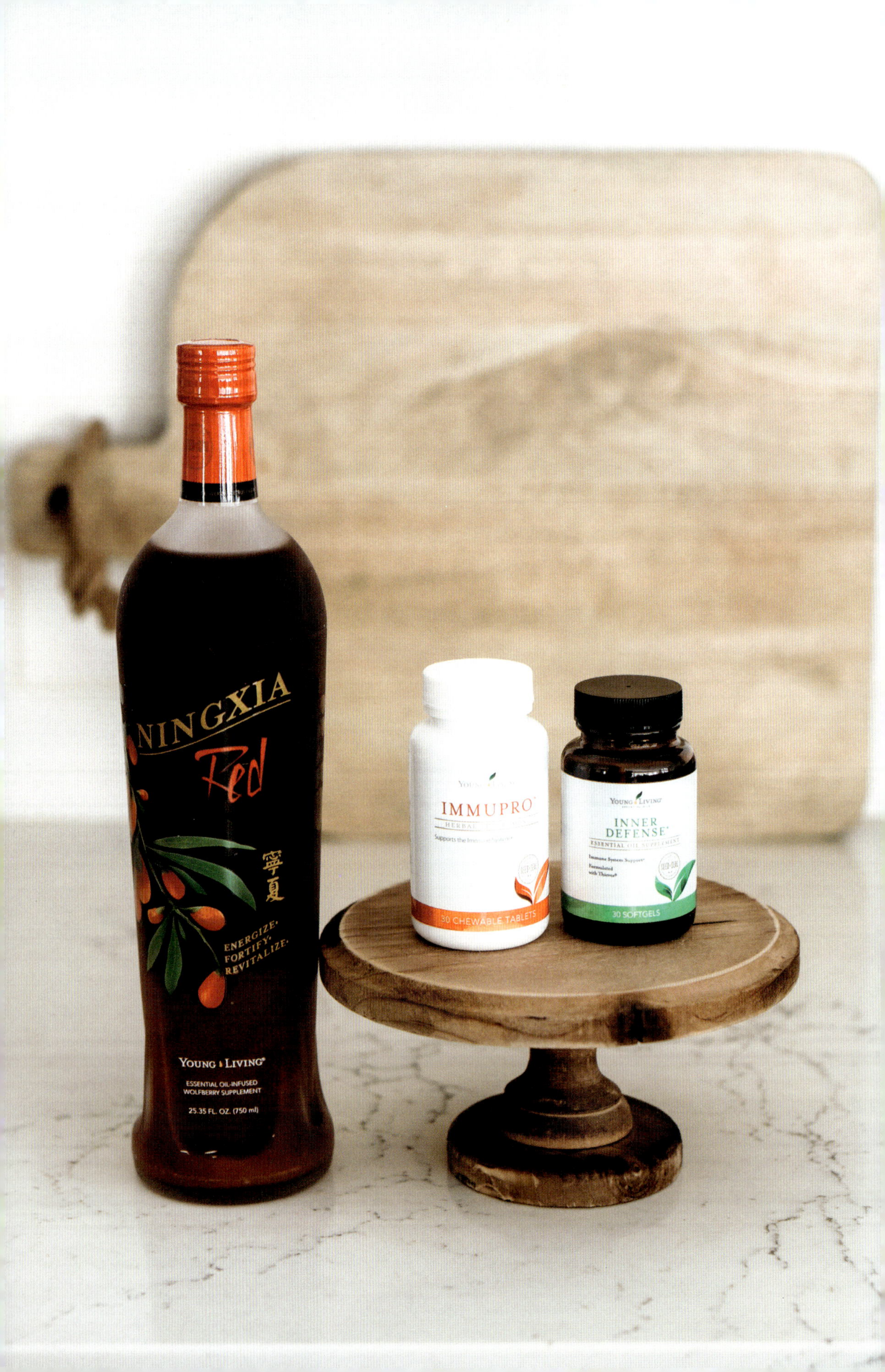
NINGXIA
Red
寧夏
ENERGIZE·
FORTIFY·
REVITALIZE·
YOUNG LIVING
ESSENTIAL OIL-INFUSED
WOLFBERRY SUPPLEMENT
25.35 FL. OZ. (750 ml)
IMMUPRO
30 CHEWABLE TABLETS
YOUNG LIVING
INNER
DEFENSE
ESSENTIAL OIL SUPPLEMENT
30 SOFTGELS

Part 2: SUPPLEMENTS FOR THE IMMUNE SYSTEM

Supplements for the immune system are some of the most popular supplements, both conventional and herbal, which makes sense. We all want to be and stay healthy, especially in this modern world. Young Living has an incredible line of immune support options that include herbs and essential oils that are known for their immunoprotective properties.

Before we dive into supplements that support the immune system, let's do a quick Immunology 101 to learn how the immune system works.

UNDERSTANDING THE IMMUNE SYSTEM

There are two types of immunity—innate and humoral. Both are essential for immune health, and the differences are simply in the types of immune cells that are involved and their actions. The human body uses both innate immunity and adaptive immunity to destroy invading pathogens and prevent re-infection.

The innate immune system is sometimes referred to as the general immune system and is what most people think of when they think of immunity. It is our first line of defense to detect danger patterns and destroy pathogens, such as viruses, bacteria, and even cancer cells. The innate immune system works quickly and responds in the same way to all invaders. When bacteria enter the body through a small skin wound, the innate immune system acts immediately to destroy the bacteria. If germs make it past the skin and mucous membranes, the innate immune system releases specialized cells to destroy the pathogens. These include macrophages, dendritic cells, granulocytes, and natural killer cells.

If the innate immune system can't control an issue, the adaptive immune system takes over. The adaptive immune system utilizes more specialized cells—T-cells, B-cells, and antigens—to launch an attack that is directed at the specific invading pathogen (versus the more generalized approach that the innate immune system utilizes). Because of this, the adaptive immune system creates a database of pathogens to which it is exposed. The relationship between B-cells, T-cells, and antibodies is somewhat complex. To put it simply, antibodies are created, they attack

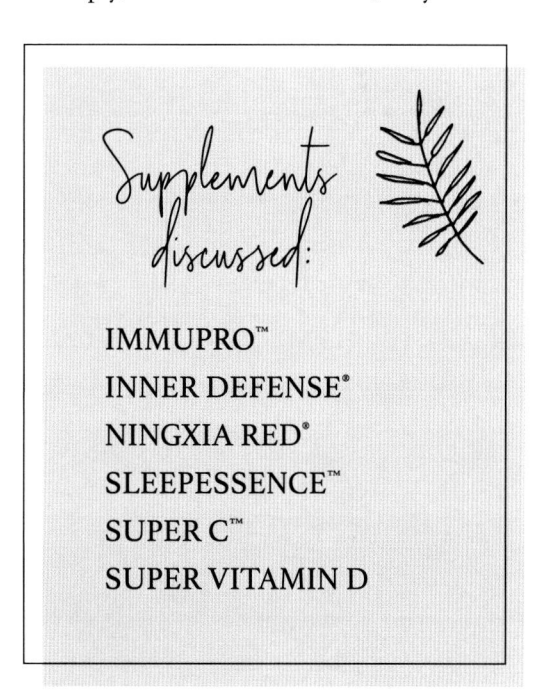

Supplements discussed:

IMMUPRO™
INNER DEFENSE®
NINGXIA RED®
SLEEPESSENCE™
SUPER C™
SUPER VITAMIN D

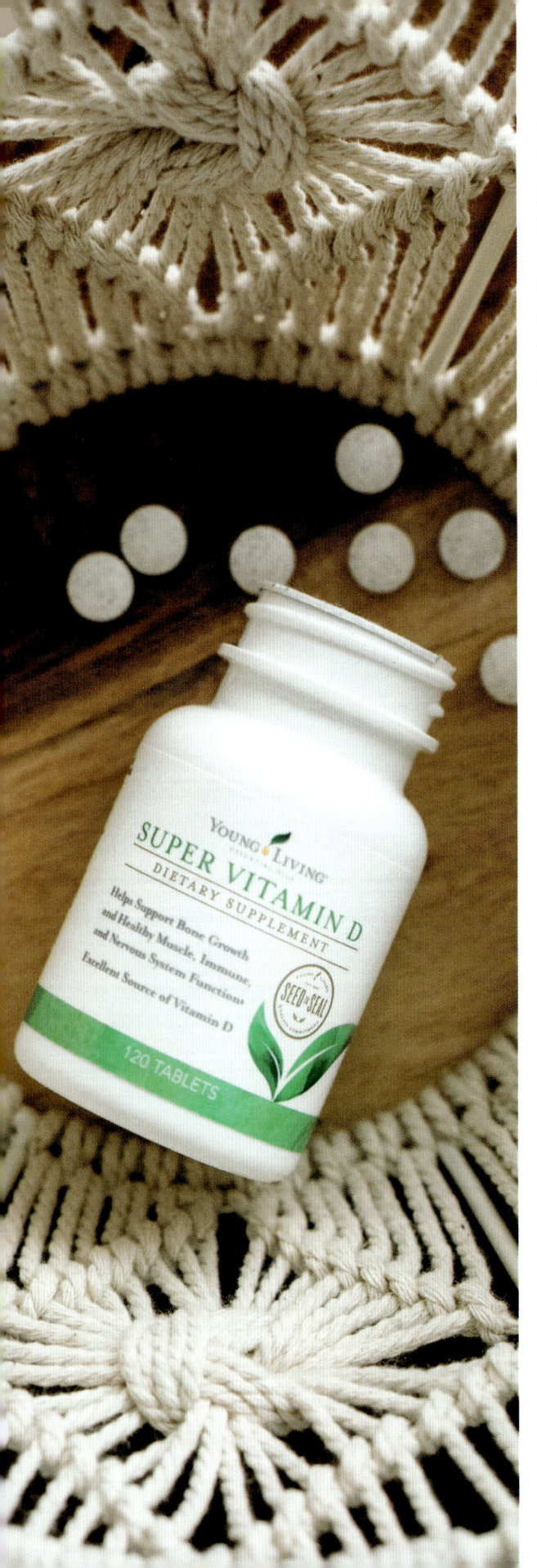

the invading germs, and then a portion of the antibody is saved so that when/if the pathogen invades again, the immune system can quickly ramp up a specific defense.

Overall, the immune system is a beautiful and complex system with multiple areas that can be supported and enhanced to bolster immunity both acutely and daily.

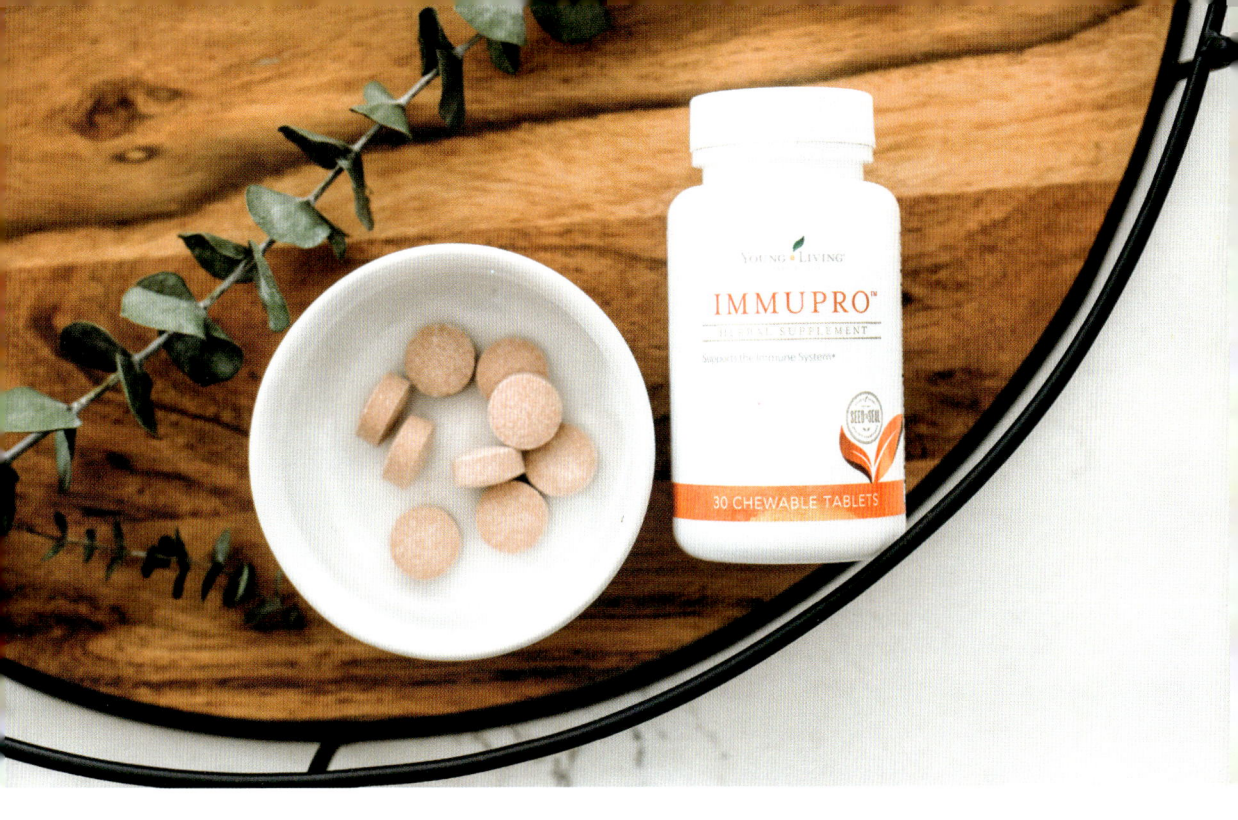

IMMUPRO™

ImmuPro™ is a power-packed supplement that combines multiple ingredients with powerful antioxidant activity. ImmuPro™ includes naturally derived NingXia wolfberry polysaccharides and a blend of reishi, maitake, agaricus blazei mushroom powders, zinc, and selenium for proper immune function, along with chelated minerals that are more easily absorbed by the body. All of these ingredients work synergistically to give the body a robust set of nutrients to bolster immunity.

ImmuPro™ also contains melatonin, a natural, endogenous hormone that our bodies release at night to help us sleep. Sleep is essential when the immune system needs to get its defenses going, and the melatonin in ImmuPro™ encourages restful sleep by promoting the body's natural sleep rhythm.

BENEFITS OF IMMUPRO™
- Stimulates both cell-mediated and humoral immunity
- Provides minerals, such as zinc, copper, and selenium, that bolster immunity
- Allows the body to rest by providing a small amount of melatonin
- Includes a mushroom blend to bolster the immune system

ImmuPro™ combines reishi, maitake, and agaricus blazei organic mushrooms with NingXia wolfberry polysaccharides and orange essential oil to create an immune-supporting supplement that is full of antioxidants. Although we've already covered how important antioxidants are, when your body's defenses go down, the role of antioxidants becomes even more important. Acute (and chronic) illness takes a physical toll on the body and causes more oxidative damage as pathogens invade cells and produce free radicals. The ingredients in ImmuPro™ can reduce the damaging effects of oxidative stress and improve immune function.

- **Reishi mushroom:** Reishi mushrooms contain many powerful constituents that improve and increase white blood cell function[97,98], protect against infections and viruses[99], and decrease inflammation. Moreover, it is an antioxidant and immune modulator[100] and restores homeostasis to the body by stabilizing the immune response and hormone levels.
- **Maitake mushroom**: Maitake mushrooms are well known for their immune support and adaptogenic properties[101]. They regulate the body's stress response, balance hormones, and boost both innate and humoral immunity[102].
- **Agaricus blazei mushroom:** This mushroom is well known for its immune modulating activities. It activates white blood cells in the innate immune system to provide protection against both bacteria and viruses[103] and is high in beta glucans, polysaccharides that promote an increase or decrease in the immune response, depending on the body's innate need[104].
- **Orange essential oil:** Orange is high in d-limonene, a constituent that is known to improve immune function through an increase in immunoglobulin and antibody levels[105]. It shows anti-inflammatory, wound-healing, and anticancer effects. D-limonene alters the signaling pathways within cancer cells in a way that stops cancer cells from multiplying and causes their death[22].
- **Melatonin:** Melatonin is widely known for its ability to regulate circadian rhythm. It modulates the immune response at various stages in the immune process and helps to regulate glutathione levels[106] (glutathione is one of the body's primary antioxidants).

When we are stressed (physically or emotionally), our bodies need sleep to allow healing to occur. Not only is the body physically tired, but there are certain immune processes that take place during sleep. Sleep is essential for T-cell production, the cells that are the front-line fighters when pathogens invade. Although we always have T-cells present, their production is ramped up during times of acute illness. Stress hormones, such as cortisol, can decrease the number of T-cells that are produced, and stress hormone levels are higher when we are awake, which makes sleep essential during times of illness.

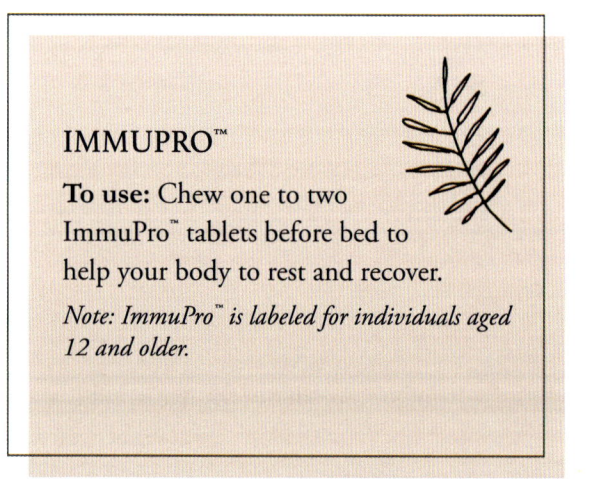

> **IMMUPRO™**
>
> **To use:** Chew one to two ImmuPro™ tablets before bed to help your body to rest and recover.
>
> Note: ImmuPro™ is labeled for individuals aged 12 and older.

Sleep can be a tricky thing to support. Although everyone has individual preferences and needs, there is much that we can do to help our bodies find deep, healthy rest. One simple way to promote healthy sleep is to create a daily bedtime routine that you use regularly, then add in extra support to specific areas (such as the immune system) when needed.

- Make a mug of "Thieves® Tea" (one drop of Thieves® Vitality™ in honey, then add hot water) to drink in the evenings.
- Draw a relaxing bath with ten drops of patchouli and five drops of clove in one cup of Epsom salt. (As a bonus, light a DIY beeswax candle and read something inspiring while you soak.)
- After your bath, apply diluted nutmeg over the adrenals to lower cortisol levels.
- Roll your wellness blend over the spine and lymph nodes (my favorite is Thieves®, frankincense, lemon, geranium, pine, and oregano in a 10 mL roller bottle with carrier).
- Chew one to two ImmuPro™ tablets.
- Fire up your diffuser with Valor®, frankincense, and lavender.
- Apply your favorite sleep-supporting oils (I love Tranquil® Roll-on) and snooze away!

INNER DEFENSE®

Inner Defense® is just what the name suggests—defense and protection from all that today's world can throw at us. This powerhouse blend of essential oils supports the immune and respiratory systems, which makes it a wonderful addition to your health routine for either daily use or when your defenses start to go down.

BENEFITS OF INNER DEFENSE®
- Reinforces natural systemic defenses
- Supports and enhances immune system activity
- Promotes healthy respiratory function
- Creates an unfriendly terrain for the growth of yeast and fungus
- Dissolves quickly for maximum results
- Highly effective at meeting the immune system's needs

So much of our modern world can take a toll on our health—environmental exposure, devitalized food, lack of sleep, abundance of psychological stress, polluted water and air, and pathogen exposure. And even exposure to these things in small quantities can add up to a cumulative dose that leaves us needing extra support. Sometimes, we need that support acutely, and other times, we need it on a more consistent basis. Either way, Inner Defense® is a great option for strengthening the body's immune defense systems.

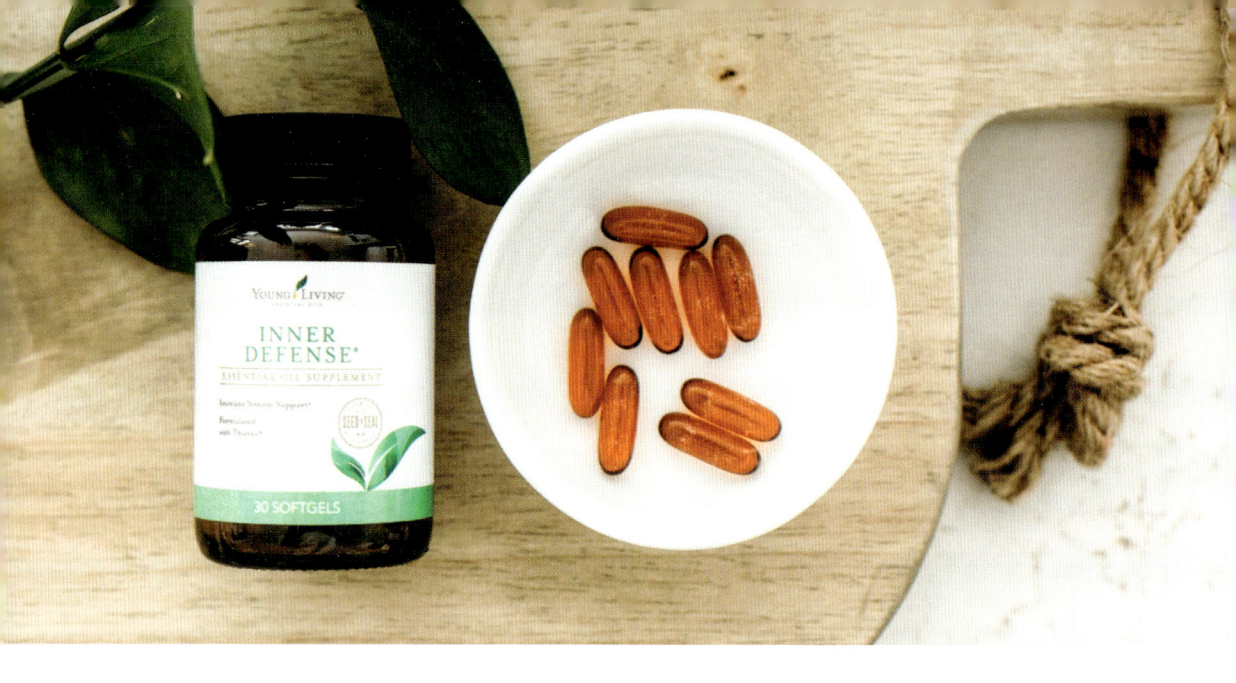

Inner Defense® is a powerhouse mix of essential oils that are well known for their antimicrobial and antioxidant activity.

- **Clove essential oil**: Clove has profound immune support and is a powerful antioxidant. It has an average ORAC value of over 290,000[19] and is effective at stopping the growth of some bacteria and fungi[20], including *Candida*[21], at higher doses.
- **Oregano essential oil**: Oregano is high in carvacrol and thymol, constituents that support the immune system through direct bacterial activity[107]. It has shown activity against antibiotic-resistant *Salmonella,* especially in combination with cinnamon bark essential oil[108].
- **Thyme essential oil**: Thyme is rich in the constituent thymol, a potent antioxidant that supports the respiratory and immune systems through direct bactericidal activity against many common pathogens[109]. It protects DHA levels and brain function, has demonstrated efficacy against antibiotic-resistant bacterial strains[23], and supports a healthy hormone balance[24]. In addition, it works as a circulatory stimulant, helping maintain healthy blood pressure and cholesterol levels[25].
- **Lemongrass essential oil**: Lemongrass is a cleansing oil with antibacterial activity, even against drug-resistant strains of *Candida*[110]. It boosts the body's response to bladder infections and calms the digestive system.
- **Lemon essential oil:** Lemon is high in limonene and supports respiration and immune function through an increase in white blood cell production[111]. It has direct bacterial effects on many common pathogens[112], acts as an antioxidant, and mitigates free radical damage within cells[113].
- **Eucalyptus radiata essential oil**: Eucalyptus is known for its support of the respiratory system. It cleanses, purifies, and supports immune function through direct bactericidal action[110].
- **Rosemary essential oil:** Rosemary cleanses, purifies, and provides immune support through direct bactericidal activity, even on certain drug-resistant bacteria and fungi[110].

- **Cinnamon bark essential oil**: Cinnamon is a potent antioxidant with antimicrobial activity. It is effective against drug-resistant bacterial strains, especially when blended with rosemary and eucalyptus essential oils[114].

INNER DEFENSE® AND EMOTIONAL HEALTH

When we begin to fall below the wellness line, our emotional and mental health is also affected. As all our body systems are interconnected, it makes sense that we often feel run down, fatigued, and exhausted on an emotional level with acute or chronic infections. Sometimes, the emotional and mental effects of illness show up first, which suggest that we need more support. When you're feeling run down, weary, vulnerable, and easily overwhelmed or triggered, stop and take inventory of your physical health. The organisms that invade our cells and bring us down affect our emotions too!

Note: Contains fish (tilapia, carp) and tree nuts (coconut).

INNER DEFENSE®

To use:
- Take one softgel three to five times daily for acute needs. Take with food and at the very first sign of illness.
- Take one softgel daily for overall immune support as desired. Many individuals choose to take Inner Defense® when traveling or during times of unusual germ exposure.
- For best results, take Inner Defense® with food (especially a healthy fat, such as peanut butter or coconut oil), and take Life 9® Probiotic approximately eight hours later.
- Parenting tip: If you'd like to use Inner Defense® for children, use a safety pin or needle to create a small hole in the gel cap, then gently squeeze and apply the contents along the spine or the bottom of the feet.

NINGXIA RED®

For more information on NingXia Red®, check out the "Foundational Supplements" section on page 41.

NingXia Red® is one of Young Living's most popular products, and for good reason. This wolfberry puree is so much more than a delicious addition to your day. NingXia Red® is a nutrient-dense fuel source for our bodies. Much like a car runs better with proper fuel, our bodies perform better when they are supplied with all the nutrients that they need.

NINGXIA RED® AND IMMUNE HEALTH

NingXia Red® is rich in ellagic acid, polyphenols, flavonoids, vitamins, and minerals. In addition, it has 18 amino acids, 21 trace minerals, beta-carotene, and vitamins B1, B2, B6, and E. It is an excellent whole-food source of nutrients that provides energy and strength to the body. Although we need these things daily, we need them even more so when our defenses go down.

NingXia Red® combines the NingXia wolfberry, blueberry, plum, cherry, pomegranate, and Aronia juices to create a supplement with a large range of antioxidants that support the entire body. This balanced approach to antioxidant supplementation makes NingXia unique and means that it can support many body systems. NingXia Red® also includes orange, tangerine, lemon, and yuzu essential oils, all of which contain the powerful constituent d-limonene, a constituent that decreases inflammation and improves immune function by increasing immunoglobulin and antibody levels[105].

NINGXIA RED®

To use: Take 2-4 oz. daily on its own or mixed with water, juice, or sparkling water. NingXia Red® can also be added to a smoothie.

NINGXIA
Red

ENERGIZE.
FORTIFY.
REVITALIZE.

宁夏

Young Living®

ESSENTIAL OIL-INFUSED
WOLFBERRY SUPPLEMENT

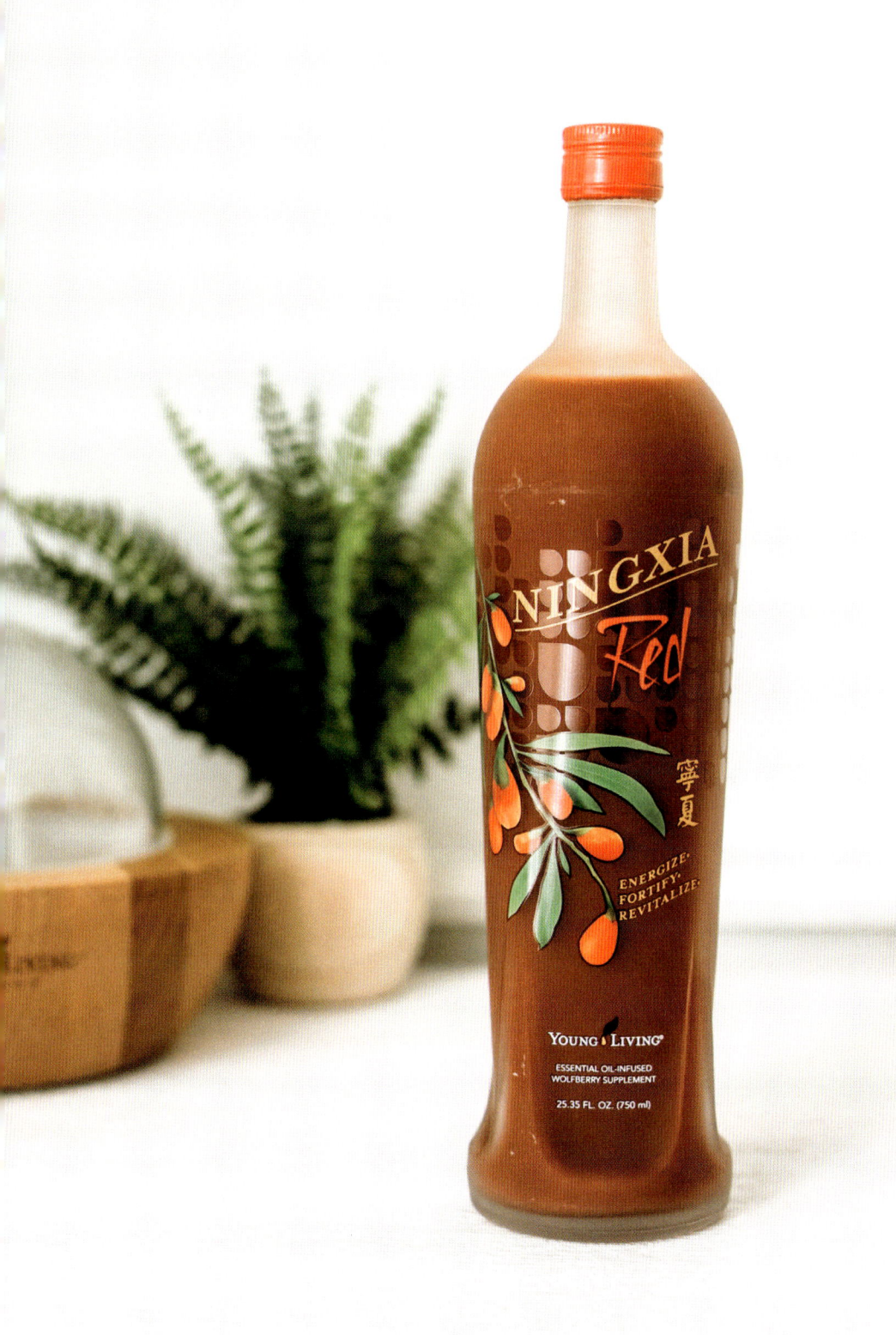

25.35 FL. OZ. (750 ml)

SLEEPESSENCE™

SleepEssence™ is a wonderful supplement that helps the body to relax into its natural, restful sleep rhythm. It contains many sleep-supporting essential oils and melatonin to help you fall asleep and sleep well.

BENEFITS OF SLEEPESSENCE™
- Formulated with lavender and valerian essential oils, which help to promote restful sleep
- Supports the body's natural sleep rhythm with melatonin
- Promotes overall well-being when used in conjunction with a healthy lifestyle

SleepEssence™ can be used whenever you need help with sleeping. As we mentioned earlier, sleep is essential when the body is run down. The body utilizes sleep to perform many immune system tasks to decrease inflammation and produce cells to fight infection.

Each ingredient in SleepEssence™ plays a powerful role that helps the body to relax physically and mentally to find restful sleep. This supplement is superior to any melatonin supplement that you'd find at a pharmacy counter because of the addition of sleep-supporting essential oils.

- **Lavender essential oil:** Lavender is well known for its ability to support physical and emotional relaxation and decrease the stress response within the body[115]. It has also shown antidepressant activity in clinical studies[116].
- **Vetiver essential oil:** Vetiver contains sesquiterpenes, constituents that reduce psychological stress and feelings of anxiety and mental fatigue, which often keep our brains from shutting off at bedtime. It helps to calm brain waves to a state more conducive to sleep.
- **Valerian essential oil:** Valerian contains constituents that act as natural modulators of GABA receptors, the receptors in our brains that are responsible for sleep and waking (commonly used pharmaceutical agents for relaxation and sleep act on these same receptors). It helps the body to relax into sleep more quickly and improves sleep quality[117].
- **Tangerine essential oil:** Tangerine is high in limonene, which bolsters the immune system, provides antioxidant support to repair free radical damage, shows anti-inflammatory effects, calms the central nervous system, and relaxes the muscles to support healthy sleep[118].
- **Rue essential oil:** This oil has been used in herbal medicine for many years for its ability to calm the nervous system. It has antioxidant properties and helps the body to repair free radical damage at a cellular level[119].

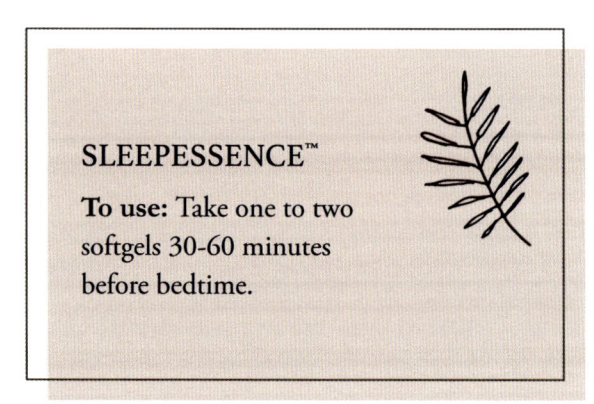

SLEEPESSENCE™
To use: Take one to two softgels 30-60 minutes before bedtime.

- **Melatonin:** Melatonin is widely known for its ability to regulate circadian rhythm. It modulates the immune response at various stages in the immune process and helps to regulate glutathione levels[106] (glutathione is one of the body's primary antioxidants).

SUPER C™ (AND SUPER C™ CHEWABLE)

For more information on Super C™ and Super C™ Chewable, check out the "Foundational Supplements" section on page 51.

We all know that vitamin C is good for us and can help boost immunity, and Young Living's Super C™ and Super C™ Chewable don't disappoint. Super C™ contains 2,166% of the recommended dietary intake of vitamin C per serving and is fortified with rutin, citrus bioflavonoids, and minerals to balance electrolytes and enhance the effectiveness and absorption of vitamin C.

Super C™ and Super C™ Chewable contain citrus essential oils, which, when combined with the other ingredients, play a role in normal immune and circulatory function, strengthen connective tissues, and promote overall health, vitality, and longevity[59].

VITAMIN C AND IMMUNE HEALTH

Because vitamin C has a well-documented role in immune health, many individuals choose to use this supplement daily. Infections significantly impact vitamin C levels because of enhanced inflammation and metabolic requirements. Therefore, when acute needs arise, higher levels of vitamin C are needed to rid the body of infection and bring things back into balance. The B- and T-cells of the adaptive immune system need high levels of vitamin C to function properly[120], and we want to give them what they need! (B- and T-cells are the part of the immune system that focus on pathogen-specific activity.)

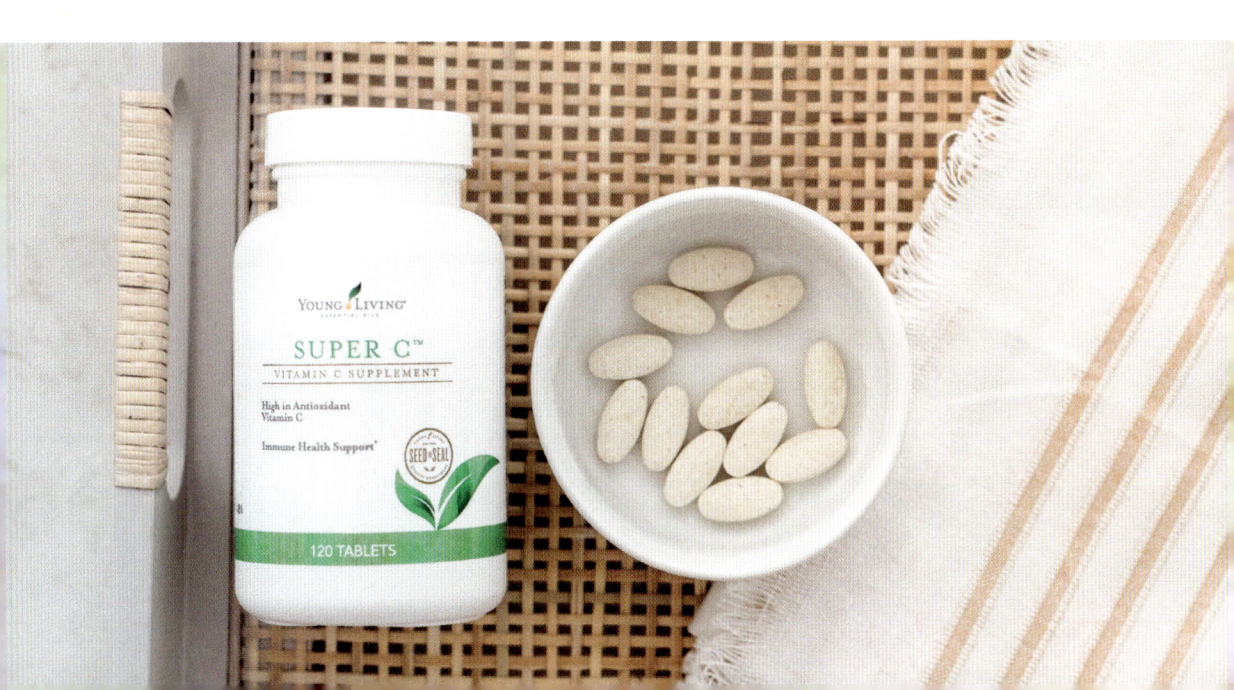

Vitamin C is primarily absorbed inside the cells, although some passive absorption occurs within the GI tract. Because the transporter that moves vitamin C into our cells can only carry so much at one time, we say that it is "saturable." This is important because it means that when taking higher doses of vitamin C for acute needs, it is preferable to take a little less each dose but dose more frequently. Adequate levels of vitamin C during acute infection should meet the saturation requirements of the cells but not exceed it. The average "high" dose of vitamin C for acute needs is 2,000-5,000 mg per dose. Although it is difficult to say how much will be absorbed at one time with higher doses, some evidence suggests that plant-based sources of vitamin C (i.e., rose hips, such as in Super C™ Chewable) may have slightly better bioavailability than ascorbic acid[121]. However, the data is not robust or conclusive enough to make a definitive statement either way.

> **SUPER C™ AND SUPER C™ CHEWABLE**
>
> **To use:**
> - For reinforcing immune strength, take up to 2,000 mg three times or more daily as desired, making sure to separate the doses by a few hours.
> - For maintenance, take approximately 1,000 mg once or twice daily. It works best when taken before meals.

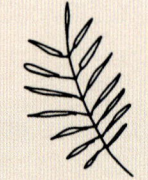

SUPER VITAMIN D

Find more information on Super Vitamin D under the "Foundational Supplements" section on page 54.

Vitamin D is a powerhouse when it comes to our health. Immune, respiratory, bone and joint, emotions, and autoimmune needs are all supported with healthy vitamin D levels. When our natural defenses go down, vitamin D is critical. Having adequate stores *before* we fall below the wellness line is ideal, as vitamin D metabolites work best in a preventative setting[122]. However, we can also supplement during times of acute needs.

Young Living's Super Vitamin D is a highly absorbable, vegan-friendly tablet made with lemon balm extract and lime and Melissa essential oils. These essential oils increase the bioavailability of vitamin D, which means that our bodies absorb more of it in the presence of the essential oils.

Melissa essential oil is a wonderful addition to Young Living's Super Vitamin D. Some studies have shown that ingesting Melissa oil can be helpful in diseases that are associated with inflammation and pain[64]. Melissa oil has also been evaluated for its ability to treat bacterial infections, including those resistant to medications[67].

VITAMIN D AND IMMUNE HEALTH

The role of vitamin D in the immune system is a newer concept in the medical and scientific world. However, the bottom line is that vitamin D has broader effects than we originally realized, including important immunomodulatory properties. Vitamin D deficiency is linked to an under-functioning immune system and a higher predisposition to autoimmune diseases[123].

Almost every cell in the immune system has a vitamin D receptor on it, both in the innate and adaptive immune systems. Although the significance of this is still under investigation, research shows that the effect of vitamin D on immune cells is complex. Some immune system cells gain higher concentrations of vitamin D when activated, while others lose their vitamin D expression when they are activated[122]. Vitamin D's effect on the immune system is one of modulating, shifting the adaptive immune system toward antigen tolerance and the innate immune system to microbial clearance[122].

Additionally, it's important to note that when we are talking about vitamin D's roles in health, we are specifically referring to 1,25-dihydroxyvitamin D3 (1,25(OH)2D3), which is the active metabolite that is most easily isolated from vitamin D3. Young Living's Super Vitamin D supplies D3, which is what we want to maximize the health benefits of vitamin D.

SUPER VITAMIN D

To use: Take one to two tablets daily with food or as directed by your physician. Place in mouth and allow to dissolve for five to ten seconds, then chew for optimal results.

Note: Each sublingual tablet contains 1,000 IU vitamin D. Use this to guide your dosing and requirements.

Protocols For Immune System Support

Daily support of the immune system with supplements and essential oils is key, as this keeps our defenses strong and capable. When we do have an acute need, we can use many of the same supplements and essential oils more frequently to help our bodies fight off illness.

IMMUNE SYSTEM (DAILY SUPPORT)
- Inner Defense® (daily as desired)
- Life 9® (separate from Inner Defense® by at least four hours, ideally eight)
- Mineral Essence™
- MultiGreens™
- NingXia Red®
- Super C™
- Super Vitamin D
- Other options for more support: Thieves® Roll-On, ImmuPower™ Essential Oil Blend

IMMUNE SYSTEM (ACUTE NEEDS)
- ImmuPro™ (take before bed)
- Inner Defense® (up to five times a day)
- Life 9® (separate from Inner Defense® by at least four hours, ideally eight)
- Mineral Essence™
- MultiGreens™
- NingXia Red® (option to increase intake during acute needs)
- Super C™ (up to three times a day)
- Super Vitamin D
- Other options for more support: Thieves® Roll-On, ImmuPower™ Essential Oil Blend, Oregano Essential Oil, Raindrop Massage (or use these oils to make a roller and/or add to an Epsom salt bath)

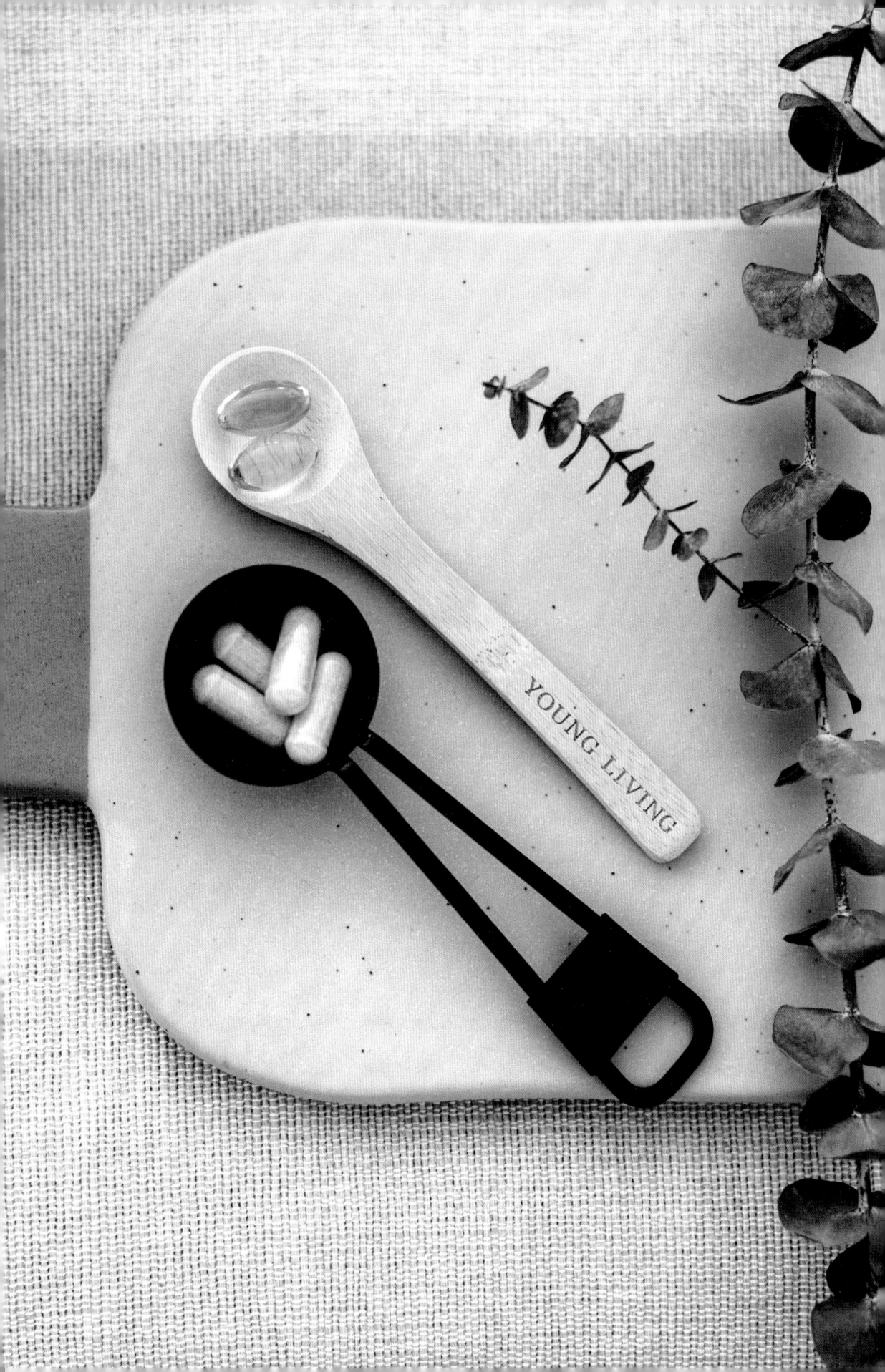

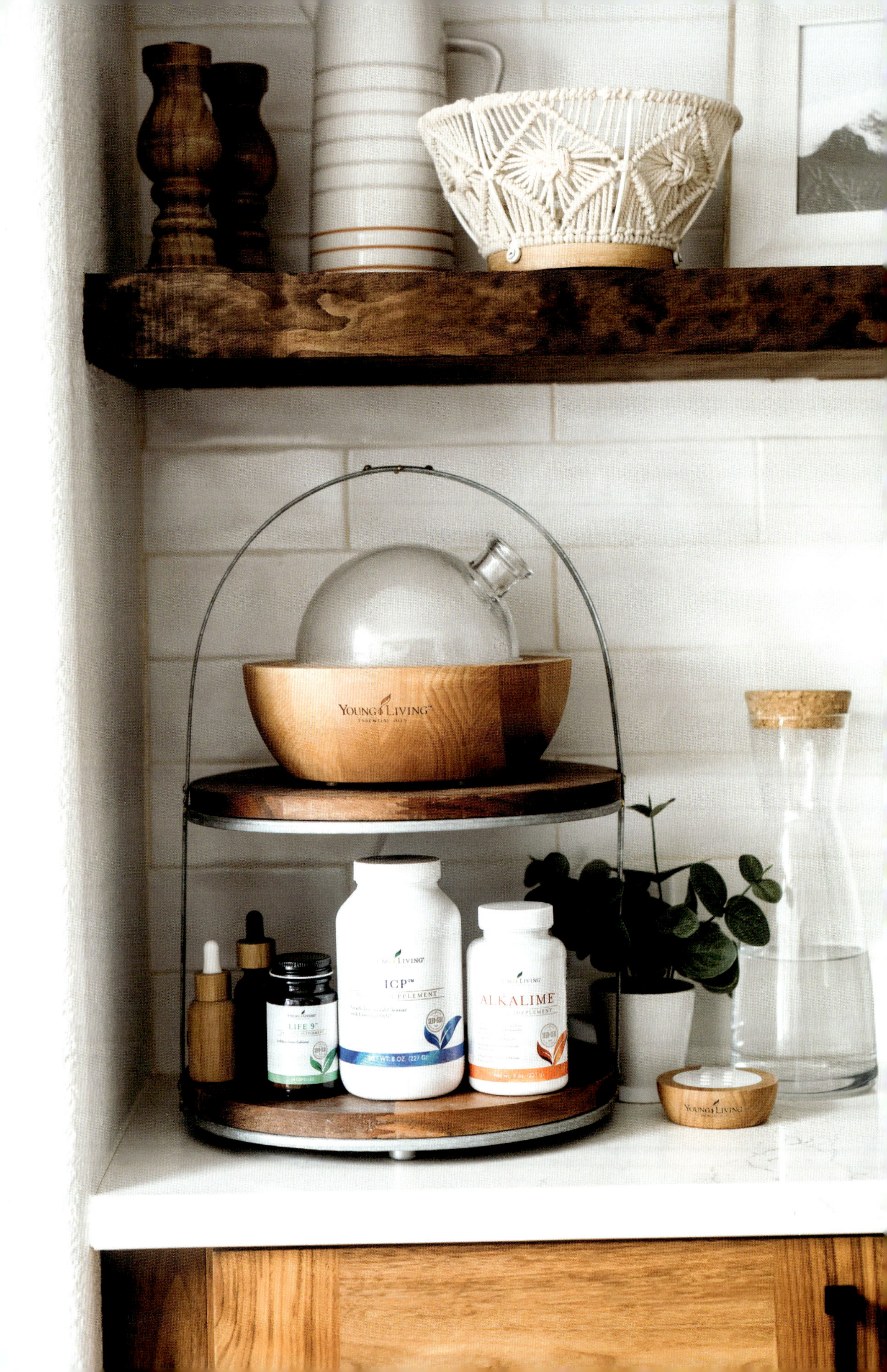
YOUNG LIVING
ICP™
ALKALIME
LIFE 9™

Part 3: DIGESTIVE SUPPLEMENTS

We've all heard how important digestive health is for overall wellness, and we are learning more about how digestion affects immunity, mood, mental clarity, and all body systems. Because it's so important, we want to support digestion well.

Did you know that over 75% of your immune system is in your gut? Or that almost 90% of all the serotonin in our bodies is produced by the gut? These are even more reasons why a healthy, happy belly is of utmost importance.

If you're thinking that you don't feel bad, don't have dietary sensitivities, and feel like your gut is just fine, you could still be experiencing symptoms of gut inflammation and imbalance (dysbiosis). Many things in our daily life can result in tiny holes in the gut lining, which creates a "leaky gut." This is a huge topic of medical study because a leaky gut can cause a whole host of symptoms. Some less straightforward symptoms include migraines, brain fog, joint pain, eczema, acne, and emotional instability.

DAILY HABITS FOR GUT HEALTH
- Eat whole, nutrient-dense foods
- Include fermented foods in your diet
- Move your body gently first thing in the morning (yoga, sun salutations, stretching)
- Avoid commercially processed seed oils (canola oil, soybean oil, etc.)
- If you eat wheat, choose Einkorn wheat and ideally consume in fermented states (sourdough)
- Take a high-quality probiotic, such as Life 9®
- Eat prebiotic foods, such as garlic, onions, and NingXia wolfberries
- Take ICP™ Daily
- Add enzymes, such as Essentialzymes-4™ or Allerzyme™, to your daily routine

THE GUT–BRAIN CONNECTION

Although it may seem strange to link gut health with emotions, there is a significant reason why these two things are connected.

We've all heard about serotonin—it is one of our "happy" hormones, along with dopamine. Serotonin is the control switch for the body and the brain's neurotransmitters. It helps us to regulate our emotions, from excited and energetic to calm and focused. When levels are too low, problems can arise.

Although lots of serotonin is produced in the brain (this is what we hear about a lot with mental health needs), a large amount is also produced in the digestive system, to the extent that our gut is called the "second brain." In fact, almost 90% of the serotonin in our bodies is produced by the peripheral nervous system in the gut.

Often, when we crave foods that are high in sugar or white flour, we are innately trying to regulate low serotonin levels. Although these foods may give us a quick energy burst, they also lead to a crash shortly after. Luckily, there are many ways that we can support the gut daily to maintain adequate serotonin (among other important things).

Many things in our daily life impact the gut's ability to produce and maintain adequate levels of serotonin, including food sensitivities and allergies, acute and chronic stress, gut flora imbalances, yeast overgrowth, acute and chronic illness, conventional medication, and antibiotic use. Some of these things are within our control to change, whereas with others, we have to simply support and rebuild the gut. Acute needs are going to require work, but the real ticket to health is in daily actions!

Bottom line? **Gut health is important for everyone, not just those with acute or chronic needs, and it impacts all areas of health.**

Supplements discussed:

ALKALIME®
COMFORTONE® CAPSULES
DIGEST & CLEANSE™
ENZYME SUPPLEMENTS:
  • ALLERZYME™
  • ESSENTIALZYME™
  • ESSENTIALZYMES-4™
ICP DAILY™
LIFE 9®

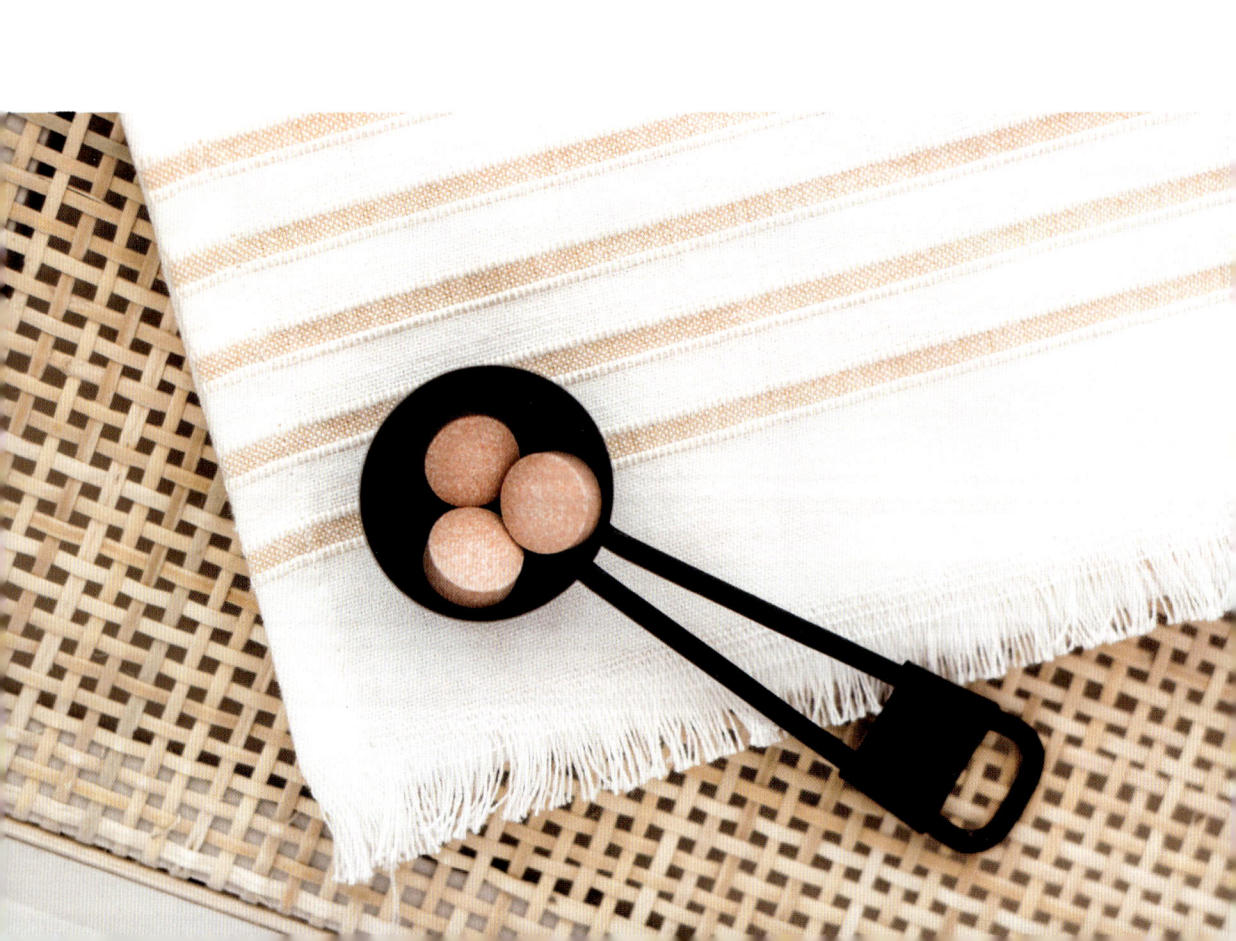

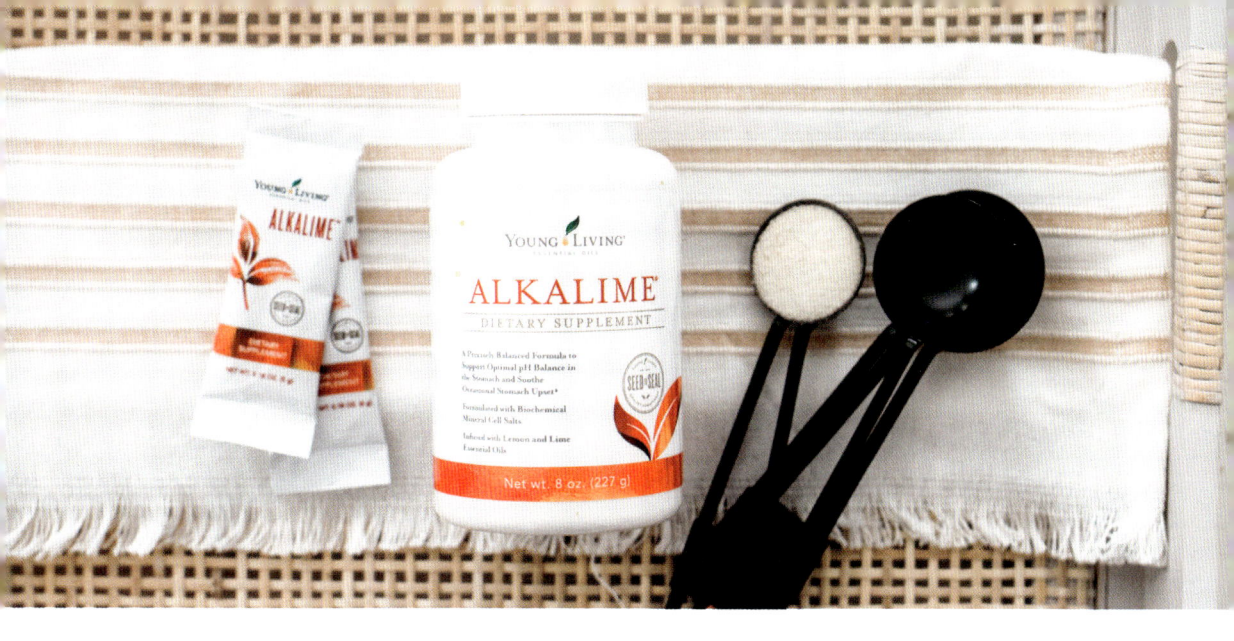

ALKALIME®

So many modern foods are loaded with (often hidden) sugars and stimulants, which impede the body's ability to foster a healthy pH balance. AlkaLime® works to combat this with its array of high-alkaline salts and other yeast-fighting elements, such as citric acid and lemon and lime essential oils. Young Living's AlkaLime® works as a natural alkalizing agent to maintain optimal pH in the stomach. This is a wonderful supplement for those who have dietary sensitivities. AlkaLime® helps the body decrease inflammation and restore balance when exposed to a food that is pro-inflammatory.

BENEFITS OF ALKALIME®
- Absorbed easily and quickly by the body
- Effervescent formula starts working right away to soothe stomach upset
- Gentle on the stomach
- Helps to maintain optimal pH in the stomach
- Free of artificial colors, flavors, or sweeteners
- Formulated with nine biochemical mineral cell salts
- Contains lemon and lime essential oils, which are high in limonene and support digestive health

By creating a more alkaline environment in the body (as opposed to an acidic environment), we can decrease the potential for yeast and fungus growth. An overgrowth of acid-based yeast and fungus can lead to many common issues, including fatigue, unexplained aches and weakness, intestinal upset, headaches, and mood swings. Creating an alkaline environment in the digestive system helps with the assimilation of nutrients and creates an environment where supplements and essential oils can work more effectively. It can also reduce the risk of bone loss[124] and soothe digestive discomfort for individuals with dietary sensitivities when they are exposed to a food that causes inflammation. AlkaLime® will work best in these situations when taken proactively, if possible.

AlkaLime® contains:
- **Biochemical mineral cell salts:** This is a mix of calcium, sodium, and potassium in various forms that balance the pH in the stomach.
- **Lime and lemon essential oils:** Lime and lemon are high in limonene, a constituent that strengthens the immune system, helps to decongest the lymphatic system, and improves nutrient absorption.

> **ALKALIME®**
>
> **To use:**
> - Add one level tsp. to 4-6 oz. of distilled water, mix thoroughly, and drink immediately.
> - Take one to three times daily, one hour before meals or retiring to bed as an aid in alkalizing.
> - Mix with water only.

Note: Keep out of reach of children. Not recommended for individuals on a sodium-restricted diet.

COMFORTONE®

ComforTone® is a gentle, effective way to promote healthy digestion through a mixture of herbs and essential oils. This supplement helps the body to eliminate waste in the colon, which enables it to function optimally and promotes consistent and easy bowel movements that can relieve hemorrhoids, bloating, and other symptoms of constipation.

BENEFITS OF COMFORTONE®
- Promotes normal digestion
- Cascara sagrada can aid in the body's natural cleansing system
- Psyllium seed provides natural fiber
- Ginger and tarragon essential oils support cleansing and digestive comfort
- Contains cleansing ingredients to remove toxins from the body
- Works well with ICP™ and Essentialzyme™, which break down residues in the colon, allowing ComforTone® to remove waste
- Usually used temporarily for gut and colon cleanses to promote normal digestion and may be stopped to allow the body to stimulate bowel movements without supplementation

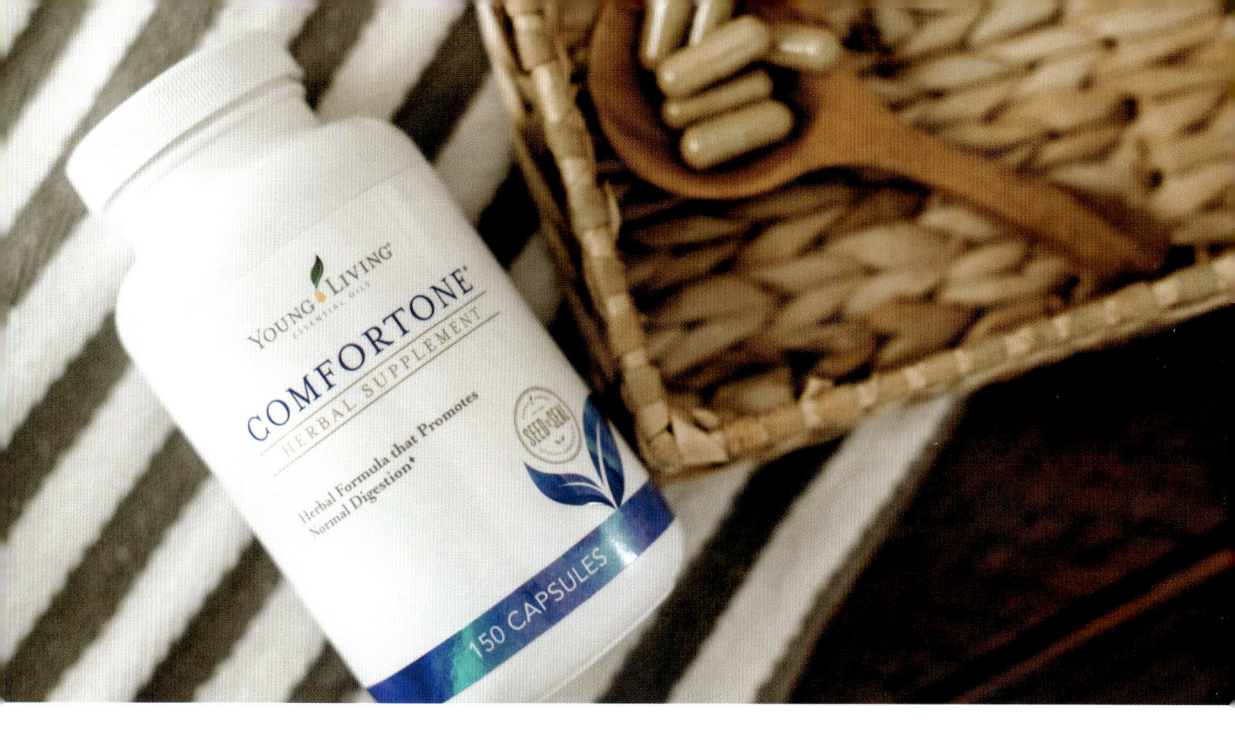

ComforTone® combines ingredients that have been shown to soothe the colon such as psyllium seed, bentonite clay, and diatomaceous earth, which bind toxins and remove them from the body. These are combined with ginger and tarragon essential oils to provide a natural solution to support the body's digestive process.

- **Cascara sagrada**: This herb cleanses the liver to move waste through the colon, supports the body's natural elimination process, and is an effective treatment for chronic constipation.
- **Psyllium seed**: This soft fiber absorbs toxins and helps to relieve digestive discomfort.
- **Fennel seed**: Fennel aids in digestion, regulates intestinal bloating, and helps to regulate intestinal flora.
- **Burdock root**: This herb helps to balance intestinal flora and absorbs toxins from the bowel.
- **Garlic**: Garlic is highly regarded for its health benefits. It aids in digestion and bolsters the immune system.
- **Barberry bark**: This herb supports healthy liver function and bile flow and strengthens the immune system.
- **Echinacea root**: Echinacea supports healthy bowel function, absorbs toxins in the colon, and stimulates the immune system.
- **Bentonite clay**: Bentonite clay is an intestinal cleansing agent that absorbs toxins and helps to transport them from the body.
- **Diatomaceous earth**: This is an intestinal cleansing agent that specifically helps to absorb mercury, pesticide residue, undigested proteins, and pathogens.
- **Ginger root**: Ginger is an anti-inflammatory herb that helps to cleanse the colon and supports healthy cholesterol levels.
- **German chamomile extract**: This herb is calming to the gut and gut lining.
- **Apple pectin**: Apple pectin supports enzyme production and proper digestive function.
- **Licorice root extract**: Licorice root supports the liver's cleansing and detoxification processes.

- **Cayenne pepper**: This herb stimulates circulation in the digestive tract.
- **Anise essential oil**: Anise supports overall digestion and circulation, may act as a diuretic, improves digestion, and has anti-inflammatory properties that help to ease intestinal cramping.
- **Ginger essential oil**: Ginger has analgesic, anti-inflammatory, antibacterial, and antioxidant properties. It soothes digestion[11], contains powerful antioxidants that can protect against oxidative stress, combats inflammation[12], and promotes liver health[13].
- **Tarragon essential oil**: Tarragon soothes and supports digestion, may support the immune system, and calms nausea.
- **Peppermint essential oil**: Peppermint supports healthy digestion, helps calm nausea, supports healthy respiratory function, and decreases inflammation through the actions of the constituents menthol and menthone.
- **Tangerine essential oil:** Tangerine supports overall cleansing, is high in limonene, which bolsters the immune system, provides antioxidant support to repair free radical damage, has anti-inflammatory effects, calms the central nervous system, and relaxes the muscles to support healthy sleep[11].
- **Rosemary essential oil**: Rosemary helps to balance the endocrine system, cleanses and purifies the liver and body overall, and provides immune support through direct bactericidal activity, even on certain drug-resistant bacteria and fungi[110].
- **Ocotea essential oil**: Ocotea contains high levels of alpha-humulene, a constituent that supports the body's response to inflammation and injury, promotes healthy blood sugar levels, and prevents the overgrowth of unhealthy intestinal flora.
- **German chamomile essential oil:** German chamomile supports the parasympathetic system and intestinal mucous levels, calming the muscles of the colon wall.

> **COMFORTONE®**
>
> **To use:**
> Take one capsule three times daily. Drink at least 64 oz. of distilled water throughout the day for best results.
>
> ComforTone® is also a key component of the Cleansing Trio™ (discussed on page 130).

DIGEST & CLEANSE™

Digest & Cleanse™ is a wonderful tool for digestive health! This essential oil based supplement calms gastrointestinal upset caused by stress, overeating, and toxins. It helps soothe the bowel, prevent gas, and stimulate stomach secretions, aiding overall digestion and nutrient absorption.

BENEFITS OF DIGEST & CLEANSE™
- Helps prevent gas and upset stomach
- Includes peppermint and caraway essential oils, which have been used for centuries to ease occasional digestive discomfort
- Formulated with lemon essential oil, which has been used as a traditional method to stimulate digestion
- Supports overall digestive health with daily use
- Helps cleanse and support the body's natural digestive processes
- A key component of the popular 5 Day Nutritive Cleanse.

Each gel capsule contains fennel, anise, and ginger essential oils to support digestion; peppermint and caraway essential oils, which help ease digestive discomfort; and lemon essential oil, which helps to stimulate digestion. These ingredients work together to support your overall digestive health, soothe inflammation and upset in the digestive tract, and improve absorption of nutrients.

- **Peppermint essential oil:** Peppermint supports healthy digestion and respiratory function, calms nausea, and decreases inflammation through the action of the constituents menthol and menthone.
- **Caraway essential oil:** Caraway is a wonderful digestive oil as it helps improve digestion, combat indigestion, relieve gas pain and pressure, and helps remove excess water from the body.
- **Lemon essential oil:** Lemon is high in limonene, a constituent that is known to strengthen the immune system and help decongest the lymphatic system. D-limonene also alters the signaling pathways within cancer cells in a way that stops cancer cells from multiplying and causes their death[22]
- **Ginger essential oil:** Ginger has analgesic, anti-inflammatory, antibacterial, and antioxidant properties, is great for soothing digestion[11], contains powerful antioxidants that can protect against oxidative stress, combats inflammation[12], and promotes liver health[13].
- **Fennel essential oil:** Fennel supports digestion, eases intestinal discomfort, supports the pancreas and liver, provides immune support, and promotes the excretion of toxins.
- **Anise essential oil:** Anise supports overall digestion and circulation, may act as a diuretic, improves digestion, and has anti-inflammatory properties that help to ease intestinal cramping.

FIVE DAY NUTRITIVE CLEANSE
When we open up our cleansing pathways (the colon, the kidneys, the lungs, and the skin via sweating), we allow the body to release toxins and chemicals that have been stored. This allows our bodies to heal as they are no longer holding onto things that are causing harm. One way to do this is with the Young Living 5 Day Nutritive Cleanse.

This cleanse combines three incredible supplements for a gentle, but effective cleanse that is great for beginners. This trio of products facilitates gentle and effective cleansing to improve overall health and will help balance the extremes of the modern diet.

- **NingXia Red®:** an energizing, replenishing, whole-wolfberry nutrient supplement drink that is full of antioxidants, vitamins and minerals.
- **Balance Complete™:** a superfood-based daily energizer and nutritive cleanser that can be used as a meal replacement shake or mixed into a smoothie.
- **Digest & Cleanse™:** an essential oil-infused supplement that soothes gastrointestinal discomfort and supports healthy digestion.

DIGEST & CLEANSE™

To use: Take 1 softgel 1-3 times daily with water 30-60 minutes prior to meals.

Note: Contains coconut products.

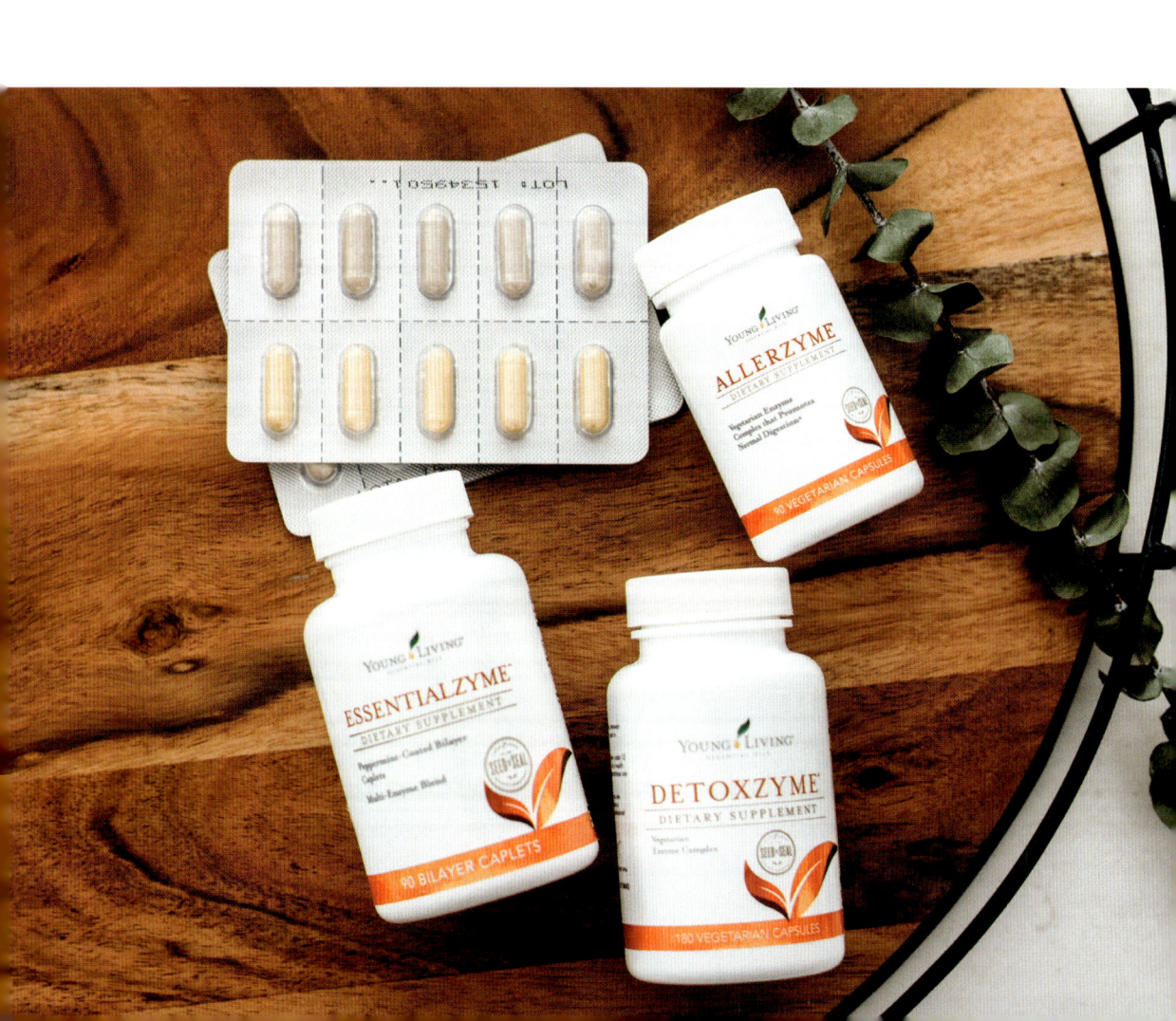

ENZYME Supplements

One way to improve digestion daily is with enzyme supplements. Enzymes work on every system in the body, and when taken with or between meals, they can help the body to break down and absorb the nutrients in foods. In addition, enzymes can help to mitigate symptoms of digestive upset, such as bloating, fullness, gas, and discomfort after eating.

There are so many areas of health that enzymes can support:
- Gut health and digestion
- Focus and attention
- Mood and disposition
- Nutrient absorption
- Energy levels

Enzymes are protein molecules that are manufactured by all plant and animal cells and are critical for those cells to perform their everyday tasks. Enzymes are essential for our bodies to function. They allow the cells to communicate with each other, assist in cell turnover (cell life, growth, and death—an essential natural process), and are responsible for every chemical reaction in our bodies. Enzymes are utilized in and support all systems in the body:
- **Digestion:** Enzymes break down the food that we eat to allow it to be absorbed.
- **Nutrient absorption:** Enzymes assist in assimilating nutrients from food into the bloodstream and transporting them to where they are needed.
- **Neurotransmitter and hormone production:** Enzymes are essential to produce all the chemical messengers within the body—thyroid hormone, estrogen, progesterone, testosterone, serotonin, dopamine, and many more.
- **Cell repair, division, and natural cell death:** Enzymes are needed to repair cells, keep cells dividing at a normal, healthy rate, and allow necessary cells to die off when appropriate.
- **Reproduction:** Enzymes are required for hormone production and cell division.
- **Respiration:** Enzymes are needed to transport oxygen between the heart and lungs and deliver oxygen to the muscles.
- **Muscle and joint health:** Enzymes help to maintain joint fluid and aid in muscle contractions.
- **Detoxification:** Enzymes in the liver process toxins and prevent waste buildup in the body.

Young Living has four different enzyme supplements available: Allerzyme™, Essentialzyme™, Essentialzymes-4™, and MightyZyme™. (MightyZyme™ is discussed in the section on children's supplements.)

ALLERZYME™

Allerzyme™ is a vegetarian enzyme complex that works with your body's natural systems to promote normal digestive function. Allerzyme™ is specifically formulated for individuals with dietary and environmental sensitivities and helps to provide relief from symptoms such as fullness, pressure, bloating, gas, pain, and/or minor cramping, which may occur after eating.

BENEFITS OF ALLERZYME™
- Vegetarian enzyme complex that promotes normal digestion
- Works with your body's natural system
- Provides relief from occasional symptoms, such as fullness, pressure, bloating, gas, pain, and/or minor cramping, that may occur after eating
- Contains plantain leaf, which is known to calm digestive inflammation
- Infused with tarragon and ginger essential oils

Each ingredient in Allerzyme™ is gentle on the system while also playing a specific support role for nutrient absorption and digestive health.
- **Amylase**: Amylase is a powerful starch-digesting enzyme that prevents the fermentation of starches in the digestive system.
- **Bromelain**: Bromelain is a proteolytic enzyme that is found in pineapples and supports carbohydrate digestion.
- **Peptidase**: Peptidase supports the formation and absorption of amino acids.
- **Protease**: Protease are protein-digesting enzymes that are stable in the varying pH conditions of the digestive tract. Additionally, they fight off bacteria, yeast, and parasites in the intestines.
- **Phytase**: This enzyme is necessary to break down minerals, such as zinc, magnesium, and potassium, that are found in grains, nuts, seeds, and other foods.
- **Lipase**: This is a fat-dissolving enzyme that is vital for the absorption of vitamins A, D, and E.
- **Lactase**: Lactase breaks down lactose into glucose, which enables it to be used for energy within the body.
- **Cellulase** Cellulase breaks down cellulose into simpler sugars for digestion.
- **Alpha-galactosidase**: This enzyme assists in the breakdown of complex carbohydrates that could otherwise cause gas, bloating, and general discomfort.
- **Malt diastase**: This helps to digest carbohydrate-rich foods.
- **Plantain leaf:** Plantain leaf is a natural diuretic that cleanses the liver and calms inflammation in the digestive tract.
- **Barley grass**: Barley is a powerful antioxidant that cleanses the digestive tract and is rich in vitamins and minerals.
- **Anise essential oil**: Anise supports overall digestion and circulation, may act as a diuretic, improves digestion, and has anti-inflammatory properties that help to ease intestinal cramping.

- **Ginger essential oil**: Ginger has analgesic, anti-inflammatory, antibacterial, and antioxidant properties, is great for soothing digestion[11], contains powerful antioxidants that can protect against oxidative stress, combats inflammation[12], and promotes liver health[13].
- **Tarragon essential oil**: Tarragon soothes and supports digestion, calms nausea, and supports the immune system.
- **Peppermint essential oil**: Peppermint supports healthy digestion, calms nausea, and decreases inflammation through the actions of the constituents menthol and menthone.
- **Juniper essential oil**: Juniper purifies and helps to detoxify the digestive system and promotes the excretion of toxins from the body.
- **Lemongrass essential oil**: Lemongrass is a cleansing oil that helps the body's clear bladder infections and calms the digestive system.
- **Patchouli essential oil**: Patchouli can combat nausea, helps to digest and expel toxins, and supports the immune system and the body's response to inflammation.
- **Fennel essential oil**: Fennel supports digestion, eases intestinal discomfort, supports the pancreas and liver, provides immune support, and promotes the excretion of toxins.

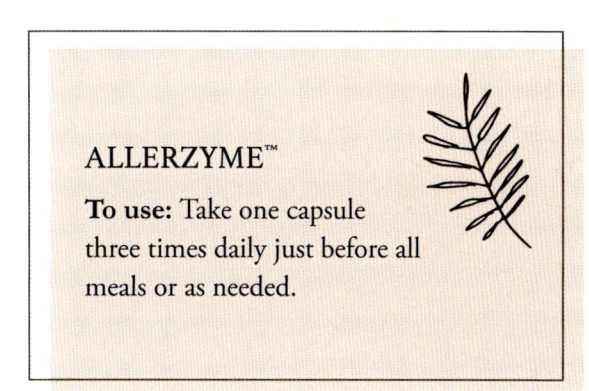

ALLERZYME™

To use: Take one capsule three times daily just before all meals or as needed.

ESSENTIALZYME™

Essentialzyme™ is another of Young Living's enzyme supplements. Essentialzyme™ is a multienzyme complex that has been formulated to support and balance digestive health and stimulate overall enzyme activity. It is best taken an hour before a meal. Essentialzyme™ contains tarragon, peppermint, anise, fennel, and clove essential oils that improve enzyme activity and support healthy pancreatic function.

BENEFITS OF ESSENTIALZYME™
- Stimulates overall enzyme activity
- Supports and balances digestive health
- Supports healthy pancreatic function
- Assists the body in breaking down and digesting food
- Infused with gut- and pancreas-supporting essential oils

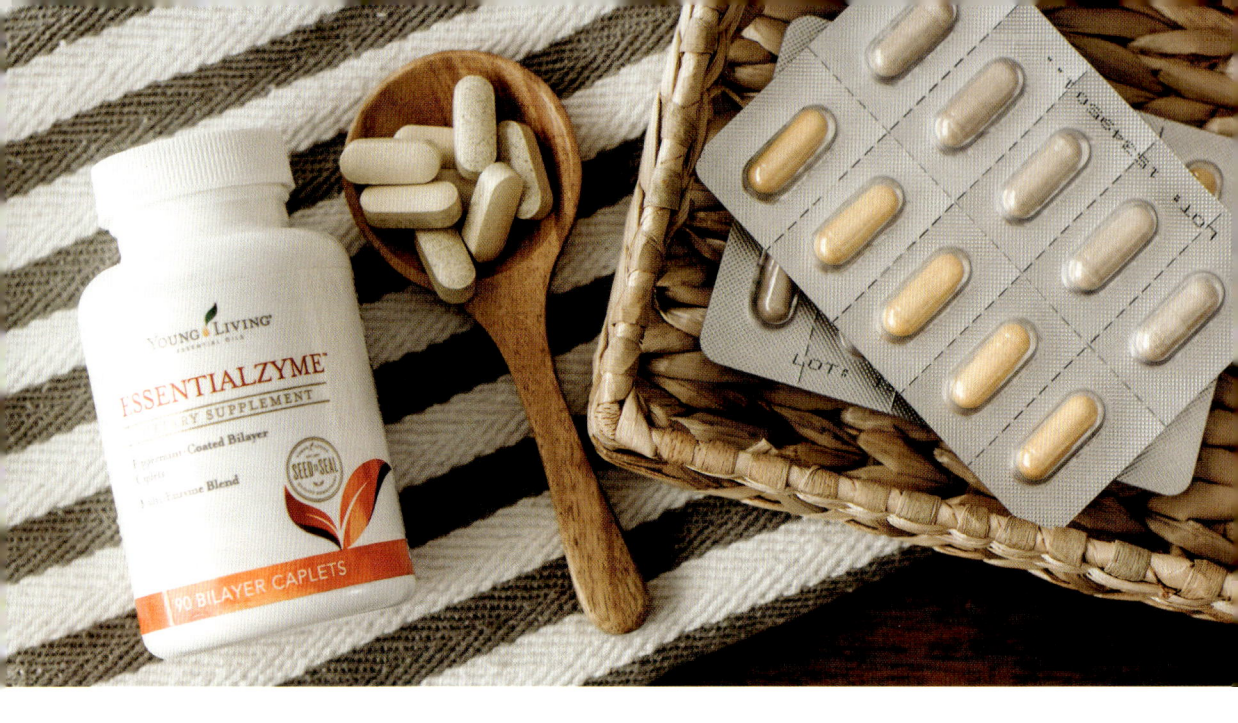

Essentialzyme™ contains a unique blend of enzymes, including pancrelipase and pancreatin, that assist the body in breaking down and digesting food, as well as essential oils that improve overall enzyme activity and support healthy pancreatic function.

- **Pancrelipase**: This is a potent pancreatic enzyme mix of amylase (breaks down starches and prevents their fermentation), lipase (breaks down dietary fats), and protease (breaks down proteins).
- **Pancreatin**: This is a less potent mix of the pancreatic enzymes amylase, lipase, and protease that works with pancrelipase to break down foods.
- **Trypsin**: Trypsin is a pancreatic enzyme that breaks down proteins into peptides and amino acids, which are then utilized by the body.
- **Betaine HCI:** Betaine is a derivative of the nutrient choline. It aids in liver function, detoxification, and cellular functioning within the body.
- **Bromelain**: Bromelain is a proteolytic enzyme found in pineapples that supports carbohydrate digestion.
- **Alfalfa:** Alfalfa is high in chlorophyll, calcium, iron, potassium, phosphorus, and vitamins C and K. It has a positive effect on blood sugar, cholesterol, and blood pressure levels[51] and is beneficial in treating arthritis, urinary tract infections, menstrual problems, and an array of other disorders[52].
- **Papain**: Papain is a vegetable enzyme that is derived from papaya that supports carbohydrate digestion.
- **Anise essential oil**: Anise supports overall digestion and circulation, may act as a diuretic, improves digestion, and has anti-inflammatory properties that help to ease intestinal cramping.
- **Fennel essential oil**: Fennel supports digestion, eases intestinal discomfort, supports the pancreas and liver, provides immune support, and promotes the excretion of toxins.
- **Tarragon essential oil**: Tarragon soothes and supports digestion, may support the immune system, and calms nausea.

- **Peppermint essential oil**: Peppermint supports healthy digestion and respiratory function, calms nausea, and decreases inflammation through the action of the constituents menthol and menthone.
- **Clove essential oil:** Clove has profound immune support and is a powerful antioxidant (ORAC value of over 290,000[19]). It cleanses the gut and can stop the growth of some bacteria and fungi[20], including *Candida*[21], at higher doses.

> **ESSENTIALZYME™**
>
> **To use:** Take one dual time release caplet one hour before your largest meal of the day for best results.

ESSENTIALZYMES-4™

Essentialzymes-4™ is a multienzyme complex with a dual capsule system that aids digestion and is formulated to take with meals. Each capsule is infused with ginger, fennel, tarragon, and anise essential oils and includes a diverse combination of enzymes to improve digestion and the assimilation of nutrients.

BENEFITS OF ESSENTIALZYMES-4™
- Aids in the digestion of dietary fats, proteins, fiber, and carbohydrates
- Releases the animal- and plant-based enzymes at separate times within the digestive tract for optimal nutrient absorption
- Formulated with a unique blend of herbal ingredients to improve digestion
- Infused with ginger, fennel, tarragon, and anise essential oils

Essentialzymes-4™ has a plant-based and an animal-based enzyme system. The plant-based enzymes are designed to release immediately upon entering the stomach, where the environment is conducive to the digestion of plant material. The animal-based enzymes are designed to target release in the lower intestine, where the environment is better suited for the digestion of animal fats and proteins.

The plant-based enzyme capsule's key ingredients are:
- **Amylase**: This is a powerful starch-digesting enzyme that prevents the fermentation of starches in the digestive tract.
- **Cellulase**: Cellulase breaks down cellulose into simpler sugars for digestion.
- **Protease**: This is a protein-digesting enzyme that is stable in the varying pH conditions of the digestive tract.

- **Lipase**: Lipase is a fat-dissolving enzyme that is vital for the absorption of vitamins A, D, and E.
- **Phytase**: This enzyme is necessary to break down minerals such as zinc, magnesium, and potassium found in grains, nuts, seeds, and other foods.
- **Bromelain**: Bromelain is a proteolytic enzyme found in pineapples that supports carbohydrate digestion.
- **Papain**: This vegetable enzyme is derived from papaya and supports carbohydrate digestion.
- **Peptidase**: This enzyme supports the formation and absorption of amino acids.
- **Vitamin B2 (Riboflavin)**: B2 is vital for metabolic processes within the cells, energy production, and cell growth.
- **Ginger essential oil:** Ginger has analgesic, anti-inflammatory, antibacterial, and antioxidant properties. It is great for soothing digestion[11], contains powerful antioxidants that can protect against oxidative stress, combats inflammation[12], and promotes liver health[13].
- **Rosemary essential oil:** Rosemary helps to balance the endocrine system, cleanses and purifies the liver, and provides immune support through direct bactericidal activity, even on certain drug-resistant bacteria and fungi[110].
- **Anise essential oil:** Anise supports overall digestion and circulation, may act as a diuretic, improves digestion, and has anti-inflammatory properties that help to ease intestinal cramping.
- **Fennel essential oil**: Fennel supports digestion, eases intestinal discomfort, supports the pancreas and liver, provides immune support, and promotes the excretion of toxins.
- **Tarragon essential oil**: Tarragon soothes and supports digestion, supports the immune system, and calms nausea

The animal-based enzyme capsule's key ingredients are:
- **Pancreatin**: This natural protein-digesting enzyme complex contains proteases, amylases, and lipases.
- **Bee pollen powder:** Bee pollen is high in protein and contains many minerals and vitamins, such as potassium, magnesium, zinc, manganese, and B vitamins.
- **Lipase**: Lipase is a fat-dissolving enzyme that is vital for the absorption of vitamins A, D, and E.
- **Rice flour** (non-GMO): Rice flour is required for capsule dilution, and it is easier to digest than other diluents such as conventional flour or starch.
- **Ginger essential oil:** Ginger has analgesic, anti-inflammatory, antibacterial, and antioxidant properties, is great for soothing digestion[11], contains powerful antioxidants that can protect against oxidative stress, combats inflammation[12], and promotes liver health[13].
- **Anise essential oil:** Anise supports overall digestion and circulation, acts as a diuretic, improves digestion, and has anti-inflammatory properties that help to ease intestinal cramping.

- **Fennel essential oil**: Fennel supports digestion, eases intestinal discomfort, supports the pancreas and liver, provides immune support, and promotes the excretion of toxins.
- **Tarragon essential oil**: Tarragon soothes and supports digestion, may support the immune system, and calms nausea.
- **Lemongrass essential oil**: Lemongrass is a cleansing oil that helps the body to clear bladder infections, calms the digestive system, and has antibacterial activity, even against drug-resistant strains of *Candida*[110].

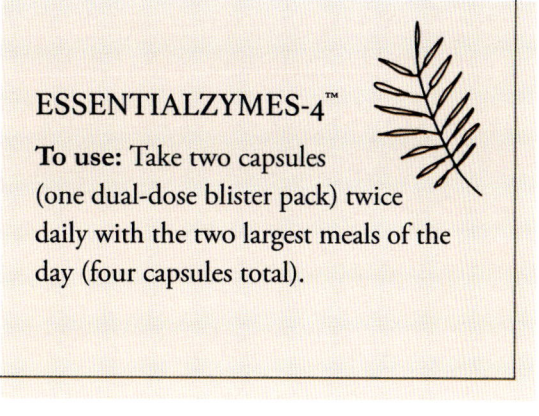

> ESSENTIALZYMES-4™
>
> **To use:** Take two capsules (one dual-dose blister pack) twice daily with the two largest meals of the day (four capsules total).

WHAT'S THE DIFFERENCE BETWEEN ALLERZYME™, ESSENTIALZYME™, AND ESSENTIALZYMES-4™?

- Allerzyme™ is specifically formulated for individuals who have known dietary sensitivities and is a good option for those wanting a vegetarian-friendly formula.
- Essentialzyme™ contains a unique blend of enzymes, such as pancrelipase and pancreatin, that assist the body in breaking down and digesting food and specifically support the pancreas. These enzymes should be taken once a day before your largest meal and are a good option for those needing more targeted pancreas support.
- Essentialzymes-4™ is a set of two dual-enzyme capsules. The plant-based enzymes are designed to release immediately upon entering the stomach, where the environment is conducive to the digestion of plant material. The animal-based enzymes are designed to target release in the lower intestine, where the environment is better suited for the digestion of animal fats and proteins. When combined, these two capsules aid in the digestion of dietary fats, proteins, fiber, and carbohydrates for optimal nutrient absorption. These enzymes should be taken with your two largest meals of the day.
- The differences between the formulations are slight, and one could be used to replace the other if needed due to stock issues. However, note that there *are* differences in both the enzyme composition and the timing of supplementation.

COMPARISON OF ALLERZYME™, ESSENTIALZYME™, AND ESSENTIALZYMES-4™

	VEGETARIAN FORMULA?	CONTAINS PANCREATIC ENZYMES?	DOSING	NOTES
ALLERZYME™	Yes	No	Three times daily, just before meals	Specifically formulated for those with dietary or environmental allergies
ESSENTIALZYME™	No	Yes	Once daily, one hour before the largest meal of the day	
ESSENTIALZYMES-4™	No	No	Twice daily with the largest meals of the day	2 capsules per dose

ICP DAILY™

Taking daily steps to build, support, detoxify, and balance gut bacteria and bolster the intestinal lining is crucial to overall health, and one simple way to do this is with ICP Daily™. ICP Daily™ is a daily prebiotic and fiber drink that is both delicious and easy on the stomach. It is a great choice for maintaining a healthy gut microbiome, as it aids the body's natural detoxification process, promotes healthy postbiotics in the gut, and helps you to feel full longer.

BENEFITS OF ICP DAILY™
- Contains 6 grams of plant-based prebiotics and 5 grams of soluble fiber
- Aids in the body's natural detoxification process
- Helps to maintain a healthy gut microbiome
- Easy on the stomach and well tolerated by those with digestive sensitivities
- Promotes healthy postbiotics in the gut
- Contains fennel, anise, tarragon, ginger, lemongrass, and rosemary essential oils
- Helps you to feel full longer
- Supports cardiovascular health and the immune system

This gentle daily formula contains 6g of plant-based prebiotics, 5g of soluble fiber, and a belly-supporting blend of essential oils, including fennel, anise, tarragon, ginger, lemongrass, and rosemary. Prebiotics and fiber are crucial for overall gut health, digestive mobility (they make it easier for things to move through, which is definitely what we want!), and cardiovascular and immune system health.

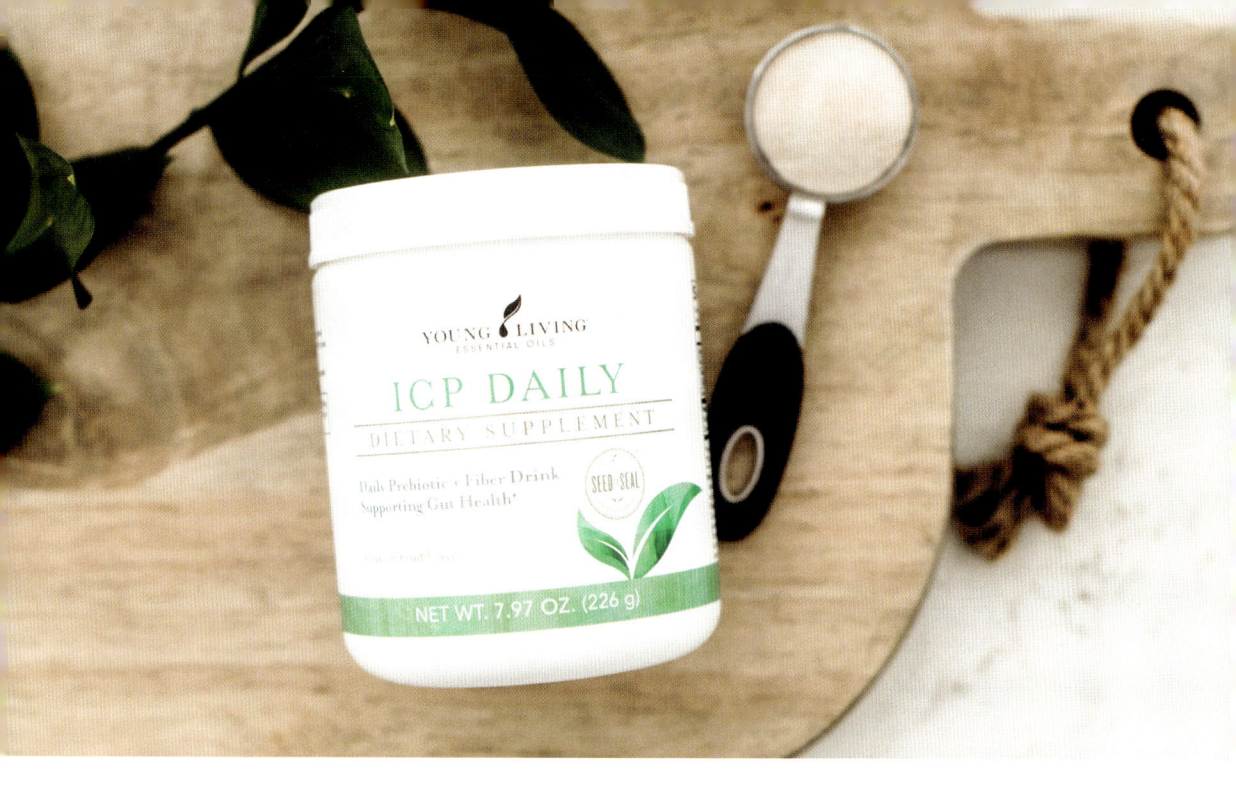

ICP Daily™ contains powerful ingredients, such as agave inulin, guar gum, and prickly pear cactus extract, that work synergistically (1+1=3) with the essential oils to detoxify the gut and promote a healthy environment for bacterial balance.
- **Agave inulin:** This is a source of fiber that is selectively metabolized in the lower gut, which enables better nutrient absorption and a gut flora balance.
- **Guar gum:** Guar gum cleanses the colon and promotes normal, easy bowel movements and an overall healthy colon function.
- **Prickly pear cactus extract:** This is a good source of fiber and vitamin C that helps to gently cleanse the system and supports healthy blood sugar levels.
- **Anise essential oil**: Anise supports overall digestion and circulation, may act as a diuretic, improves digestion, and has anti-inflammatory properties that help to ease intestinal cramping.
- **Ginger essential oil**: Ginger has analgesic, anti-inflammatory, antibacterial, and antioxidant properties, is great for soothing digestion[11], contains powerful antioxidants that can protect against oxidative stress, combats inflammation[12], and promotes liver health[13].
- **Tarragon essential oil**: Tarragon soothes and supports digestion, may support the immune system, and calms nausea.
- **Lemongrass essential oil**: Lemongrass is a cleansing oil that helps the body's cleanse bladder infections, calms the digestive system, and shows antibacterial activity, even against drug-resistant strains of *Candida*[110].

- **Fennel essential oil:** Fennel supports digestion, eases intestinal discomfort, supports the pancreas and liver, provides immune support, and promotes the excretion of toxins.
- **Rosemary essential oil:** Rosemary helps to balance the endocrine system, supports heart health, cleanses and purifies the liver, and provides immune support through direct bactericidal activity, even on certain drug-resistant bacteria and fungi[110].

Safety notes: If you are pregnant, nursing, taking medication, or have a medical condition, consult a healthcare professional before use.

ICP DAILY™

To use:
- Mix one scoop in 8 oz. of water, NingXia Red®, or juice once daily.
- Take in the morning (30 minutes before meals) on an empty stomach.
- Pairing ICP Daily™ with Life 9® is ideal, as ICP Daily™ creates a clean, happy home for the diverse bacteria of the Life 9® probiotic.

LIFE 9®

For more information on Life 9®, see the "Foundational Supplements" section on page 25

Life 9® is Young Living's high-potency probiotic and is one of Young Living's most popular supplements. Many health experts (myself included!) consider a high-quality, diverse probiotic to be a cornerstone of overall health. Research shows that a healthy gut is key to brain, immune, and skin health and emotional regulation.

Many components of our modern lifestyle, such as medications, chlorinated water, contaminated water supplies, sugar consumption, a lack of dietary fiber, and mental and emotional stress, increase our need to supplement with healthy bacteria. Although much of this is within our control, even with the best habits, we still need extra support.

Your body contains approximately 100 trillion bacteria, which is more than ten times the number of cells you have in your entire body. Research has shown that the type and quantity of the microorganisms in your gut interact with your body in ways that can either prevent or encourage the development of many diseases. This means that maintaining an ideal bacterial balance is key. The ideal ratio between the bacteria in your gut is 85% "good" and 15% "bad," and it is attainable through simple, daily habits.

Life 9® includes nine probiotic strains for full-spectrum gut support throughout the entire digestive tract.

There are Bifidobacterium that populate the entire gut, lactobacillus that populate the small intestine, and Streptococcus thermophilus that populate the intestines.

BENEFITS OF LIFE 9®
- Daily use supports overall health and wellness and a healthy, diverse gut microbiome
- Contains a diverse set of bacteria that work synergistically towards gut health
- Aids in healthy digestion and assists in digestive distress
- Helps to maintain immune health
- Helps with emotional health

A high-quality probiotic is always a cornerstone of health, but it is especially important to repopulate the gut with diverse, supportive bacteria after using antibiotics. I recommend taking Life 9® while on an antibiotic regimen (herbal, oil-based, or conventional) or you can start Life 9® after completing the regimen. If you choose to use Life 9® during the course of an antibiotic, separate the two by at least four hours.

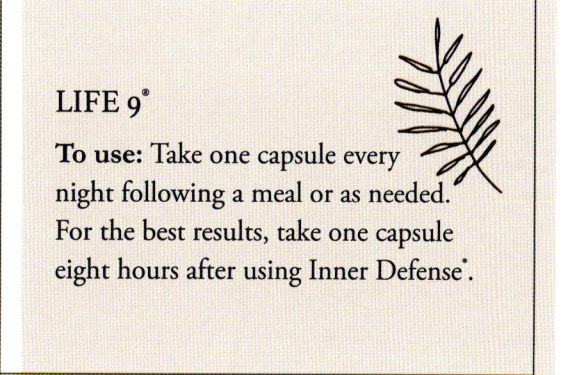

> **LIFE 9®**
>
> **To use:** Take one capsule every night following a meal or as needed. For the best results, take one capsule eight hours after using Inner Defense®.

Safety notes: If you are pregnant, nursing, taking medication, or have a medical condition, consult a health professional before use.

Protocols For Digestive Health

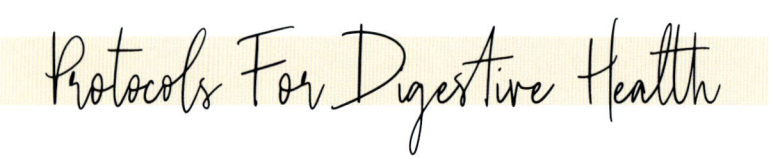

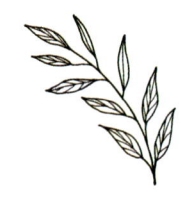

Digestive health is a multifactorial support area and one that is unique to each person. Therefore, keeping track of symptoms, emotions, diet, supplement, etc. is going to be very helpful when dealing with digestive issues. Here are a few starting points for overall digestive health and acute needs.

OVERALL DIGESTIVE HEALTH (FOR MOST ADULTS)
- Digest & Cleanse™
- Essentialzymes-4™ (or Essentialzyme™)
- ICP Daily™
- Life 9®
- Mineral Essence™
- NingXia Red®
- Other options for more support: DiGize™ Vitality™ Essential Oil Blend, Ocotea Vitality™ Essential Oil (great for battling *Candida*)

TARGETED DIGESTIVE HEALTH
- AlkaLime® (especially helpful for those with dietary sensitivities)
- Allerzyme™ (especially helpful for those with dietary or environmental sensitivities)
- ComforTone®
- Digest & Cleanse™
- Essentialzymes-4™ (or Essentialzyme™)
- ICP Daily™
- Life 9®
- Mineral Essence™
- NingXia Red®
- Other options for more support: DiGize™ Vitality™ Essential Oil Blend, Ocotea Vitality™ Essential Oil (great for battling *Candida*)

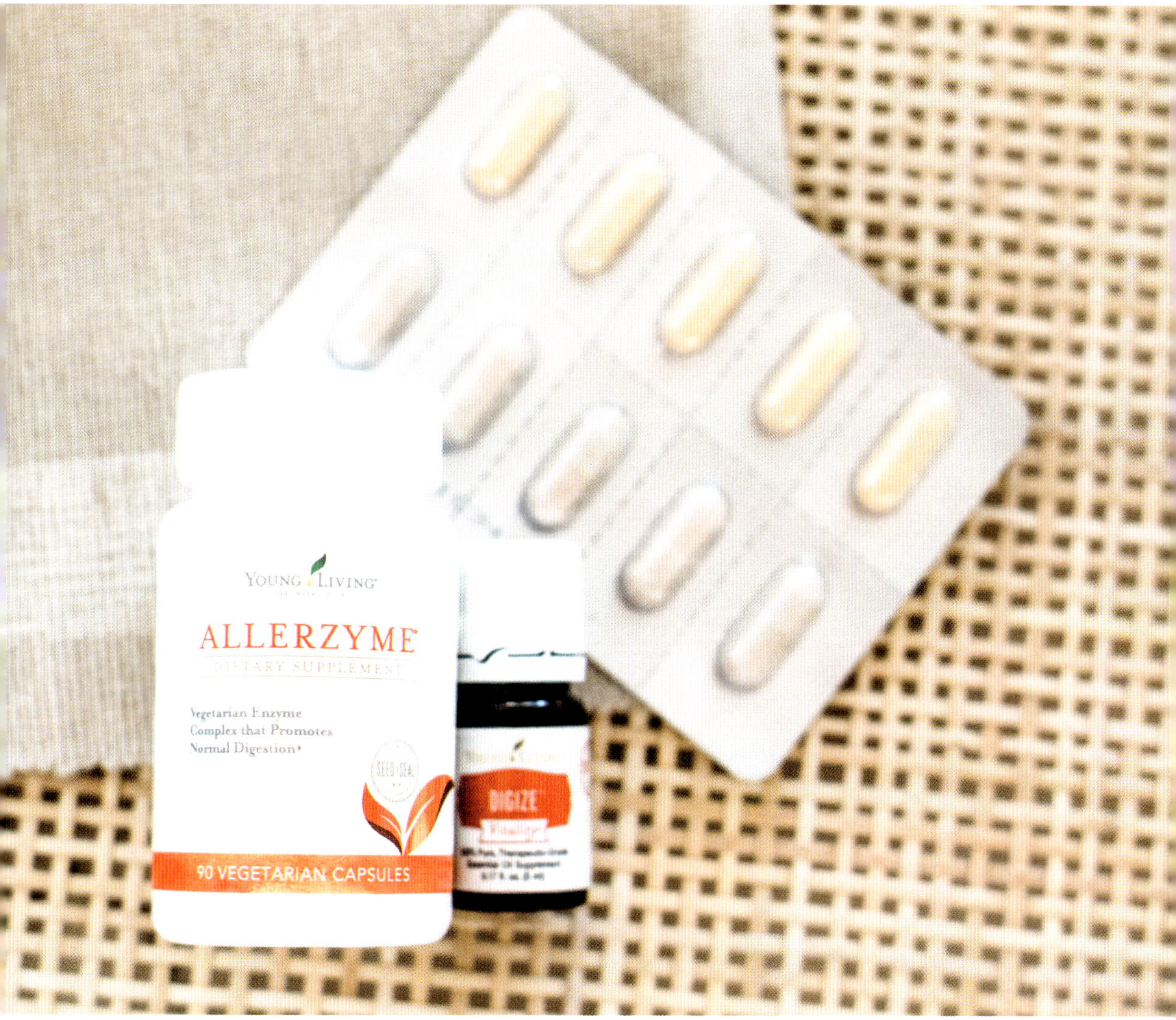
YOUNG LIVING
ALLERZYME
DIETARY SUPPLEMENT
Vegetarian Enzyme
Complex that Promotes
Normal Digestion
90 VEGETARIAN CAPSULES
DIGIZE

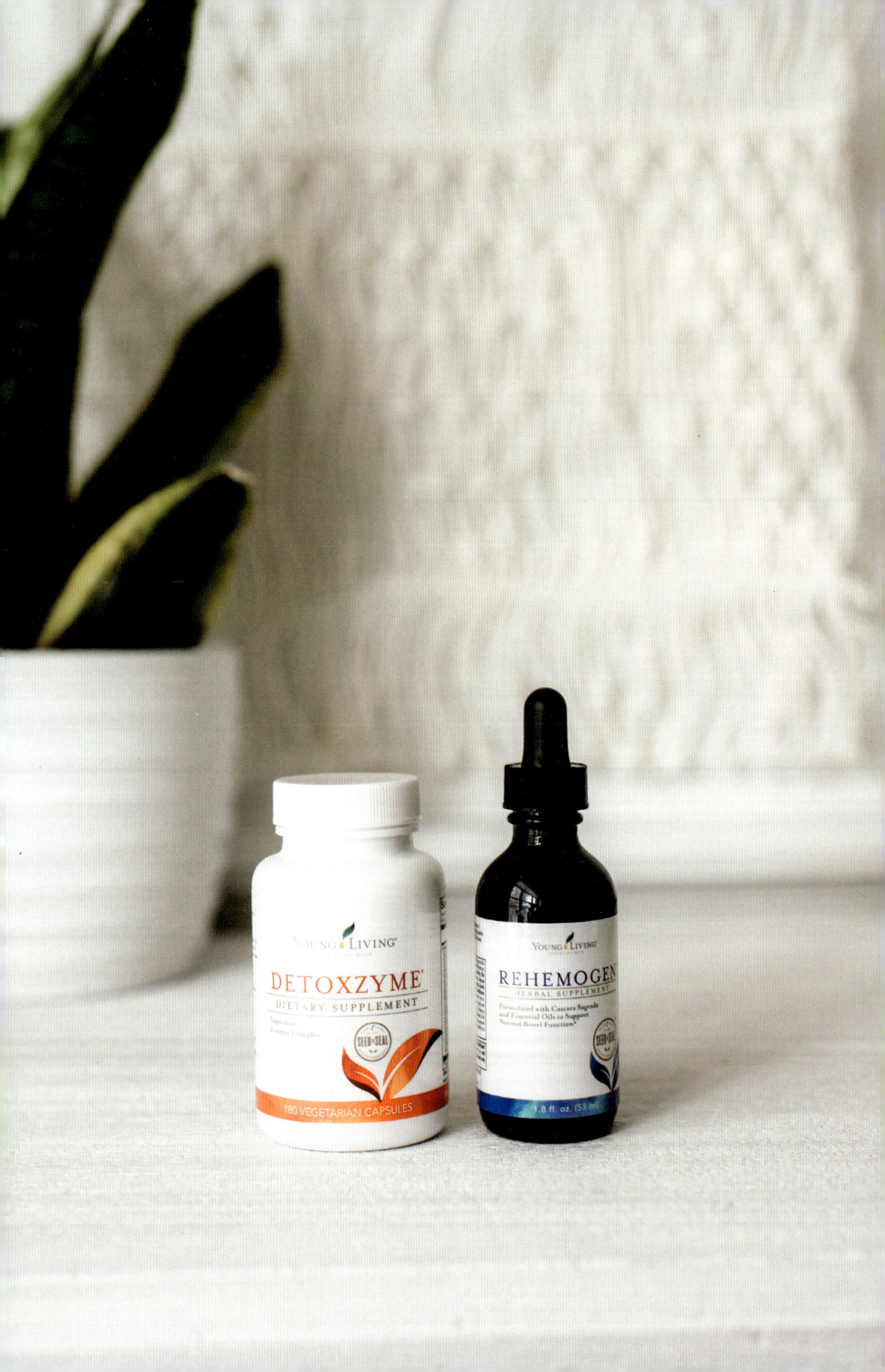
YOUNG LIVING
DETOXZYME
DIETARY SUPPLEMENT
180 VEGETARIAN CAPSULES
YOUNG LIVING
REHEMOGEN
HERBAL SUPPLEMENT
Formulated with Cascara Sagrada
and Essential Oils to Support
Normal Bowel Function*
1.8 fl. oz. (53 ml)

Part 4: CLEANSING & LIVER SUPPORT SUPPLEMENTS

We are all exposed to a myriad of toxins in our day-to-day life—heavy metals, chemicals, and pollutants are in everything from the air that we breathe to the food on our plates. Even with the most pure, low-tox lifestyle, it's impossible to prevent all the buildup from occurring. Lifestyle factors, such as chronic stress, lack of sleep, and physical inactivity, can stress our liver and digestive system, which makes it harder for our bodies to remove toxins from our system.

The body is naturally equipped with a detoxification system to remove the unwanted compounds, which is why daily support is key (I'm looking at you Longevity™, NingXia Red®, JuvaPower®...). Diet, lifestyle, and good supplements go a long way toward supporting our natural detox pathways. However, another great way to give your body a reset and flush out all the buildup is through cleansing.

A body cleanse or detox plan that involves cutting out junk foods and increasing your intake of nutritious whole foods, along with a few good supplements, can be an easy way to help your body to remove the buildup and hit the reset button. Young Living's Cleansing Trio™ would be a great option for this.

CLEANSING AND EMOTIONAL HEALTH

When our bodies are overloaded with toxins or weighed down from constantly filtering everything that we throw at it, things become sluggish. This not only affects our physical health; it also takes a toll on us emotionally. This often manifests as feeling lethargic, sluggish, unmotivated, not enjoying the things that we normally would, or simply feeling down. Cleansing and detoxing our systems can have profound effects on our emotional health.

Doing a more intense cleanse every so often is a good health habit, and it is more effective for overall health when we add good habits to our everyday lifestyle. Adding in high-quality support supplements, such as Life 9®, ICP™ Daily, and NingXia Red®, give the body the things that it needs each day to maintain normal function and promote longevity.

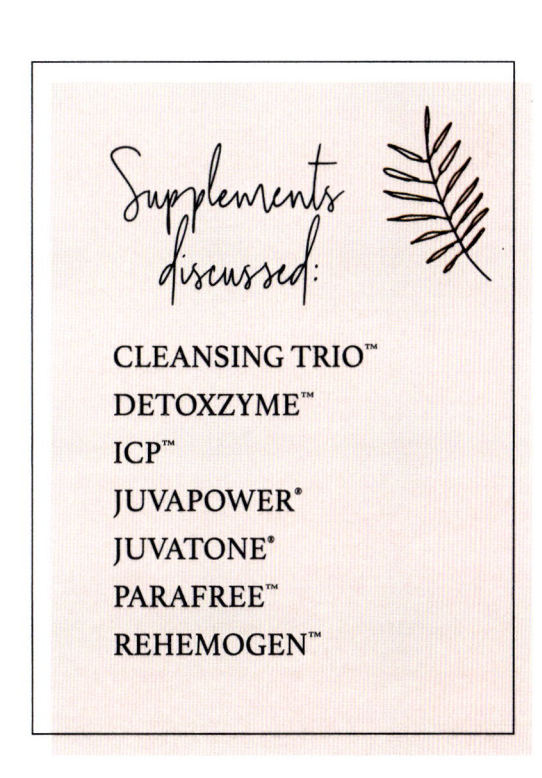

Supplements discussed:

CLEANSING TRIO™
DETOXZYME™
ICP™
JUVAPOWER®
JUVATONE®
PARAFREE™
REHEMOGEN™

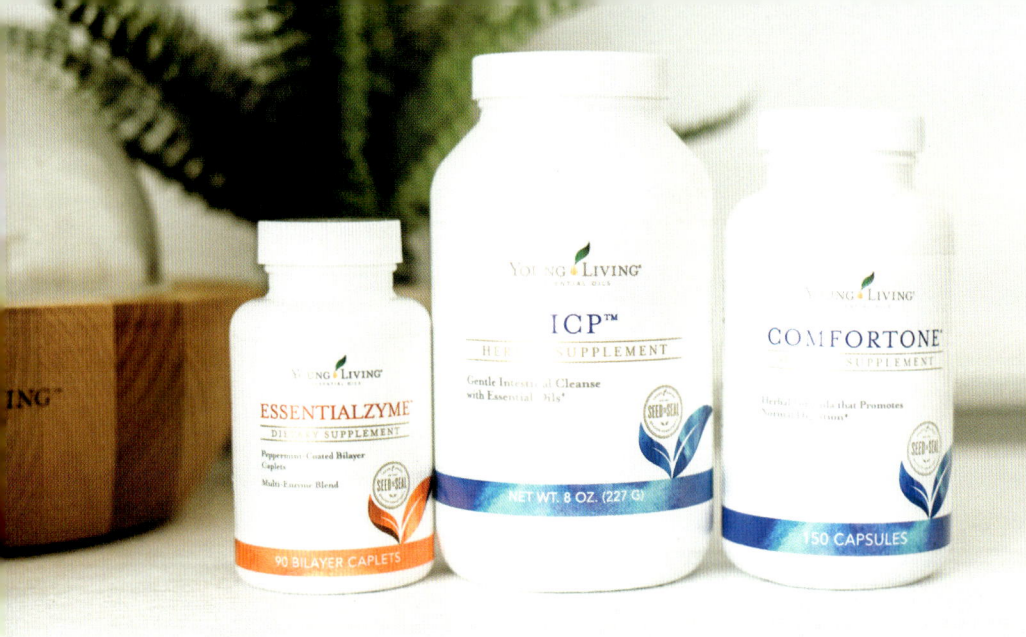

CLEANSING TRIO™

The Cleansing Trio™ Kit contains the products that you need to cleanse your system and eliminate built-up waste, while specifically supporting normal liver function. Each individual supplement is augmented with herbs that are rich in vitamins, minerals, enzymes, amino acids, fiber, and essential oils, and when used in combination, these supplements cleanse the digestive system to provide the body with renewed energy and a sense of well-being.

ICP™, ComforTone®, and Essentialzyme™ were paired together as an excellent means of cleansing the body's system and to support healthy liver function, as Essentialzyme™ stimulates natural enzyme activity in the body, ICP™ introduces a unique blend of fibers that assist in eliminating waste, and ComforTone® gently boosts the colon to easily and effectively remove toxins.

BENEFITS OF THE CLEANSING TRIO™
- ComforTone® provides a combination of cascara sagrada, psyllium seed, and ginger and tarragon essential oils that gently cleanse the colon.
- Essentialzyme™ stimulates overall enzyme activity and supports and balances digestive health to combat the modern diet.
- ICP™ is a gentle intestinal cleanse that uses an advanced mix of fibers and essential oils to improve nutrient absorption, decrease the buildup of wastes, and help to maintain a healthy heart.

COMFORTONE®
ComforTone® is a gentle, effective way to help promote healthy digestion through a mixture of herbs and essential oils. This supplement helps the body to eliminate waste in the colon, which allows it to function optimally. ComforTone® helps to promote consistent and easy bowel movements that can relieve hemorrhoids, bloating, and other symptoms of constipation.

ComforTone® is usually recommended for temporary use for cleanses and to get the body functioning normally. It is then stopped so that the body learns to stimulate bowel movements on its own.

ESSENTIALZYME™

Essentialzyme™ is a multienzyme complex that has been formulated to support and balance digestive health and stimulate overall enzyme activity. Essentialzyme™ contains the pancreatic enzymes pancrelipase and pancreatin and tarragon, peppermint, anise, fennel, and clove essential oils that improve enzyme activity and support healthy pancreatic function.

ICP™

ICP™ helps to keep your colon clean with an advanced mix of fibers to remove residues. A healthy digestive system is important for the proper functioning of all other systems because the digestive system absorbs all the nutrients that are used throughout the body.

ICP™ works best when paired with ComforTone® to get the bowels moving and Essentialzyme™ to break down what is caked and hardened in the colon.

CLEANSING TRIO™ PROTOCOL

- ComforTone®: Take one capsule three times daily. Drink at least 64 oz. of distilled water throughout the day for best results.
- Essentialzyme™: Take one dual time-release caplet one hour before your largest meal of the day for best results.
- ICP™: Mix two rounded tsp. with at least 8 oz. of juice or water three times daily. Drink immediately, as this product tends to thicken quickly when added to liquid. It tastes best in carrot juice, apple juice, NingXia Red®, or smoothies.

Safety notes: This product contains cascara sagrada bark. Read and follow the directions carefully. Women who are pregnant or nursing and those who have a medical condition should not use this product, except under the direction of a physician. Children under 12 should not use this product. Discontinue use and consult a physician if you have or develop abdominal pain, diarrhea, nausea, or vomiting. Do not exceed the recommended dosage. Not for long-term use. Not to be used as a weight-loss product. Keep out of reach of children. Do not give this product to children under the age of six, except under the supervision of a health professional. If discomfort persists, discontinue use of this product and consult a health professional. Keep out of reach of children. If you are pregnant, nursing, taking medication, or have a medical condition, consult a health practitioner before use. Using this product without enough liquid may cause choking. Do not use this product if you have difficulty swallowing. This product contains aloe vera (A. barbadensis) leaf. Do not use if you have or develop diarrhea, loose stools, or abdominal pain. Consult your physician if you have frequent diarrhea.

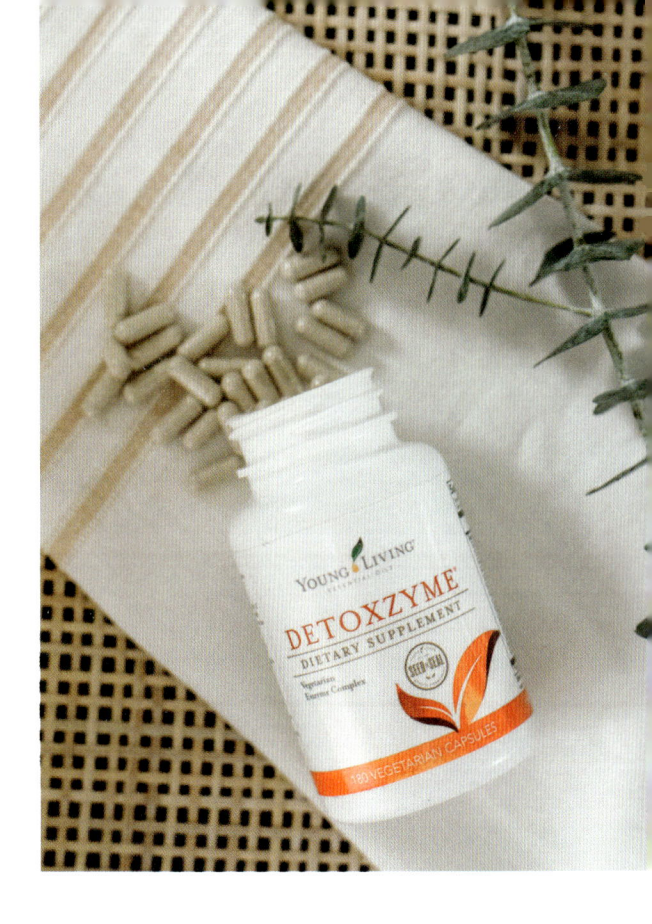

DETOXZYME™

Detoxzyme™ is a blend of enzymes and essential oils that have been formulated to promote detoxification and cleansing, which support normal digestive function. Detoxzyme™ contains powerful essential oils, such as cumin, anise, and fennel, that work synergistically with fast-acting, powerful enzymes to help to break down food, assimilate nutrients, and mitigate symptoms of digestive upset.

BENEFITS OF DETOXZYME™
- Promotes detoxification and cleansing
- Vegetarian-friendly formula
- Helps to relieve fullness, pressure, bloating, gas, pain, and/or minor cramping
- Works synergistically with a cleansing program
- Helps the body to get rid of toxins, parasites, and yeast overgrowth

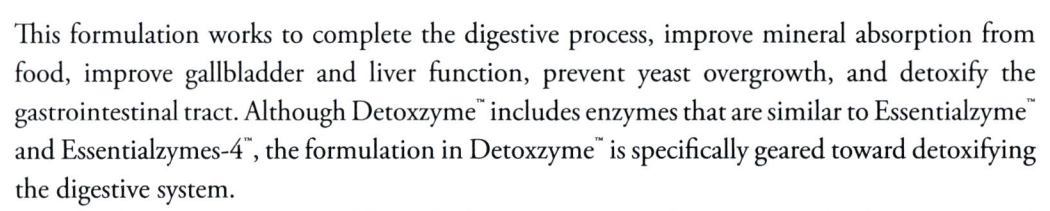

This formulation works to complete the digestive process, improve mineral absorption from food, improve gallbladder and liver function, prevent yeast overgrowth, and detoxify the gastrointestinal tract. Although Detoxzyme™ includes enzymes that are similar to Essentialzyme™ and Essentialzymes-4™, the formulation in Detoxzyme™ is specifically geared toward detoxifying the digestive system.

- **Amylase**: This is a powerful starch-digesting enzyme that prevents the fermentation of starches in the digestive system.
- **Invertase:** Invertase splits the sugar sucrose into glucose and fructose so that it can be utilized within the body.
- **Protease 4.5**: This is a blend of protein-digesting enzymes that are stable in the varying pH conditions of the digestive tract. They combat bacteria, yeast, and parasites in the intestines.
- **Glucoamylase:** This digestive enzyme breaks down starches into glucose and helps with symptoms of Chron's and Irritable Bowel Syndrome.

DETOXZYME™
To use: Take two capsules three times daily between meals or as needed.

- **Bromelain**: This proteolytic enzyme is found in pineapples and supports carbohydrate digestion.
- **Phytase**: Phytase is an enzyme necessary to break down minerals such as zinc, magnesium, and potassium, which are found in grains, nuts, seeds, and other foods.
- **Lipase**: Lipase is a fat-dissolving enzyme that promotes the excretion of toxins.

Safety notes: Do not give this product to children under 12 years of age, except under the supervision of a healthcare professional. If discomfort persists, discontinue use of this product, and consult your physician. Keep out of reach of children. If you are pregnant, nursing, taking medication, or have a medical condition, consult a healthcare professional before use.

ICP™

ICP™ is a gentle intestinal cleanse that uses a mix of fibers and essential oils to improve nutrient absorption, decrease the buildup of waste, and help to maintain a healthy heart. Although ICP™ works best when used with ComforTone® and Essentialzyme™ as part of a cleanse, it can also be used on its own.

BENEFITS OF ICP™
- Gentle intestinal cleanse infused with essential oils
- Helps to maintain a healthy heart
- Improves nutrient absorption
- Decreases the buildup of waste
- Removes buildup in the colon

ICP™ is an intestinal cleanse that features a blend of soluble and insoluble fibers that are sourced from psyllium, oat bran, and flax and fennel seeds. The formula is enhanced with digestion-supporting essential oils that also cleanse and purify the system. These ingredients work together for a gentle cleanse that improves nutrient absorption, decreases the buildup of waste, and helps to maintain a healthy heart.
- **Psyllium seed powder**: This soft fiber absorbs toxins and helps to relieve digestive discomfort.
- **Oat bran powder:** Oat bran is high in beta-glycans, which support the immune system. It is a source of fiber and helps to clean the system and bind fat from foods.
- **Flax seed powder**: Flax seed is high in fiber and omega-3 fatty acids, which help to promote heart health and intestinal motility. It also stimulates the release of digestive enzymes from the pancreas.
- **Fennel seed powder:** Fennel stimulates the digestive tract, helps to improve symptoms of nausea and gas, and improves pancreatic function.

- **Rice bran:** Rice bran is high in antioxidants, trace minerals, and essential fatty acids that support overall health and wellness.
- **Guar gum seed powder**: Guar gum helps to cleanse the colon and promotes healthy colon function.
- **Yucca root powder:** Yucca naturally contains digestive enzymes that aid in nutrient absorption and cleanse the digestive tract.
- **Aloe vera leaf extract**: Aloe vera is a natural laxative that promotes motility in the digestive tract and helps to relax the colon.
- **Lipase, protease 4.5, protease 3.0, protease 6.0, phytase, peptidase**: These enzymes break down fat, protein, and starch and are essential for mineral absorption.
- **Fennel essential oil**: Fennel supports digestion, eases intestinal discomfort, supports the pancreas and liver, provides immune support, and promotes the excretion of toxins.
- **Anise essential oil**: Anise supports overall digestion and circulation, acts as a diuretic, improves digestion, and has anti-inflammatory properties that help to ease intestinal cramping.
- **Ginger essential oil**: Ginger has analgesic, anti-inflammatory, antibacterial, and antioxidant properties, is great for soothing digestion[11], contains powerful antioxidants that can protect against oxidative stress, combats inflammation[12], and promotes liver health[13].

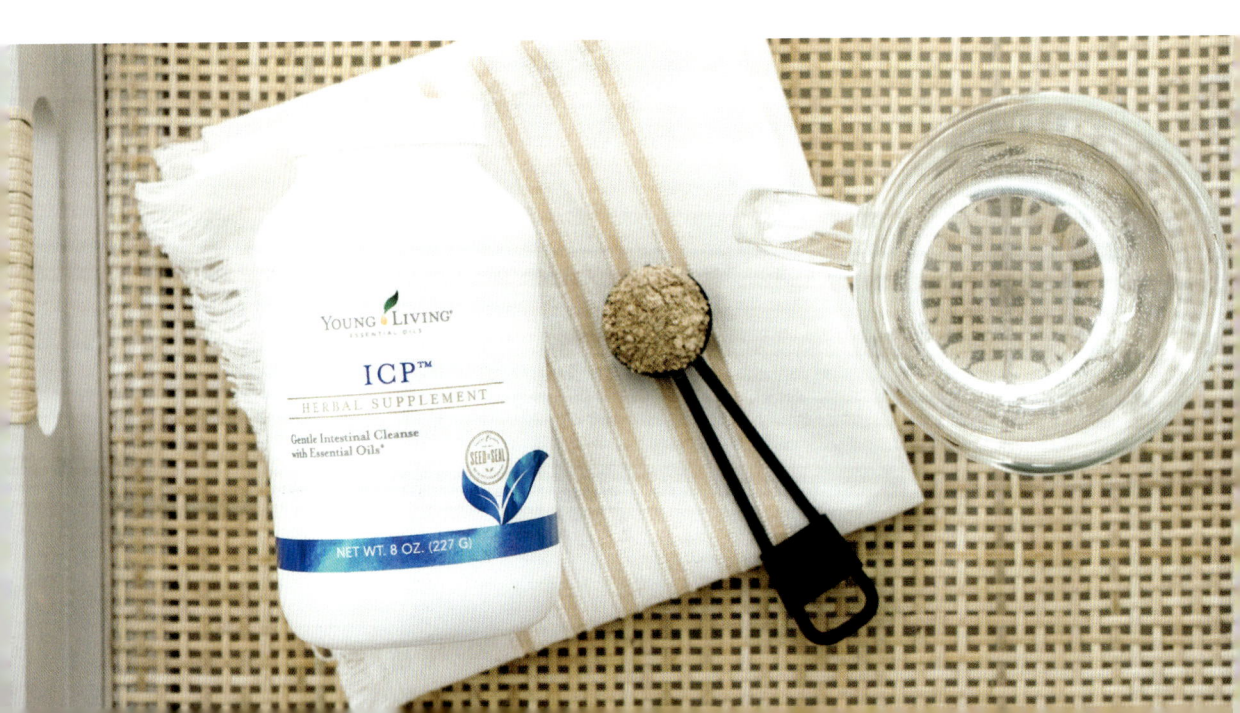

ICP™

To use: Mix two rounded tsp. with at least 8 oz. of juice or water. If cleansing or eating a high-protein diet, use three times daily. If eating a low-protein diet, use once daily. Drink immediately, as this product tends to thicken quickly when added to liquid. It tastes best in carrot juice, apple juice, or smoothies.

- **Lemongrass essential oil**: Lemongrass is a cleansing oil that helps the body's clear bladder infections, calms the digestive system, and shows antibacterial activity, even against drug-resistant strains of *Candida*[110].
- **Rosemary essential oil:** Rosemary helps to balance the endocrine system, supports heart health, cleanses and purifies the liver, and provides immune support through direct bactericidal activity, even on certain drug-resistant bacteria and fungi[110].

Safety notes: Keep out of reach of children. If you are pregnant, nursing, taking medication, or have a medical condition, consult a health professional before use. Using this product without enough liquid may cause choking. Do not use this product if you have difficulty swallowing. This product may cause an allergic reaction in people who are sensitive to psyllium. This product contains aloe vera (A. barbadensis) leaf. Read and follow the directions carefully. Do not use if you have or develop diarrhea, loose stools, or abdominal pain. Consult your physician if you have frequent diarrhea. Some ingredients are manufactured in a facility that also processes wheat.

JUVAPOWER®

JuvaPower® is a daily liver support supplement that combines vegetable powders with essential oils. JuvaPower® provides the body with nutrients and antioxidants that cleanse the intestines and promote a healthy liver, which is essential for filtering everything that goes into the body.

BENEFITS OF JUVAPOWER®
- Rich in antioxidants from whole-food vegetable powders
- Promotes internal cleansing and healthy liver function
- Appropriate for daily liver support
- Infused with liver-supporting essential oils
- Helps to bind acids in the digestive tract

JuvaPower® is a great supplement to use daily to cleanse and support the colon and liver, especially with all the potential toxins that we are exposed to daily. Ingredients such as spinach, broccoli, and beetroot powder provide whole-food antioxidants and acid binders to help to maintain balance within the body.
- **Rice seed bran:** Rice bran provides magnesium, selenium, antioxidants, and essential fatty acids.
- **Spinach leaf powder**: Spinach leaf helps to bolster the immune system, improve energy levels, and provide the body with whole-food nutrients.
- **Tomato fruit flakes:** This is high in potassium and lycopene, which is a powerful, immune-boosting antioxidant.
- **Beetroot powder:** Beetroot cleanses and nourishes the liver and supports cardiovascular health.

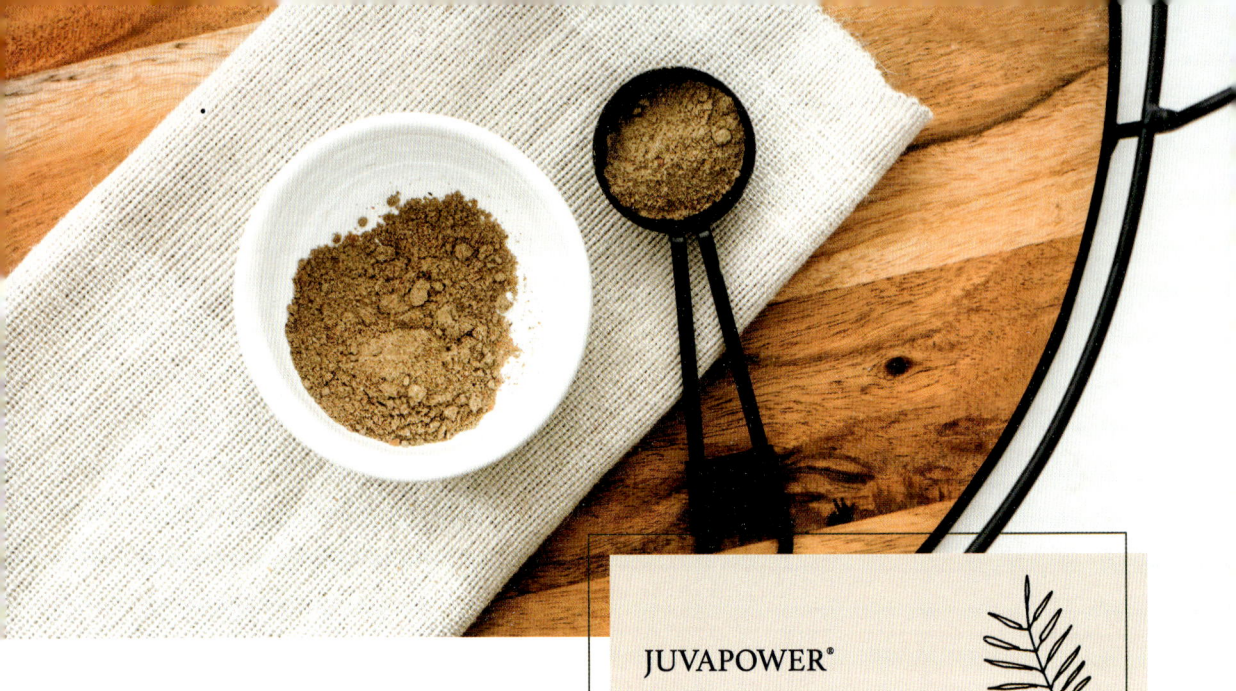

> **JUVAPOWER®**
>
> **To use:**
> - Sprinkle 7.5 g (1 Tbsp.) on food (i.e., baked potato, salad, rice, eggs) or add to 4-8 oz. purified water or rice/almond milk and drink.
> - Use three times daily for maximum benefits.

- **Flaxseed powder:** Flaxseed is a rich source of omega-3s and fiber. It cleanses the intestines, regulates cholesterol, and balances blood sugar levels[125].
- **Oat powder:** Oat powder helps bind fat for elimination, is an excellent source of antioxidants, including polyphenols, lowers cholesterol, and aids in digestion.
- **Broccoli powder:** Broccoli powder is high in fiber, antioxidants, vitamins, and nutrients, including vitamin C, which is a potent antioxidant that supports digestive, heart, and immune health.
- **Cucumber fruit powder:** Cucumber is high in fiber and minerals, promotes intestinal cleansing, and removes toxins.
- **Dill seed powder:** Dill seed exhibits anti-inflammatory and analgesic properties that fight free radical damage[126].
- **Sprouted barley seed powder**: This is a nutrient-rich superfood that is loaded with vitamins and antioxidants. In addition, it acts as a powerful cleansing agent and is an excellent source of both soluble and insoluble fiber. Insoluble fiber feeds the good bacteria in the gut and helps with digestion and intestinal health. Soluble fiber helps the stomach to absorb sugar more slowly, keeping blood sugar and cholesterol levels low.
- **Ginger root powder:** Ginger has anti-inflammatory properties that soothe the digestive tract. It aids in the elimination of toxins and waste.
- **Slippery elm bark:** Slippery elm is high in antioxidants that soothe inflammation and coat the GI tract. It increases levels of beneficial gut bacteria, promotes a healthy intestinal lining, and helps to remove toxins from the intestines.

- **L-Taurine:** This amino acid is essential to produce bile acid and protect the liver.
- **Psyllium seed**: This is a soft fiber that absorbs toxins and helps to relieve digestive discomfort.
- **Anise seed powder:** Anise has anti-inflammatory properties that help to ease intestinal cramping and improve digestion.
- **Fennel seed powder:** Fennel stimulates the digestive tract, helps to improve symptoms of nausea and gas, and improves pancreatic function.
- **Aloe vera leaf extract:** Aloe vera is a natural laxative that promotes motility in the digestive tract and helps to relax the colon.
- **Anise essential oil**: Anise supports overall digestion and circulation, acts as a diuretic, improves digestion, and has anti-inflammatory properties that help to ease intestinal cramping.
- **Fennel essential oil**: Fennel supports digestion, eases intestinal discomfort, supports the pancreas and liver, provides immune support, and promotes the excretion of toxins.
- **Peppermint leaf powder**: Peppermint is commonly used in herbal medicine for digestive needs, helps to ease inflammation, soothes nausea, and is high in antioxidants.

Safety notes: If you are pregnant, nursing, taking medication, or have a medical condition, consult a health practitioner before use. Keep out of reach of children. Eating this product without enough liquid may cause choking. Do not eat this product if you have difficulty in swallowing. Warning: This product may cause an allergic reaction in people who are sensitive to inhaled or ingested psyllium.

JUVATONE®

JuvaTone® combines phytonutrients and herbs, such as beetroot, dandelion, and alfalfa, with essential oils to create a supplement that promotes healthy liver function. This supplement contains nutrients that support the liver, which is responsible for filtering everything that is put into the body and converting carbohydrates into energy. Supporting the liver is essential for overall health.

BENEFITS OF JUVATONE®
- Promotes healthy liver function with herbs and essential oils
- Excellent source of choline, which is an essential micronutrient
- Contains dl-methionine, which helps to recycle glutathione, a natural antioxidant that is crucial for normal liver function
- Contains Oregon grape root, which is a source of the liver-supporting compound berberine
- Contains bee propolis, a powerful health tool
- Infused with liver-supporting essential oils

The liver is the filtering organ of the body and is responsible for removing toxins. As toxins build up from diet, environmental exposure, illness, etc., the liver becomes sluggish and stressed. When this happens, everything from eczema to digestive upset, irritability, and brain fog can occur. JuvaTone® is a great option for when you want to cleanse and tone the liver.

JuvaTone® is an excellent source of choline and dl-methionine, which help the body to recycle glutathione and promote normal filtering and excretion. In addition, it contains Oregon grape root, which provides the liver-supporting compound berberine, and cleansing essential oils for a well-rounded liver supplement.

- **Choline**: Choline is an essential micronutrient that is necessary for numerous bodily processes, including nerve function, cholesterol processing, brain development, muscle mobility, and liver function. It ensures and stimulates a healthy metabolism, supports energy, and aids brain function and communication between nerves and muscular movement, along with numerous other bodily processes. Additionally, it is required for cardiovascular health, proper focus, and memory function and helps to maintain low levels of inflammation throughout the body.
- **Dl-methionine:** This is an amino acid and powerful antioxidant that aids in the detoxification in the liver.
- **Beetroot powder:** Beetroot helps to cleanse and nourish the liver and supports cardiovascular health.
- **Dandelion root:** Dandelion root is commonly used in herbal teas and supplements for digestive support and is helpful for promoting healthy bile flow and liver health.
- **L-Cysteine:** This is a precursor for glutathione, which is the body's main antioxidant. It is involved in many necessary functions, especially those that promote detoxification and longevity.
- **Alfalfa sprout powder:** Alfalfa is high in chlorophyll, calcium, iron, potassium, phosphorus, vitamin C, and vitamin K. It is beneficial in treating diabetes, high cholesterol, arthritis, urinary tract infections, menstrual problems, and an array of other disorders[52], and has a positive effect on blood sugar levels, cholesterol levels, and blood pressure[51].
- **Oregon grape root**: Oregon grape root was historically used to cleanse the liver and gallbladder to optimize bile flow and improve the elimination of toxins.
- **Parsley leaf powder:** Parsley leaf is commonly used in herbal medicine to cleanse and purify the urinary tract and is high in antioxidants, which support liver health.
- **Bee propolis:** This resin is made by honeybees and has incredible health benefits. It has been used medicinally since ancient times for its antimicrobial, antioxidative, and anti-tumor properties[127].
- **Echinacea purpurea root**: Echinacea is known to help fight viral infections[128] and reduce inflammation[129].
- **Lemon essential oil**: Lemon is high in limonene, an antioxidant that mitigates free radical damage within cells[113]. It cleanses and soothes the digestive system.
- **German chamomile essential oil**: German chamomile is a powerful antioxidant that supports healthy cholesterol levels, the liver, gallbladder, and the body's natural response to inflammation.

- **Geranium essential oil:** Geranium promotes healthy hormone balance and aids circulation. It is a natural diuretic with anti-inflammatory and antimicrobial properties.
- **Rosemary essential oil:** Rosemary helps to balance the endocrine system, cleanses the liver, and supports cardiovascular health. It cleanses, purifies, and provides immune support through direct bactericidal activity, even on certain drug-resistant bacteria and fungi[110].
- **Myrtle essential oil:** Myrtle balances thyroid hormones, has positive effects on glandular imbalances, and supports detoxification in the liver.
- **Blue tansy essential oil:** Blue tansy has anti-inflammatory properties that help to cleanse the liver and lymphatic system and calms the nervous system.

> **JUVATONE®**
>
> **To use:** Take two tablets twice daily. Increase as needed, up to four tablets four times daily. For best results, take between meals.

Safety notes: If you are pregnant, nursing, taking medication, or have a medical condition, consult a health practitioner before use.

	KEY INGREDIENTS	FUNCTION	NOTES
JUVAPOWER®	Whole-food plant sources of antioxidants (beet, tomato, oat, broccoli, and more)	Provides antioxidants to the body and helps to bind toxins in the liver and digestive tract	Powder to be sprinkled over food or added to water three times daily
JUVATONE®	Choline, dl-methionine, berberine, Oregon grape root, cleansing essential oils	Promotes glutathione (primary antioxidant) recycling within the body, gently cleanses the liver of toxins, and supports overall liver health	Tablets taken twice daily (can be used up to four times daily as needed) between meals

NOTE: JuvaPower® and JuvaTone® can be used together for a wonderful, targeted liver support protocol. JuvaPower® is a whole-food support powder that provides antioxidants and helps to bind toxins in the digestive tract. JuvaTone® provides the body with choline and dl-methionine, which help the body to recycle glutathione, which is the main antioxidant of the body. JuvaTone® also provides other liver-supporting herbs and essential oils. The two supplements work synergistically to support the liver from multiple angles.

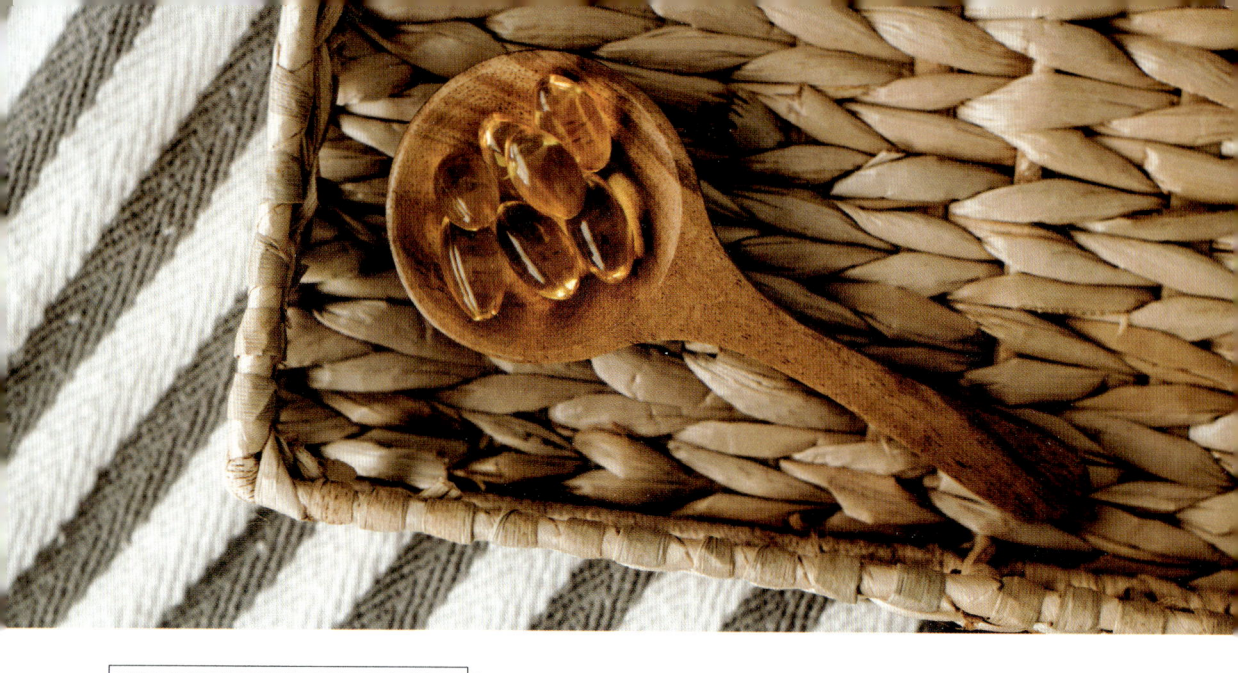

PARAFREE™

ParaFree™ is formulated with an advanced blend of some of the strongest essential oils that have been studied for their cleansing abilities. This formulation is specifically helpful for ridding the body of parasites.

BENEFITS OF PARAFREE™
- Helps to rid the body of parasites and unwanted pathogens
- Formulated to support digestion and gut health
- Helps to rid the body of toxins and unwanted microbes
- Contains powerful cleansing essential oils

ParaFree™ is a powerful blend of cleansing oils that supports the removal of toxins, parasites, and unwanted microbes from the digestive tract.
- **Sesame seed oil**: Sesame seed is high in essential fatty acids and helps to dilute the essential oils.
- **Olive fruit oil:** Olive fruit is a natural phytochemical with strong antioxidant and antimicrobial properties that provides immune support.
- **Cumin seed oil:** Cumin supports cleansing and immune function and has antiparasitic properties.
- **Anise essential oil**: Anise supports overall digestion and circulation, removes parasites, acts as a diuretic, and has anti-inflammatory properties that help to ease intestinal cramping.
- **Fennel essential oil**: Fennel supports digestion, eases intestinal discomfort, supports the pancreas and liver, provides immune support, and promotes the excretion of toxins.
- **Vetiver essential oil:** Vetiver supports the immune system, helps to mitigate intestinal spasms, cleanses, and detoxifies.

- **Bay laurel (Laurus nobilis) essential oil**: Bay laurel cleanses and detoxifies and has antiparasitic properties.
- **Nutmeg essential oil:** Nutmeg is a cleansing oil that supports healthy digestion and the body's stress response and lowers cortisol levels.
- **Tea tree essential oil:** Tea tree has well-documented antimicrobial activity, which makes it one of the most widely used essential oils for cleansing and purifying[130].
- **Thyme essential oil**: Thyme is rich in the constituent thymol, a potent antioxidant that has direct bactericidal activity against many common pathogens[109]. It protects DHA levels and brain function, has demonstrated efficacy against antibiotic-resistant bacterial strains[23], and supports a healthy hormone balance[24]. In addition, it works as a circulatory stimulant by helping to maintain healthy blood pressure and cholesterol levels[25].
- **Clove essential oil:** Clove has profound immune support and is a powerful antioxidant (ORAC value of over 290,000[19]). It cleanses the gut and can stop the growth of some bacteria and fungi[20], including *Candida*[21], at higher doses.
- **Ocotea essential oil:** Ocotea contains high levels of alpha-humulene, which supports the body's response to inflammation and injury. In addition, it supports healthy blood sugar levels and prevents the overgrowth of unhealthy bacteria in the gut.
- **Dorado azul essential oil:** Dorado azul has antioxidant and anti-inflammatory properties, is beneficial for digestion, and fights *Candida* overgrowth, as well as other intestinal microbes. In addition, it supports the respiratory system.
- **Tarragon essential oil:** Tarragon soothes and supports digestion, may support the immune system, and calms nausea.
- **Ginger essential oil**: Ginger has analgesic, anti-inflammatory, antibacterial, and antioxidant properties. It is great for soothing digestion[11], contains powerful antioxidants that can protect against oxidative stress, combats inflammation[12], and promotes liver health[13].
- **Peppermint essential oil**: Peppermint contains the constituents menthol and menthone, which soothe the stomach and aid in digestion, have anti-inflammatory properties, and improve absorption of other ingredients.
- **Juniper essential oil**: Juniper naturally cleanses the urinary tract, is high in antioxidants, promotes healthy filtration in the kidneys, purifies and detoxifies the digestive system, and acts as a diuretic to promote the excretion of toxins from the body.

PARAFREE™

To use: Take three softgels twice daily or as needed. For best results, take for 21 days and rest for seven days.

The cycle may be repeated three times. Take on an empty stomach for maximum results.

- **Lemongrass essential oil**: Lemongrass is a cleansing oil that helps the body's clear bladder infections, calms the digestive system, and shows antibacterial activity, even against drug-resistant strains of *Candida*[110].
- **Patchouli essential oil**: Patchouli acts as a cleanser and digestive aid and has antimicrobial and anti-inflammatory properties.

Safety notes: If you are pregnant, nursing, taking medication, or have a medical condition, consult a health practitioner before use. Keep out of reach of children. Contains fish (tilapia, carp).

REHEMOGEN™

Rehemogen™ is an herbal tincture that contains powerful botanicals that were traditionally used by Native Americans to cleanse and purify the body and blood. This formula includes cascara sagrada, red clover, sarsaparilla root, burdock root, and prickly ash, among other herbs with cleansing properties. In addition, Rehemogen™ includes a unique blend of essential thyme, Roman chamomile, rosemary, and tea tree essential oils.

BENEFITS OF REHEMOGEN™
- Supports healthy digestion
- Formulated with natural herbs and essential oils that are designed to enhance digestion and support bowel function
- Made with Cascara sagrada, red clover, poke root, prickly ash bar, and burdock root, which have been historically used for their cleansing and rebuilding properties

This supplement is specifically supportive of a healthy liver, which is an essential component of cleansing and digestion. The herbs and essential oils that are included create a tincture that can be used intermittently to purify the system as a whole and is especially beneficial for rebuilding the blood.

- **Red clover blossom**: Red clover is a potent source of minerals with purifying properties that help to reduce inflammation and boost liver health. It promotes efficient cholesterol production in the liver, lowers LDL ("bad" cholesterol) levels, and supports both male and female reproductive health[131].
- **Licorice root**: Licorice root is an adaptogenic herb that helps to mitigate unhealthy stress responses, has anti-inflammatory properties, helps to improve digestion, and acts as a mild cleansing agent.
- **Poke root**: Poke root has been used traditionally for centuries to boost the immune system and improve lymphatic drainage. It has anti-inflammatory properties and helps the body eliminate toxins.

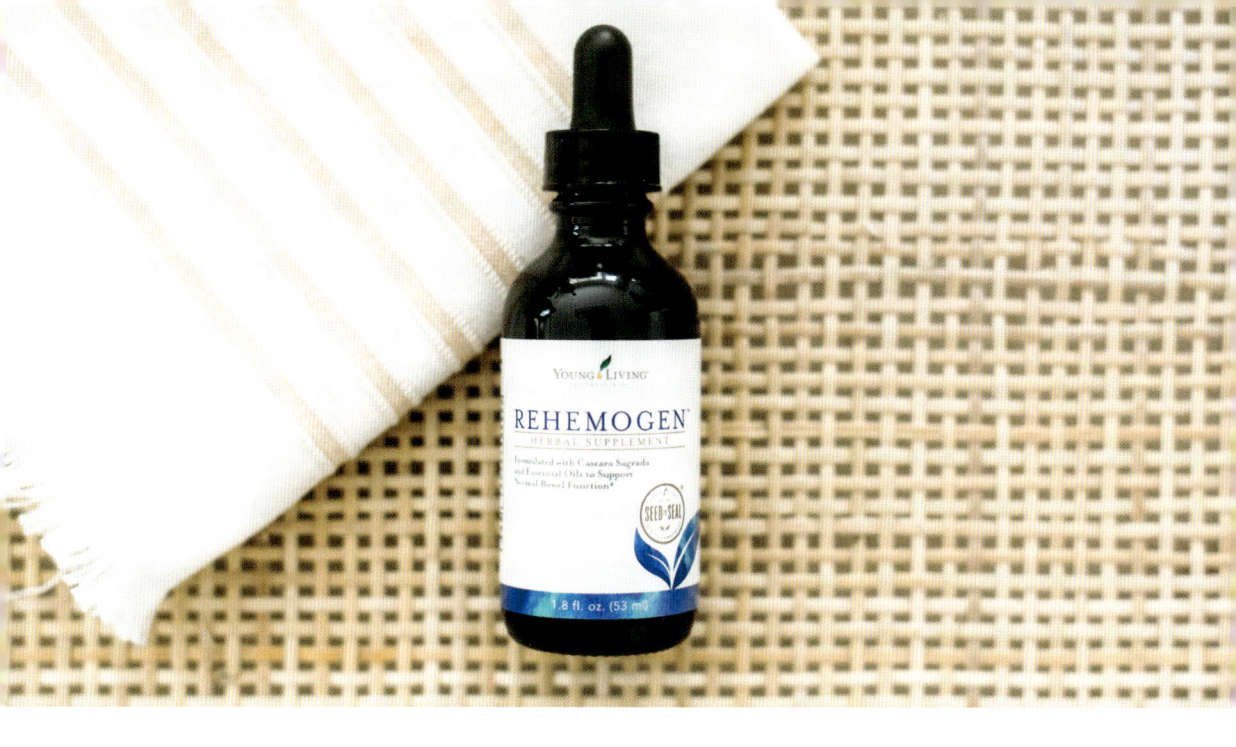

- **Oregon grape root**: Oregon grape root has historically been used to cleanse the liver and gallbladder to optimize bile flow and improve the elimination of toxins.
- **Peach tree bark**: Peach tree bark contains antioxidants and helps the body to eliminate toxin buildup.
- **Cascara sagrada**: Cascara sagrada helps to cleanse the liver to move waste through the colon and supports the body's natural elimination process. It is an effective treatment for chronic constipation.
- **Stillingia root**: Stillingia root was used traditionally in Native American medicine to support skin health and occasional constipation. It helps to remove toxins from the body and boosts blood immunity.
- **Sarsaparilla root:** This is commonly used to balance hormones, reduce fluid retention, and improve overall immune function. It contains saponins, which are molecules that help to neutralize toxins from bacteria and fungi.
- **Buckthorn bark:** Buckthorn bark was traditionally used as a diuretic and blood cleanser. It helps to ease constipation and is similar to Cascara sagrada.
- **Burdock bark:** Burdock bark is a good source of micronutrients (vitamin B6, vitamin C, calcium, iron magnesium, potassium, folate), is high in the powerful, health-promoting antioxidants quercetin and luteolin, has natural anti-inflammatory properties, and acts as a diuretic and blood cleanser.
- **Prickly ash**: This is often used in alternative medicine for tooth pain. It acts as an anti-inflammatory agent and a digestive aid.
- **Roman chamomile essential oil:** Roman chamomile contains antioxidants that promote heart[132] and digestive health and healthy bile flow. It is an essential component of detoxification in the liver and has anti-inflammatory properties that may be beneficial for kidney stones and infections.

- **Rosemary essential oil:** Rosemary cleanses, purifies, and provides immune support through direct bactericidal activity, even on certain drug-resistant bacteria and fungi[110]. It helps to balance the endocrine system and cleanse the liver, reduces free radical damage, lowers cortisol (stress hormone)[162], promotes heart health, and helps to maintain healthy blood sugar levels[163].
- **Thyme essential oil:** Thyme is rich in the constituent thymol, a potent antioxidant that supports the respiratory and immune systems through direct bactericidal activity against many common pathogens[109]. It protects DHA levels and brain function, has demonstrated efficacy against antibiotic-resistant bacterial strains[23], and helps to support healthy hormone balance[24]. In addition, it acts as a circulatory stimulant, helping to maintain healthy blood pressure and cholesterol levels[25].
- **Tea tree essential oil:** Tea tree has well-documented antimicrobial activity, which makes it one of the most widely used essential oils for cleansing and purifying[130].

> **REHEMOGEN™**
>
> **To use:** Take three half droppers (3 mL) three times daily in distilled water just before or with meals containing protein. This product is not intended for long-term use.

Safety notes: Shake well before using. Refrigerate after opening. Keep in a cool, dry place. Keep out of reach of children. Do not expose to excessive heat or direct sunlight. If pregnant or under a doctor's care, consult your physician or healthcare provider. Women who are pregnant or nursing, or anyone with a medical condition, should not use this product, except under the direction of a physician. This product contains cascara sagrada bark. Read and follow the label directions carefully. Children under 12 should not use this product. Discontinue use and consult a physician if you have or develop abdominal pain, diarrhea, nausea, or vomiting. Do not exceed the recommended dosage. This product is not intended for long-term use. It should not be used as a weight-loss product.

Protocols For Cleansing & Liver Health

Cleansing and liver support are cornerstones of overall health. The liver is the filtering organ in the body and can easily get clogged up with everything that we are exposed to daily. Like other areas of health, daily support is ideal, and adding in periodic cleanses further enhances liver and digestive health.

CLEANSING
- Cleansing Trio™ (use annually or as desired for a more cleanse)
- Detoxzyme™
- Digest & Cleanse™
- ICP™
- NingXia Red®
- Rehemogen™ (use as needed/desired for cleansing)

DAILY LIVER SUPPORT
- Balance Complete™ (use as a gently daily cleanse/meal replacement)
- ICP Daily™
- Life 9®
- Longevity™
- NingXia Red®
- JuvaPower®
- JuvaTone®
- Options for additional support: JuvaFlex™ Vitality™ Essential Oil, Lemon/Lemon Vitality™ Essential Oil, Purification® Essential Oil Blend

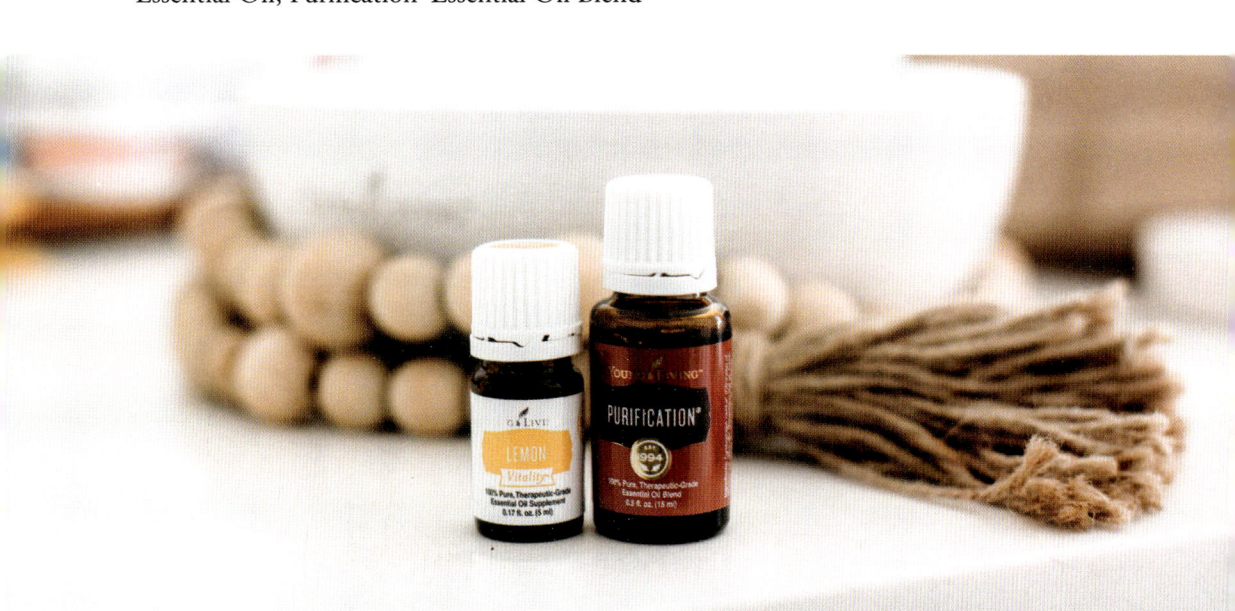

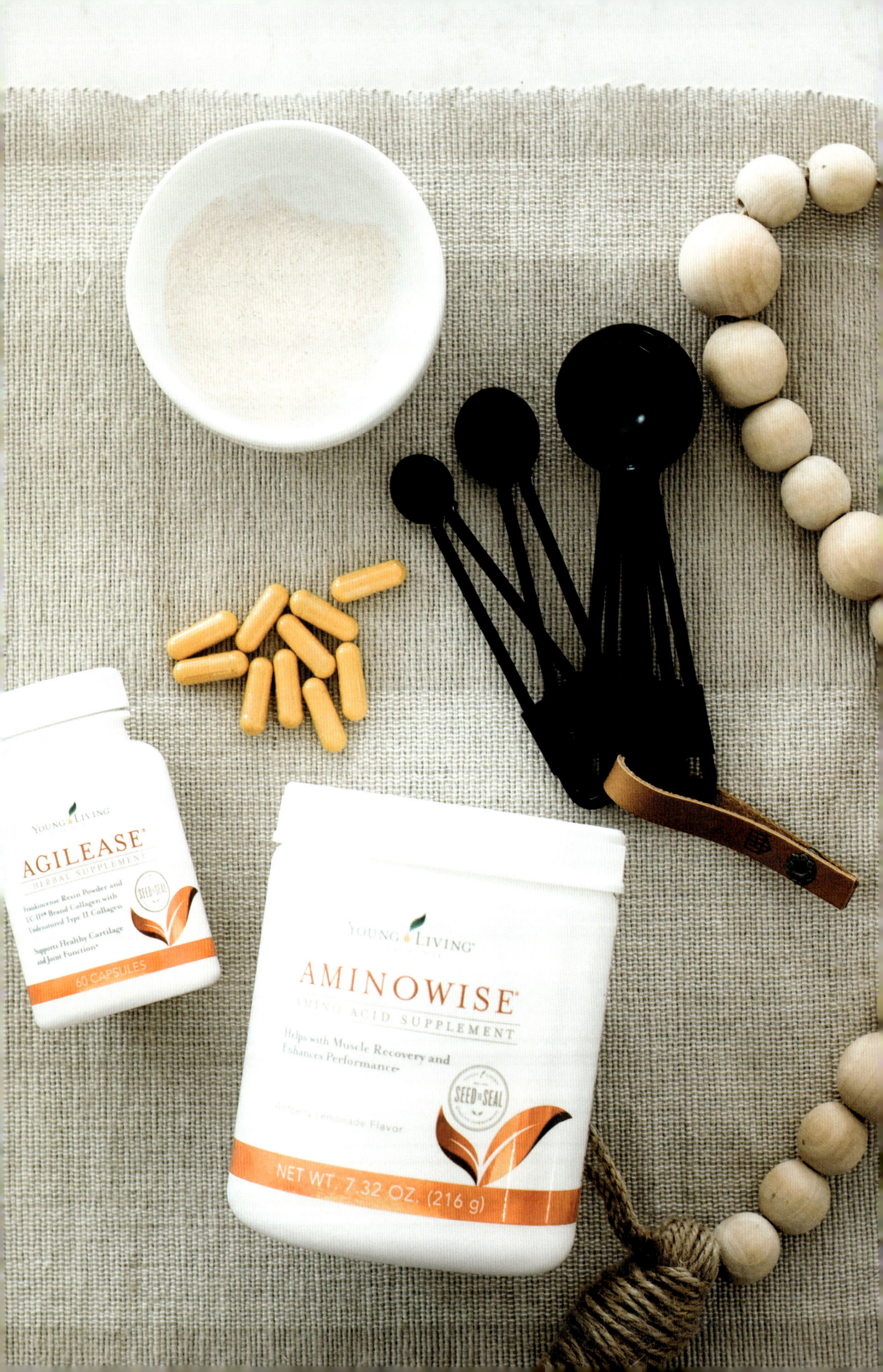
YOUNG LIVING
AGILEASE
HERBAL SUPPLEMENT
60 CAPSULES
YOUNG LIVING
AMINOWISE
AMINO ACID SUPPLEMENT
Helps with Muscle Recovery and
Enhances Performance
NET WT. 7.32 OZ. (216 g)

Part 5: SUPPLEMENTS FOR BONE & MUSCLE SUPPORT

Because our muscles and bones literally support us daily, muscle and bone health is essential, especially as we age. We want to take care of our physical bodies with exercise and proper nutrition, and adding supplements to your routine is one more layer of support for the system.

Supplements discussed:

AGILEASE®
AMINOWISE™
BLM™
GOLDEN TURMERIC™
MEGACAL™
SULFURZYME®
SUPER CAL PLUS™
SUPER VITAMIN D

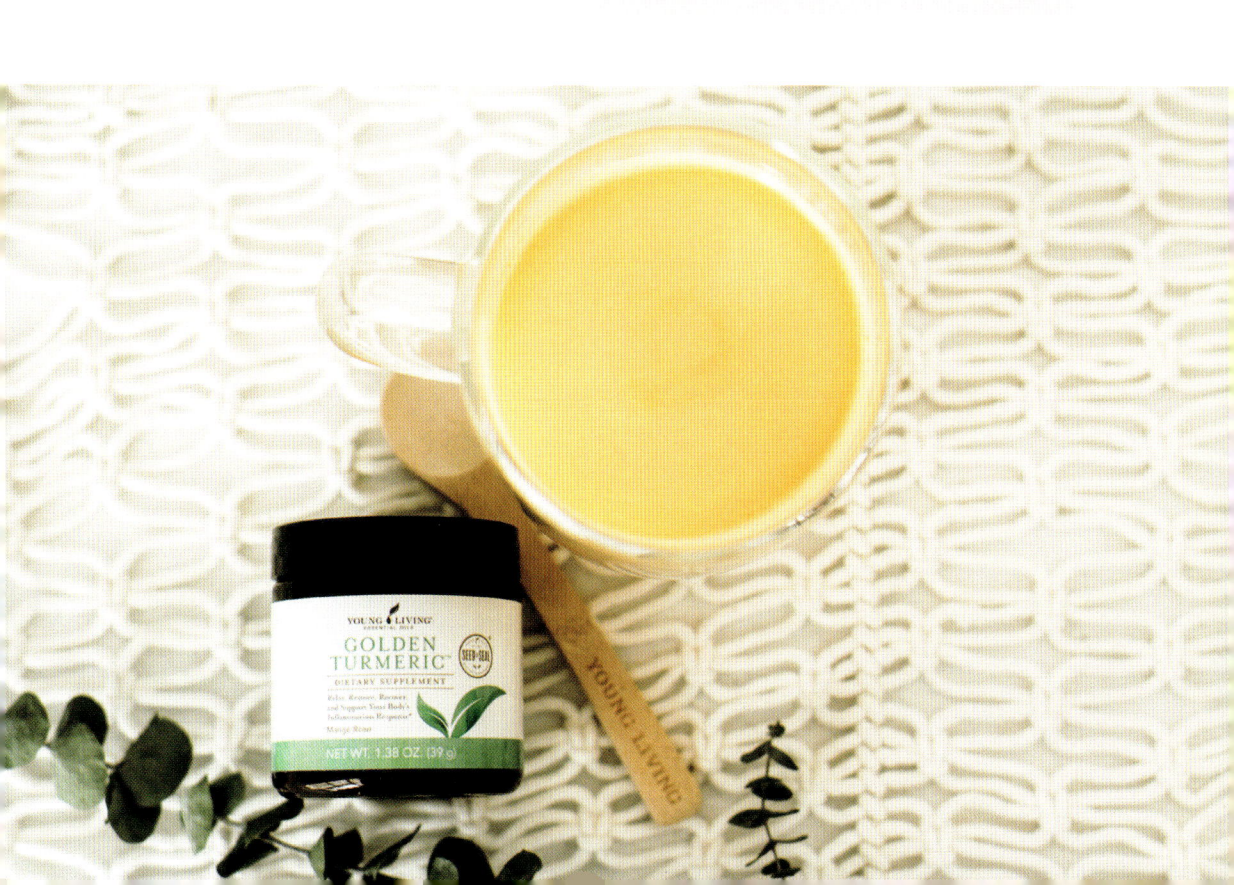

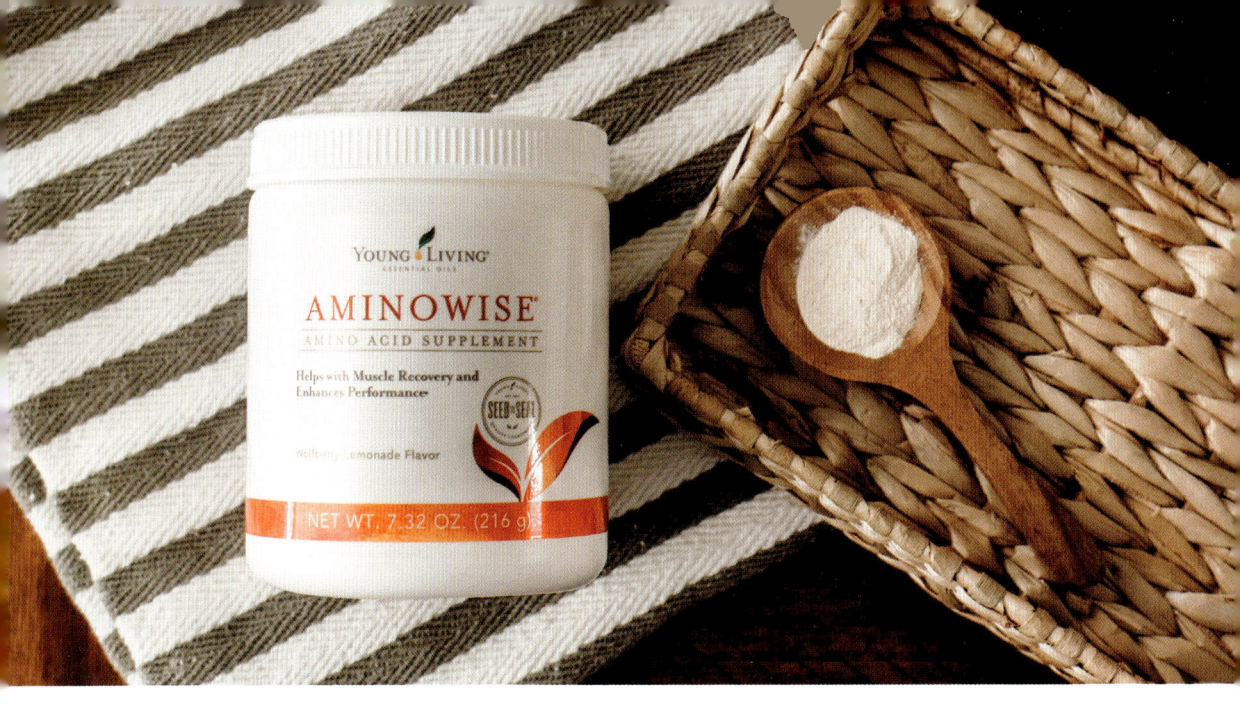

AMINOWISE™

AminoWise™ is a wolfberry lemonade-flavored drink mix that contains branched-chain amino acids (BCAAs), antioxidants, and minerals to provide the nutrients that you need to optimize workout recovery. Think of this as a natural Gatorade! AminoWise™ enhances muscle performance, reduces fatigue, and supports muscles during and after exercise.

BENEFITS OF AMINOWISE™
- Contains amino acids and antioxidants that help with fatigue and enhance muscle recovery
- Aids in reducing muscle fatigue by reducing exercise-induced lactic acid
- Supports the production of nitric oxide, which can improve vascular blood flow and enhance recovery and performance
- Contains BCAAs, which have been shown to aid in preventing muscle catabolism from exercise
- Supports hydration by replenishing important minerals that are lost during exercise
- Good source of vitamin E and zinc

WHY ARE AMINO ACIDS IMPORTANT?
Amino acids are classified as non-essential amino acids (you produce them on your own), conditionally essential amino acids (can usually be produced by your body), and essential amino acids (cannot be made by the body, so you must obtain them through diet or supplementation). Of the essential amino acids, the following three BCAAs are superstars: leucine, isoleucine, and valine. BCAAs comprise approximately 35% of your muscle tissue.

Your ability to build and maintain lean body mass is based on the levels of protein synthesis and protein breakdown throughout the day. As you age, protein breakdown tends to accelerate. To slow the rate of protein breakdown, you can eat more high-quality protein and supplement with essential amino acids.

Because your level of muscle mass plays a significant role in longevity, anything that increases protein synthesis or decreases protein breakdown can support your quality of life throughout your lifespan. Since amino acids play such an essential role in building and maintaining lean body mass, they must be a consistent part of a healthy diet[133].

AminoWise™ contains all the good stuff that we want and none of the bad, and it still tastes great. It's formulated with BCAAs and contains three key blends that combine to support your muscles during and after exercise, fight fatigue, and enhance your recovery.
- **Muscle performance blend**: This lend includes the BCAAs that help to build and repair muscles.
    - **Leucine**: This BCAA improves muscle growth and athletic performance[134], promotes muscle recovery[135], and helps to regulate blood sugar levels[136].
    - **Isoleucine**: This BCAA is required for protein formation, adequate energy levels, and blood sugar regulation and can help to decrease post-workout muscle strain and soreness.
    - **Valine**: Valine is a BCAA that supports muscle growth and tissue repair, aids in muscle strength coordination, and promotes a calm emotional state.
    - **L-citrulline**: L-citrulline is a highly absorbable precursor to L-arginine that improves the use of BCAAs[137] within the body and helps to maintain protein balance[138].
    - **L-glutamine**: L-glutamine improves muscle hydration, aids in muscle recovery, boosts the immune system, and helps to reduce inflammation and the stress of overtraining[139].
    - **B-alanine**: This amino acid aids in the production of carnosine, a compound that is involved in muscle endurance and regulates lactic acid buildup.
    - **L-arginine**: L-arginine is a precursor for nitrous oxide, which is a compound that plays a role in development, learning, and memory. It protects against brain injury and modulates stress within the body.
    - **L-taurine**: This amino acid is essential for production of bile acid and protects the liver.
- **Recovery blend**: This blend includes NingXia wolfberry powder and lemon and lime essential oils that help to reduce lactic acid buildup.
    - **NingXia wolfberry powder**: This is high in antioxidants that mitigate and repair DNA damage. Additionally, it acts as a prebiotic.
    - **Lime fruit powder:** Lime is high in vitamin C and antioxidants that help to enhance iron absorption, boost immune function, and burn fat.
    - **Zinc**: Zinc is an essential trace element that helps to strengthen the immune system, is required for calcium uptake, supports muscle health, and improves energy levels.

- **Vitamin E:** Vitamin E is a natural antioxidant that minimizes free radical damage within the body, promoting healthy cell function and overall health.
- **Lemon and lime essential oils:** These citrus oils are high in limonene, a constituent with anti-inflammatory, wound-healing, and anticancer effects. It strengthens the immune system, helps to decongest the lymphatic system, and improves nutrient absorption.
- **Hydration blend:** This blend features electrolytes that replace vital minerals that are lost during exercise.
  - **Sodium, potassium, calcium, and magnesium:** These are essential electrolytes that play a vital role in many body processes, including fluid balance, heart health, mental clarity, and nerve and muscle function.

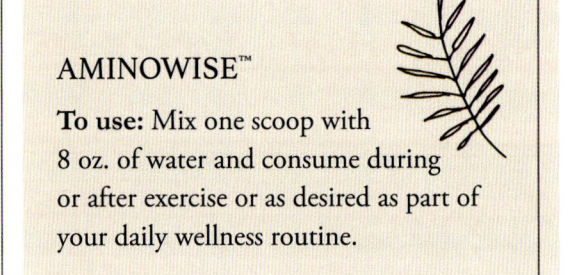

> **AMINOWISE™**
>
> **To use:** Mix one scoop with 8 oz. of water and consume during or after exercise or as desired as part of your daily wellness routine.

Safety notes: Keep out of reach of children. If you are pregnant, nursing, taking medication, or have a medical condition, consult a health professional before use.

AGILEASE®

If you have joints, you will want to add AgilEase® to your routine! This joint health supplement helps you to gain greater mobility and flexibility by reducing inflammation. AgilEase® is especially beneficial for those with an active lifestyle, athletes, and aging individuals who may experience natural, acute inflammation in their joints after exercise. Whether it is running, weightlifting, working on your feet all day, or any other physical activity, AgilEase® can provide your body with the support that it needs to recover.

BENEFITS OF AGILEASE®
- Supports and protects healthy cartilage and joints
- Supports the body's natural response to exercise in healthy individuals
- Helps to support healthy joint flexibility and mobility
- Contains undenatured collagen, turmeric, and frankincense powder
- Helps with joint discomfort to improve your quality of life
- Beneficial for athletes and active individuals of all ages who want to support and protect their joints and cartilage

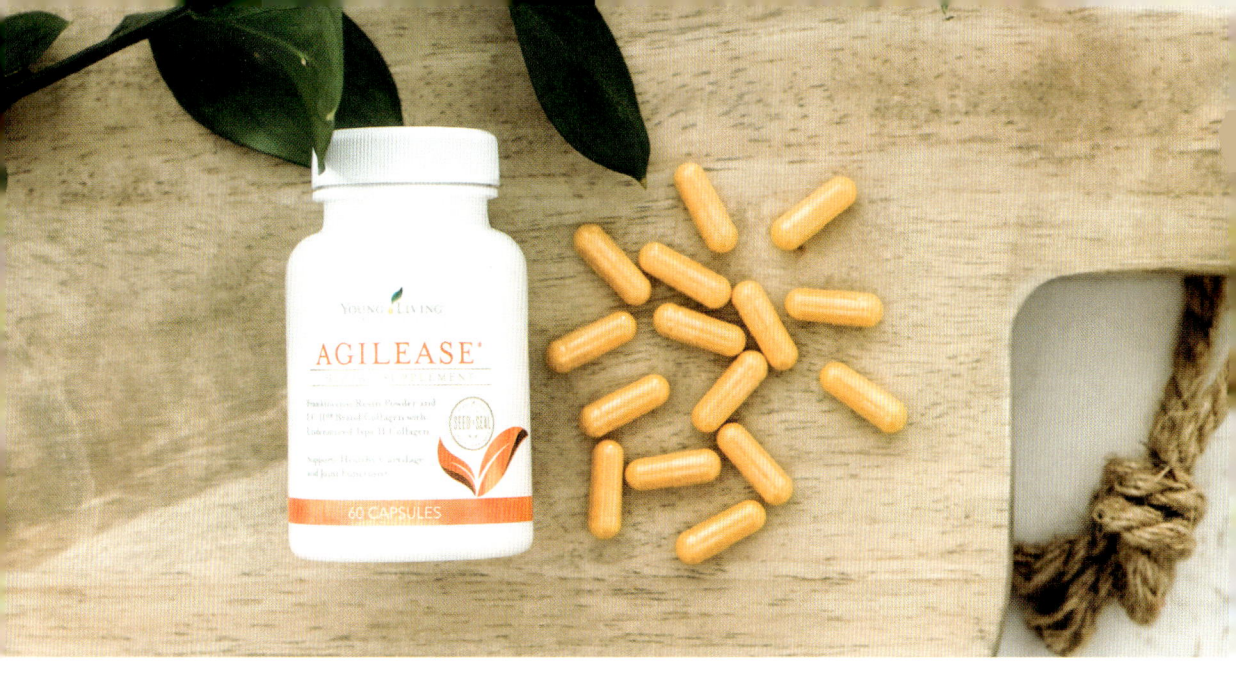

AgilEase® capsules support healthy exercise recovery. This powerful blend of ingredients can help you to protect your joint and cartilage health and gain greater mobility and flexibility. It is full of powerful ingredients that support overall joint health.

- **Frankincense resin powder**: Frankincense is a strong antioxidant that helps to repair oxidative damage at a cellular level. It promotes immune health and muscle recovery and supports the body as we age.
- **UC-II undenatured collagen**: Collagen supports the body's natural collagen production, cushions the joints, promotes healthy hair, skin, and nails, assists the body during times of inflammation, and plays a role in gut health.
- **Hyaluronic acid**: Hyaluronic acid assists the growth and development of joint cartilage and bone by promoting the growth of new cells and tissues.
- **Calcium**: Calcium is an essential mineral for healthy bones and muscles and is involved in muscle contraction and heart health.
- **Turmeric**: Turmeric has strong anti-inflammatory properties[2] that match the effectiveness of some anti-inflammatory drugs[3,4]. It is a potent antioxidant that can neutralize free radicals[5] and boosts the activity of the body's own antioxidant enzymes[6].
- **Wintergreen essential oil**: Commonly known as methyl salicylate, wintergreen supports the body's response to inflammation and eases pain.
- **Copaiba essential oil**: Copaiba is a natural anti-inflammatory agent that acts like a fire extinguisher to help put out fires within the body. It is gentle but effective.
- **Clove essential oil**: Clove has high antioxidant activity, with an average ORAC value of over 290,000[19]. It can be effective at stopping the growth of some bacteria and fungi[20] and is high in the constituent eugenol, which boasts well-documented neuroprotective, antioxidant, anti-inflammatory, antipyretic, analgesic, antiparasitic, and antimicrobial properties. It protects the brain, heart, lungs, immune system, and the body as a whole[18].
- **Northern Lights black spruce essential oil**: Black spruce supports the body's response to pain and injury and helps to calm the natural inflammation process.

These oils are known for their joint health benefits, and when used together, they work synergistically to support the body (1+1=3!).

You can use AgilEase® to support joints as you exercise or as a preventative measure to protect joint and cartilage health overall. It is a wonderful addition to a healthy lifestyle to assist with inflammation and recovery after running, yoga, weightlifting, or even just those long days of parenting or adulting (because sometimes adulting feels like an Olympic sport).

> **AGILEASE®**
>
> **To use:** Take two capsules daily to support joint health or as a preventative measure to protect joint and cartilage health.

Safety notes: Keep out of reach of children. If you are pregnant, nursing, taking medication, or have a medical condition, consult a healthcare professional before use.

BLM™

BLM™ is a powerful combination of type II collagen, MSM, glucosamine sulfate, manganese citrate and essential oils. These ingredients have been shown to support healthy cell function and encourage joint health and fluid movement. This supplement is a wonderful choice for those suffering from osteoarthritis, muscle inflammation, or anyone looking for help with cartilage production and joint health.

BENEFITS OF BLM™
- Offers nutritional support for bones, ligaments, and muscles
- Helps to ease inflammation and joint pain
- Supports joint mobility and cartilage formation
- Supports healthy cell function
- Encourages joint health and fluid movement
- Provides an excellent source of glucosamine, MSM, and collagen
- Infused with joint supportive essential oils

As we age, the amount of cartilage in the joints naturally declines. This decline is often expedited by chronic inflammation and develops into conditions, such as osteoarthritis. Glucosamine, MSM, and collagen have all been studied both for preventative and acute measures regarding arthritis and joint health because these ingredients work synergistically to reduce joint pain, lower inflammation, and cushion the joints through increased cartilage production[140].

- **Glucosamine sulfate:** Glucosamine is a well-studied proteoglycan that rebuilds cartilage, supports damaged joints, and reduces symptoms of inflammation.
- **Collagen type II**: This specific collagen is derived from avian cartilage and contains high levels of proteoglycans, which are the building blocks of joints. Additionally, it cushions the joints and reduces oxidative damage from inflammation, promotes healthy hair, skin and nails, and plays a role in gut health.
- **MSM**: MSM helps to control inflammation, reduces pain, and acts as a bioavailable source of sulfur, which is necessary for joint health. It helps to fortify muscles and soothe the stress that is placed on joints, which improves general muscular function. Additionally, it contains antioxidants that tackle the free radicals that damage your immune system[141].
- **Manganese:** Manganese is a cofactor that is required for enzyme activity in the body. It plays a role in amino acids, cholesterol, glucose, and carbohydrate metabolism, reactive oxygen species scavenging, bone formation, reproduction, and the immune response.
- **Balsam Canada essential oil:** This essential oil supports the body's response to inflammation, helps to reduce swelling, and eases joint pain.
- **Wintergreen essential oil**: Commonly known as methyl salicylate, wintergreen supports the body's response to inflammation and eases pain.
- **Clove essential oil:** Clove has high antioxidant activity, with an average ORAC value of over 290,000[19]. It can be effective at stopping the growth of some bacteria and fungi[20] and is high in the constituent eugenol, which boasts well-documented neuroprotective, antioxidant, anti-inflammatory, antipyretic, analgesic, antiparasitic, and antimicrobial properties. Moreover, it protects the brain, heart, lungs, immune system, and the whole body[18].

Think of BLM™ as a better, more powerful version of the glucosamine/chondroitin supplements that you often see in pharmacies or health food stores. Young Living doesn't add anything to their supplements that doesn't need to be there or use excessive fillers, colors, or dyes, so you know that what you're taking is the best possible option.

BLM™

To use: If you weigh less than 120 lbs., take one capsule three times daily. If you weigh 120-200 lbs., take one capsule four times daily. If you weigh over 200 lbs., take one capsule five times daily.

Allow four to eight weeks of daily use before expecting noticeable results.

Safety notes: Keep in a cool, dry place. Keep out of reach of children. Do not expose to excessive heat or direct sunlight. If you are pregnant or under a doctor's care, consult your physician. Contains shellfish (crab, shrimp).

WHAT IS THE DIFFERENCE BETWEEN AGILEASE® AND BLM™?

The biggest difference between these two joint supplements is the addition of glucosamine and MSM in BLM™. AgilEase® is a great choice for individuals who want daily support to maintain healthy joints due to an active lifestyle. BLM™ would be a better choice for individuals who have already suffered damage to their joints and cartilage, such as in the presence of osteoarthritis. BLM™ would be a great replacement for the common glucosamine/chondroitin supplements that you find in conventional health stores.

However, if your supplement of choice is out of stock, it would be worth replacing with the other.

GOLDEN TURMERIC™

Find more information on Golden Turmeric™ in the "Foundational Supplements" section on page 23.

Turmeric is no stranger to the health scene. This golden spice is well known for its ability to help the body during times of inflammation, both acute and chronic. Young Living's Golden Turmeric™ powder combines turmeric, boswellia resin, and ginger, which work synergistically to support the body's natural response to inflammation, immune response, joint health, mobility, and physical recovery.

BENEFITS OF GOLDEN TURMERIC™
- Supports the body's natural response to inflammation
- Bolsters immune response, joint health, mobility, and recovery after physical exertion
- 24 times more bioavailable than standard turmeric extract
- Contains prebiotics to support both healthy digestion and the gut-brain axis
- Contains naturally occurring curcuminoids that support joint mobility

Golden Turmeric™ powder is an excellent source of curcuminoids, which support overall wellness in the body. Chronic, low-level inflammation plays a major role in almost every Western disease from high cholesterol to heart disease, arthritis, and others. Therefore, anything that can help to fight chronic inflammation is of potential importance in preventing and treating these diseases and bolstering overall health.

- **Turmeric extract (Curcuma longa):** Turmeric has strong anti-inflammatory properties[2] that match the effectiveness of some anti-inflammatory drugs[3,4]. It is a potent antioxidant that neutralizes free radicals[5] and boosts the activity of the body's own antioxidant enzymes[6].

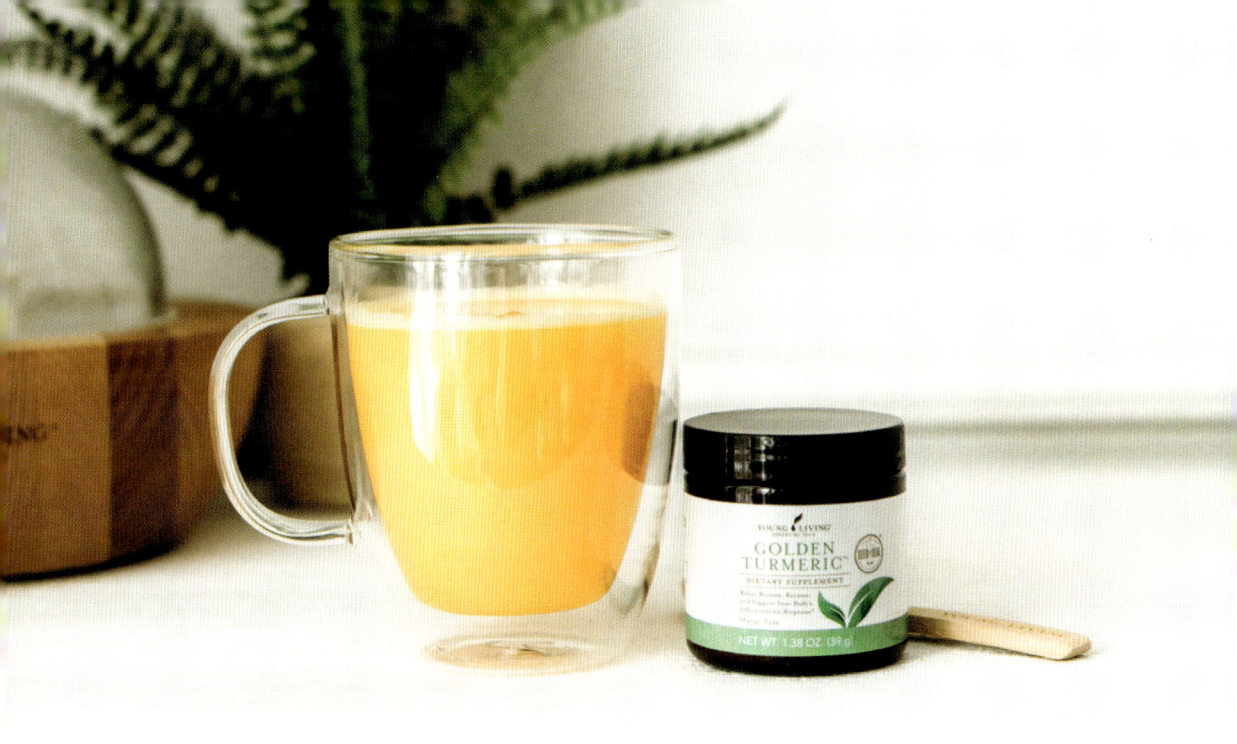

- **Boswellia resin extract**: Boswellia has both anti-inflammatory and antioxidant properties[7] that add to the effects of curcumin. It has been long revered for its health properties, including strong immune-enhancing effects[8] and the ability to improve cognition and memory[9]. Additionally, it may have anti-inflammatory and anti-tumor effects[10] due to its antioxidant property.
- **Ginger essential oil**: Ginger has analgesic, anti-inflammatory, antibacterial, and antioxidant properties. It is great for soothing digestion[11], contains powerful antioxidants that can protect against oxidative stress, combats inflammation[12], and promotes liver health[13].
- **Lime essential oil:** Lime is high in limonene, a constituent that is known to strengthen the immune system and helps to decongest the lymphatic system.

Young Living's Golden Turmeric™ powder is a great choice for just about anyone, whether you have chronic health needs, are an athlete or avid exerciser who is prone to inflammation, or a health-conscious adult wanting to do everything you can to promote overall health, wellness, and vitality.

Safety notes: Keep out of reach of children. If you are pregnant, nursing, taking medication, or have a medical condition, consult a healthcare professional before use.

GOLDEN TURMERIC™

To use: Mix 1/2 tsp. in 6-8 oz. of water, juice, herbal tea, a smoothie, NingXia Red®, or milk of choice once daily.

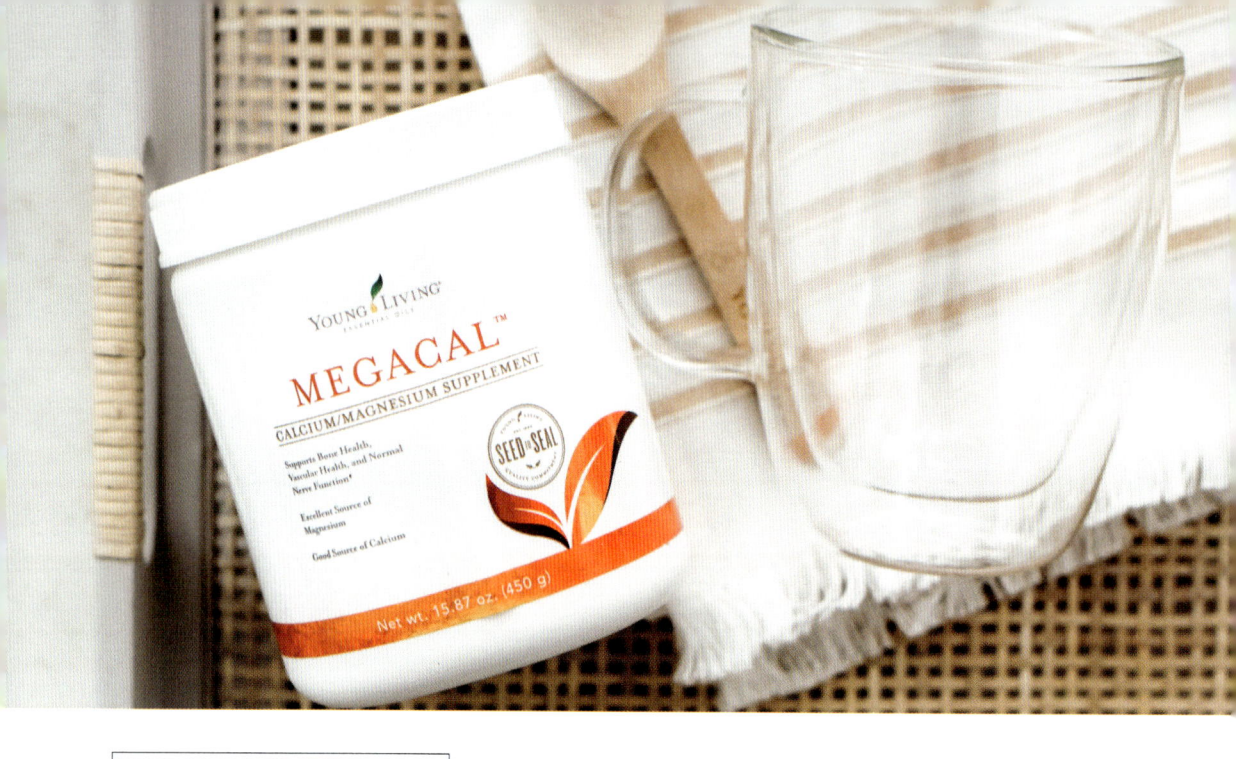

MEGACAL™

MegaCal™ is a calcium and mineral complex that supports healthy bones, heart, and nerve function with a 1:1 calcium to magnesium ratio. Additionally, the formula contains minerals such as zinc, copper, and manganese, which are required for the body to absorb and assimilate calcium.

BENEFITS OF MEGACAL™
- An excellent source of calcium, magnesium, and vitamin C
- Supports a healthy heart, bones, and nervous system
- Contains 207 mg of calcium and 188 mg of magnesium per serving
- Balances calcium with minerals, such as zinc, copper, and manganese
- Supports healthy energy levels and muscle function

Calcium and magnesium are both required to maintain healthy bones and teeth and play a role in energy levels and muscle tone. These two essential nutrients keep nerves and muscles functioning properly, including the heart muscle.
- **Vitamin C**: Vitamin C is a potent antioxidant that is essential for the growth and repair of tissues, wound healing, and the repair and maintenance of cartilage, bones, and teeth.
- **Calcium** (carbonate): Calcium assists in blood clotting, muscle contraction, cholesterol metabolism, healthy blood pressure levels, and nerve transmission. It enables normal bodily movement by keeping tissue rigid, strong, and flexible and is essential for healthy bones and teeth.
- **Magnesium** (sulfate and carbonate): Magnesium is essential for more than 300 enzyme systems within the body to regulate everything: from protein synthesis to muscle and

nerve function, blood glucose levels, and blood pressure. It contributes to the structural development of bone and is required for energy production and the synthesis of DNA, RNA, and glutathione, the body's primary antioxidant. Additionally, it plays a role in muscle contraction and helps to maintain a normal heart rhythm.
- **Zinc**: Zinc is an essential trace element that helps to strengthen the immune system, is required for calcium uptake, and supports muscle health and energy levels.
- **Manganese:** Manganese is a cofactor that is required for enzyme activity in the body. It plays a role in amino acid, cholesterol, glucose, and carbohydrate metabolism, reactive oxygen species scavenging, bone formation, reproduction, and immune response
- **Lemon and lime essential oils:** These oils are high in limonene, a constituent that strengthens the immune system, helps to decongest the lymphatic system and improves nutrient absorption.

MegaCal™ makes a great substitute for powdered magnesium supplements that are often used to promote healthy sleep, encourage muscle relaxation and recovery, and ease stress.

> **MEGACAL™**
>
> **To use:** Take one scoop (1 tsp.) with one cup (240 mL) of water or juice daily, one hour after a meal or taking medication or an hour before bedtime. Do not exceed three servings daily.

Safety notes: For human consumption only. Keep out of reach of children. If you are pregnant, nursing, taking medications, or have a medical condition, consult a health practitioner before use. Not suitable for pets.

SULFURZYME®

Sulfurzyme® supports overall wellness by bolstering your joints, aiding your immune system, and supporting normal metabolic function, circulation, and bone, hair, and skin health. This supplement is a unique combination of MSM (the protein-building compound that is found in breast milk, fresh fruits, and vegetables) and NingXia wolfberry. Together, they create a new concept by balancing the immune system and supporting almost every major function of the body.

BENEFITS OF SULFURZYME®
- Promotes healthy hair, skin, and nails
- Wonderful source of MSM, which helps with inflammation
- Bolsters the immune system

- Supports joints and muscles and helps to improve muscle recovery[142]
- Works synergistically when combined with other joint supplements
- May be beneficial for inflammatory skin and gut issues, such as eczema, Crohn's disease, and IBD

Sulfurzyme® is a wonderful choice for everyone because none of us are getting enough MSM in our diets. The MSM that we do get is likely less robust and not as bioavailable as that found in Sulfurzyme®. Weak and brittle nails, hair that doesn't grow or seems dull, joints that are painful, and skin issues can all be signs that you need more MSM in your diet or supplement routine. Skin that is ultra-sensitive to the topical use of oils (even diluted) can be another telltale sign that MSM would be beneficial. Sulfurzyme® is one supplement that can help you to benefit from everything else that you are doing to increase overall vitality.

HEALTH BENEFITS OF MSM

- *Helps to treat arthritis symptoms*: MSM helps to control inflammation, reduces pain, and acts as a source of sulfur, which is needed for joint health[141].
- *Makes skin healthier*: Hair, skin, and nail cells all contain large amounts of keratin and require sulfur to stay strong and healthy. MSM provides the necessary support to protect against accelerated aging, stretch marks, and sunburn and helps the skin to heal faster[143].
- *Eases menstrual cycle pain*: MSM can reduce inflammation and soothe the pain that is associated with menstrual cycles.
- *Helps to treat IBD:* Studies show that MSM is an effective treatment against certain inflammatory bowel diseases, such as Crohn's disease and colitis.
- *Improves immune function*: The sulfur in MSM helps to fortify muscles and soothes the stress that is placed on joints, which improves muscular function. Additionally, it contains antioxidants that help to tackle the free radicals that damage the immune system.

"What makes this product different from the other products is the exceptional purity of the MSM that we use. This pharmaceutical-grade MSM in Sulfurzyme® is light years away from the low-grade material imported from Asia. Unfortunately, a great deal of the MSM sold in the US originates from Asia. I believe that the key ingredient that makes Sulfurzyme® so effective is the Chinese wolfberry. With over 18 amino acids and 21 minerals, the wolfberry is one of the most nutrient-dense foods known. Few people realize that in order for us and our pets to properly metabolize the sulfur in MSM, the body requires minerals like molybdenum.

SULFURZYME®

To use: For the capsules: Take two capsules once daily, one hour before or after meals.

For the powder: Mix 1/2 tsp. with juice or distilled water and take twice daily, one hour before or after meals. Keep in a cool dry place. Do not expose to excessive heat or direct sunlight.

When these are missing, MSM does not work as well. This is why wolfberry is so important."
—D. Gary Young, founder of Young Living

Sulfurzyme® powder and capsules combine the power of MSM with the NingXia wolfberry, which is a nutrient powerhouse. The addition of the wolfberry provides the antioxidants, minerals, and co-enzymes that are required for sulfur metabolism and absorption.

FAQ

Q: Can pregnant and nursing women take this supplement?

A: Most believe that it is safe and beneficial for both the mother and baby. Please do your own research and decide based on what you feel is best as the mother.

Q: Can kids or pets take this supplement?

A: Yes! And with great benefit. The powder version is easy to slip into other foods or drinks.

Q: What's the difference between the powder and the capsule?

A: The only difference is that the powder contains stevia as a sweetener to enhance the taste.

Safety notes: Keep out of reach of children. If you are pregnant, nursing, taking medication, or have a medical condition, consult a healthcare professional before use.

SUPER CAL PLUS™

We have all heard how important calcium is for bone and muscle health, and evidence shows that adequate calcium and vitamin D intake can help prevent bone loss[148]. Unfortunately, conventional over-the-counter supplements are incomplete in their formulations or are full of less-than-ideal ingredients. Super Cal Plus™ from Young Living has been formulated as more than just a calcium supplement—it is a full-spectrum bone health supplement.

BENEFITS OF SUPER CAL PLUS™
- A synergistic blend of bioavailable calcium, magnesium, and other trace minerals that are derived from sustainably sourced red algae
- Helps to maintain and support the structure, integrity, and density of bones
- Supports the body's ability to resorb bone tissue (osteoclasts) and deposit new bone tissue (osteoblasts)
- An excellent source of calcium, magnesium, vitamin K, and vitamin D

Calcium is the most abundant mineral in the body because it is involved in so many processes. Calcium is needed for proper blood circulation, heart health, muscle movement, healthy teeth, and the release of hormones. Calcium helps to carry messages from the brain to all the parts of the body and is required to keep bones strong and dense. To say that it is important is a vast understatement.

CALCIUM AND BONE HEALTH

If calcium levels are low, the body will take stored calcium from the bones to release into the blood. Our innate survival system will prioritize the use of available calcium for nerve and muscle function to keep the heart pumping blood. Therefore, calcium is required for bone health, especially as we age. If we don't have enough of it, our bones will pay the price.

As we age, our bodies tend to resorb bones faster than the new tissue can be deposited, which is a big reason why calcium, magnesium, and vitamin D supplementation is incredibly important. This is even more important for individuals with risk factors for bone density issues and those with chronic illness, as these place a physical toll on the body. Adding Super Cal Plus™ to your daily wellness routine is a wonderful way to support a healthy bone structure, especially as we age.

Finding a good calcium supplement isn't easy. We want something that is readily absorbed, sustainably sourced from nature (not made in a lab), and combined with other essential vitamins and nutrients, such as magnesium and vitamin D. When added together, these components create a true bone health supplement that can support healthy bones from multiple angles.

Super Cal Plus™ is more than just calcium. This product combines a synergistic blend of bioavailable calcium, magnesium, and other trace minerals that are derived from red algae with essential oils to create a true bone health supplement. Super Cal Plus™ helps the body to maintain healthy bones by supporting the body's ability to resorb bone tissue (osteoclasts) and deposit new bone tissue (osteoblasts)—a process that happens naturally but often becomes out of balance with age. Moreover, adequate calcium and vitamin D intake throughout life in combination with a well-balanced diet and gentle exercise helps to reduce the risk of osteoporosis[148].

- **Vitamin D**: Vitamin D is essential for calcium absorption, supports optimal brain health, hormone levels, bone, teeth, and joint health, and overall well-being, and plays a role in mood regulation and immunity.
- **Vitamin K**: Vitamin K helps to regulate normal blood clotting and kidney function and assists in the absorption of other vitamins and minerals.
- **Calcium**: Calcium assists in blood clotting, muscle contraction, cholesterol metabolism, healthy blood pressure levels, and nerve transmission. It is required to keep the heart pumping, allows normal bodily movement by keeping tissue rigid, strong, and flexible, and is essential for healthy bones and teeth.

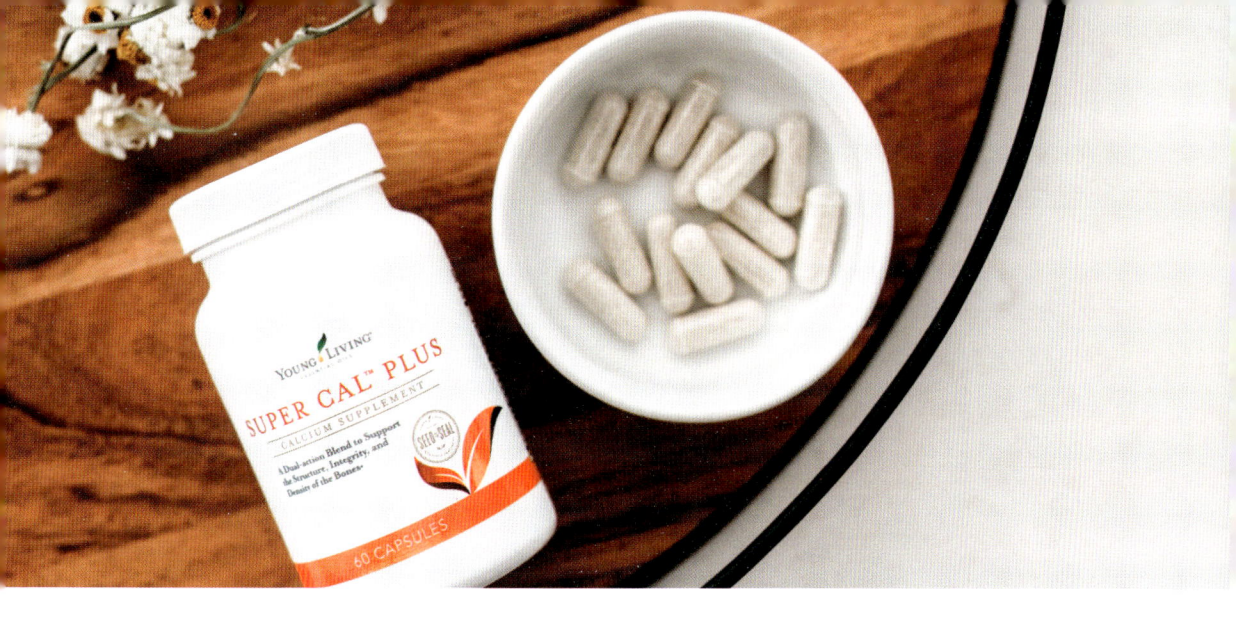

- **Magnesium**: Magnesium works alongside calcium to promote healthy teeth and bones, is crucial for enzyme function and muscle contractions, and supports healthy blood pressure levels.
- **Black spruce and Idaho blue spruce essential oils**: Blue and black spruce support the body's pain response to inflammation and injury, specifically within the joints, and are high in alpha-pinene, a constituent that reduces inflammation and oxidative stress. Alpha-pinene prevents bone resorption[146], supports hormone balance, and helps the body to reduce pain signals[87].
- **Copaiba essential oil**: Copaiba is high in sesquiterpenes, which have anti-inflammatory properties[147] that help the body to recover from injury. Additionally, it supports bone and joint health.
- **Vetiver essential oil**: Vetiver is high in sesquiterpenes which have anti-inflammatory properties[147] and aid in conditions such as arthritis. It has historically been used to treat inflammation.
- **Peppermint essential oil**: Peppermint soothes digestion, supports muscles and tendons, helps the body to absorb minerals, and supports the body's response to inflammation.

WHAT IS OSTEOPOROSIS?

Bone is living tissue that is constantly being broken down and replaced. Osteoporosis occurs when the creation of new bone doesn't keep up with the loss of old bone.

Although osteoporosis affects both men and women, out of 10 million Americans with osteoporosis, approximately 80% are women. According to the International Osteoporosis Foundation, osteoporosis and low bone mass affect approximately 44 million women and men over the age of 50 in the US, and approximately one in two women over the age of 50 will break a bone because of osteoporosis. That means that **a little over half the population aged 50 and older experience osteoporosis**[144]. To say that this is an important area of support is an understatement. However, there is a lot that we can do to help keep our bones strong and healthy.

Several factors can contribute to osteoporosis. According to the Mayo Clinic[145], some of the most common are:
- *Family tree:* If you have a family member, such as a sibling or parent, with osteoporosis, you are more likely to have the disease yourself.
- *Age:* Osteoporosis is more prevalent among people who are aged 50 years and older.
- *Small frames:* Because women and men with small body frames have less bone mass to lose, they are at higher risk for osteoporosis due to the decrease in bone mass over time.
- *Insufficient calcium intake:* A lack of calcium across a lifetime can cause reduced bone density.
- *Lack of exercise:* Those who tend to sit all day, such as at desk jobs, or who don't exercise enough are more prone to osteoporosis.

We often think about building our muscles, but what about the structure that supports us? Caring for your bones while you're young will give you the best results; however, there is hope for everyone, regardless of age. Follow these tips by the National Institute of Arthritis and Musculoskeletal and Skin Disease to help keep your bones healthy and strong.
- *Get enough calcium and vitamin D*: Eating a well-balanced diet and getting enough calcium and vitamin D will greatly improve your chances of avoiding osteoporosis.
- *Get up and move*: The more you move, the stronger your bones will become. Weight-bearing exercises, such as walking, running, dancing, and tennis, are typically best for creating and maintaining strong and healthy bones.
- *Quit smoking and limit drinking*: Smoking negatively affects your bones, heart, and lungs. If you smoke, you may absorb less calcium from the foods that you eat. An excessive consumption of alcohol may also affect bone health. Limit your alcohol intake; your bones will thank you.

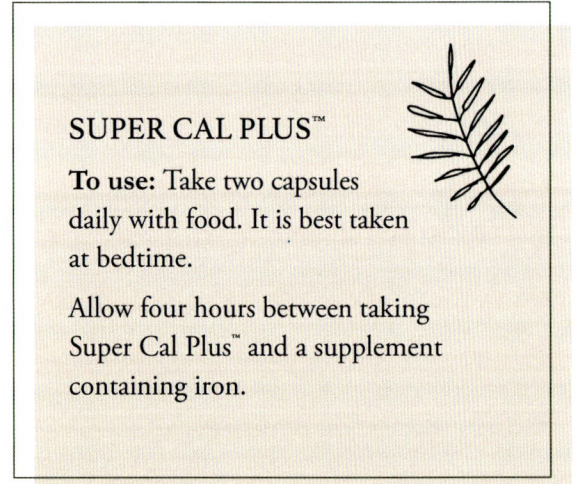

SUPER CAL PLUS™

To use: Take two capsules daily with food. It is best taken at bedtime.

Allow four hours between taking Super Cal Plus™ and a supplement containing iron.

Safety notes: Keep out of reach of children. If you are pregnant or nursing, taking medication, or have a medical condition, consult a health professional before use.

SUPER VITAMIN D

Find more information on Super Vitamin D in the "Foundational Supplements" section on page 54.

Vitamin D is one of those supplements that gets a lot of hype, and for good reason. It's estimated that between 40% and 70% of the US population is deficient in vitamin D[63], and this vitamin is a powerhouse when it comes to our health. Immune, respiratory, bone, and joint health, emotions, and autoimmune needs are all supported with healthy vitamin D levels.

"The Vitamin D Council—a scientist-led group promoting vitamin D deficiency awareness—suggests vitamin D treatment might be found helpful in treating or preventing autoimmune disease, chronic pain, depression, diabetes, heart disease, high blood pressure, flu, and osteoporosis."—WebMD

VITAMIN D AND BONE HEALTH

When it comes to healthy bones, calcium is likely to be the nutrient that you think of first. However, vitamin D is just as important for keeping bones strong and preventing osteoporosis[148]. Vitamin D helps your intestines to absorb calcium from the food that you eat, so getting enough of both nutrients is an important part of making sure that your bones are dense and strong. Low calcium and vitamin D levels often occur together, since absorption of calcium is connected to vitamin D and vice versa.

Young Living's Super Vitamin D is a highly absorbable, vegan-friendly tablet that is made with lemon balm extract and lime and Melissa essential oils. These essential oils help to increase the bioavailability of vitamin D and support mood and hormone regulation. Furthermore, vitamin D is supplied as D3, which is an important designation. This active metabolite is responsible for all the wonderful health benefits that we want.

> **SUPER VITAMIN D**
>
> **To use:** Take one to two tablets daily with food. Place in the mouth and allow to dissolve for five to ten seconds, then chew for optimal results. Note: Each sublingual tablet contains 1,000 IU vitamin D.

Safety notes: Keep out of reach of children. If you are pregnant, nursing, taking medication, or have a medical condition, consult a healthcare professional before use.

Protocols For Bone & Muscle Health

Whether you are looking for general support for an active lifestyle or need more acute support for specific bone and muscle needs, these protocols are a great place to start.

MUSCLE & BONE HEALTH
- AgilEase® or BLM™
- Golden Turmeric™
- NingXia Red®
- Sulfurzyme®
- Super Cal Plus™
- Super Vitamin D
- Options for more support: AminoWise™, MegaCal™, Pure Protein Complete™

PHYSICAL FITNESS & PERFORMANCE
- AgilEase® or BLM™
- AminoWise™
- Golden Turmeric™
- Master Formula™
- NingXia Red®
- PowerGize™
- Pure Protein Complete™
- Sulfurzyme®
- Super B™
- Super Vitamin D

AGING SUPPORT SUPPORT
- BLM™ (or AgilEase® if necessary)
- Super Cal Plus™
- Golden Turmeric™
- Longevity™
- Life 9®
- NingXia Red®
- OmegaGize³®
- Sulfurzyme®

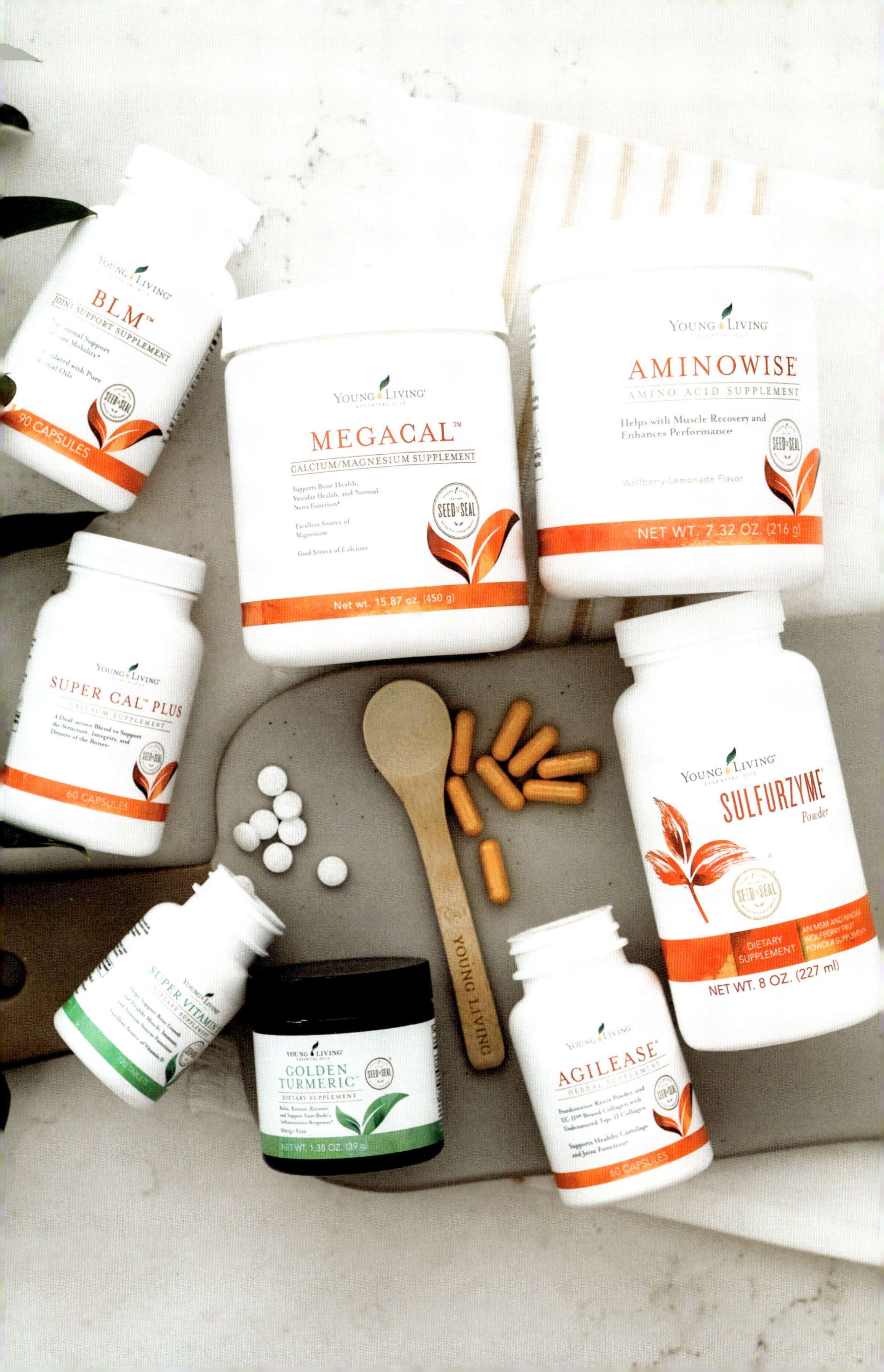
YOUNG LIVING
BLM™
JOINT SUPPORT SUPPLEMENT
90 CAPSULES
YOUNG LIVING
MEGACAL™
CALCIUM/MAGNESIUM SUPPLEMENT
Supports Bone Health, Vascular Health, and Normal Nerve Function*
Excellent Source of Magnesium
Good Source of Calcium
Net wt. 15.87 oz. (450 g)
YOUNG LIVING
AMINOWISE
AMINO ACID SUPPLEMENT
Helps with Muscle Recovery and Enhances Performance
Wolfberry-Lemonade Flavor
NET WT. 7.32 OZ. (216 g)
YOUNG LIVING
SUPER CAL™ PLUS
CALCIUM SUPPLEMENT
A Dual-action Blend to Support the Structure, Integrity, and Density of the Bones*
60 CAPSULES
YOUNG LIVING
SULFURZYME
Powder
DIETARY SUPPLEMENT
NET WT. 8 OZ. (227 ml)
YOUNG LIVING
YOUNG LIVING
GOLDEN TURMERIC™
DIETARY SUPPLEMENT
Mango Rose
NET WT. 1.38 OZ. (39 g)
YOUNG LIVING
AGILEASE
HERBAL SUPPLEMENT
60 CAPSULES

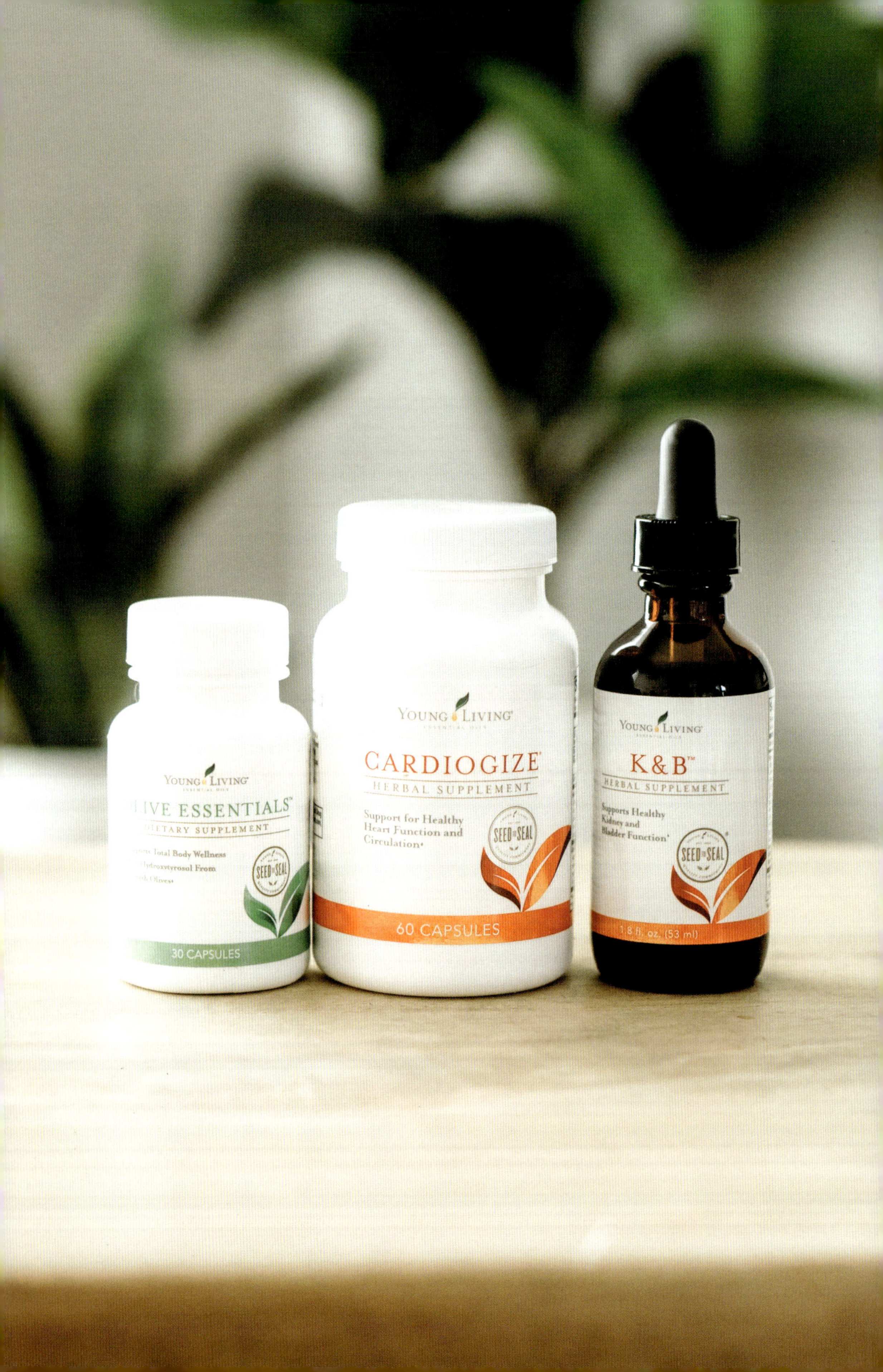
Young Living
30 CAPSULES
Young Living
CARDIOGIZE
HERBAL SUPPLEMENT
Support for Healthy Heart Function and Circulation*
60 CAPSULES
Young Living
K&B
HERBAL SUPPLEMENT
Supports Healthy Kidney and Bladder Function*
1.8 fl. oz. (53 ml)

Part 6: OTHER TARGETED SUPPLEMENTS (HEART, BLADDER, EYES, BRAIN)

One of the things that I love about Young Living supplements is the availability of options for targeted support. This is something that is hard to find elsewhere because many health food stores contain an overabundance of options with unclear designations. Additionally, the ingredients that are used in Young Living supplements are high quality and add value to the formulation, so you can be confident knowing that you're supporting these targeted areas.

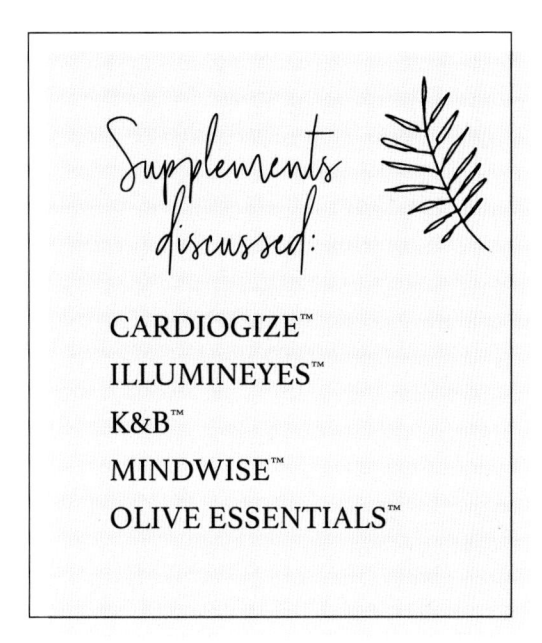

Supplements discussed:

CARDIOGIZE™
ILLUMINEYES™
K&B™
MINDWISE™
OLIVE ESSENTIALS™

CARDIOGIZE™

CardioGize™ is a daily supplement that is formulated with powerful ingredients, such as CoQ10, selenium, garlic, astragalus, dong quai, motherwort, and hawthorn berry, that support the cardiovascular system. These compounds are combined with essential oils and more to promote heart and vascular health and improve circulation.

BENEFITS OF CARDIOGIZE™
- Supports healthy heart function and blood circulation
- Features astragalus and dong quai, which have been used traditionally in China for their synergistic properties to support the cardiovascular system
- Includes motherwort and hawthorn berry, which have been used traditionally to support the cardiovascular system
- Contains deodorized garlic extract and CoQ10 to promote healthy circulation
- Supports vascular health with vitamin K2

Finding a good heart health supplement can be daunting, as there are a lot of great herbs that support blood pressure, circulation, and cholesterol levels. The combination of ingredients in CardioGize™ works synergistically to improve all these areas and more to create an overall heart health supplement.
- **Garlic bulb extract**: Garlic helps to reduce cholesterol and blood pressure levels[149,150], prevents plaque buildup in the arteries[151], bolsters the immune system, and acts as an antioxidant.
- **CoQ10**: CoQ10 is a powerful antioxidant that supports every cell in the body. It acts as a battery for our cells, helping with the production and exchange of energy and helps to facilitate the production of ATP, which is the energy currency within the body.
- **Astragalus root powder**: Astragalus root is an adaptogenic herb with anti-inflammatory and antioxidant properties. It is high in flavonoids, which prevent plaque buildup and lower cholesterol and blood pressure levels[152].
- **Dong quai root powder**: This herb was traditionally used in Chinese medicine to help lower triglyceride[153] and blood pressure levels and support hormone balance and healthy insulin levels[154].
- **Motherwort powder:** Motherwort helps to calm nervous tension and lowers an elevated heart rate.
- **Cat's claw powder:** Cat's claw has antiviral, anti-inflammatory, anti-mutagenic, and antioxidant properties. It helps to prevent the formation of blood clots[155] and lowers blood pressure[156].
- **Hawthorne berry powder**: Hawthorne berry is a potent antioxidant that is high in flavonoids, which decrease inflammation while boosting immune function. It has long been used for its cardioprotective properties to help tone the heart and provides relief from symptoms of heart failure, heart disease, and angina[157]. Additionally, it helps to lower blood pressure and cholesterol levels[158].

- **Cactus cladode powder:** This herb is high in phenols and fiber, which support overall heart health and help to lower cholesterol levels.
- **Cardamom seed powder**: Cardamom helps to lower blood pressure[159] and is high in manganese, which helps to regulate blood sugar levels.
- **Angelica essential oil:** Angelica has natural diuretic properties, which help to lower blood pressure. It calms the cardiovascular and nervous systems.
- **Cardamom essential oil:** Cardamom is another potent antioxidant with heart protective effects[30] that helps to stimulate healthy digestion. It contains the constituent 1,8-cineole, which has been shown to be highly beneficial for its antimicrobial ability.
- **Cypress essential oil:** Cypress is high in antioxidants that naturally lower cholesterol, purify the liver, and promote the removal of toxins[160]. It stimulates healthy circulation and blood flow.
- **Lavender essential oil:** Lavender increases the activity of endogenous antioxidants, such as glutathione. Additionally, it calms the body and mind, helps to reduce the negative effects of oxidative stress[161], supports physical and emotional relaxation, decreases the stress response within the body[115], and has shown antidepressant activity in clinical studies[116].
- **Helichrysum essential oil:** Helichrysum is powerful antioxidant that lowers inflammation, boosts immunity, and acts as a natural diuretic to support cardiovascular health.
- **Rosemary essential oil**: Rosemary helps to balance the endocrine system, cleanses the liver, reduces free radical damage, lowers cortisol (stress hormone)[162], promotes heart health, and helps to maintain healthy blood sugar levels[163].
- **Cinnamon bark essential oil**: Cinnamon bark supports healthy blood sugar levels, provides immune support through its antimicrobial activity, and acts as an antioxidant. Additionally, it contains high levels of phenols, which are oxygenating compounds that function as catalysts for essential enzyme function.

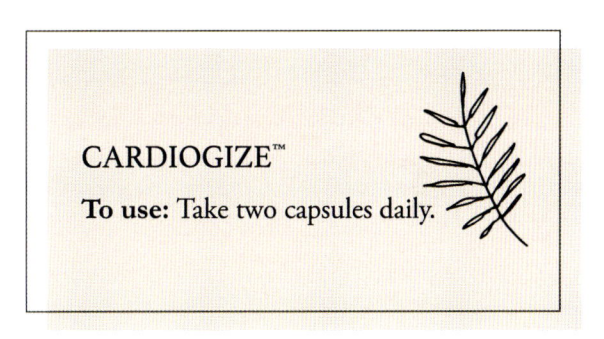

CARDIOGIZE™
To use: Take two capsules daily.

Safety notes: Keep out of reach of children. If you are pregnant, nursing, taking medication, or have a medical condition, consult a health professional before use.

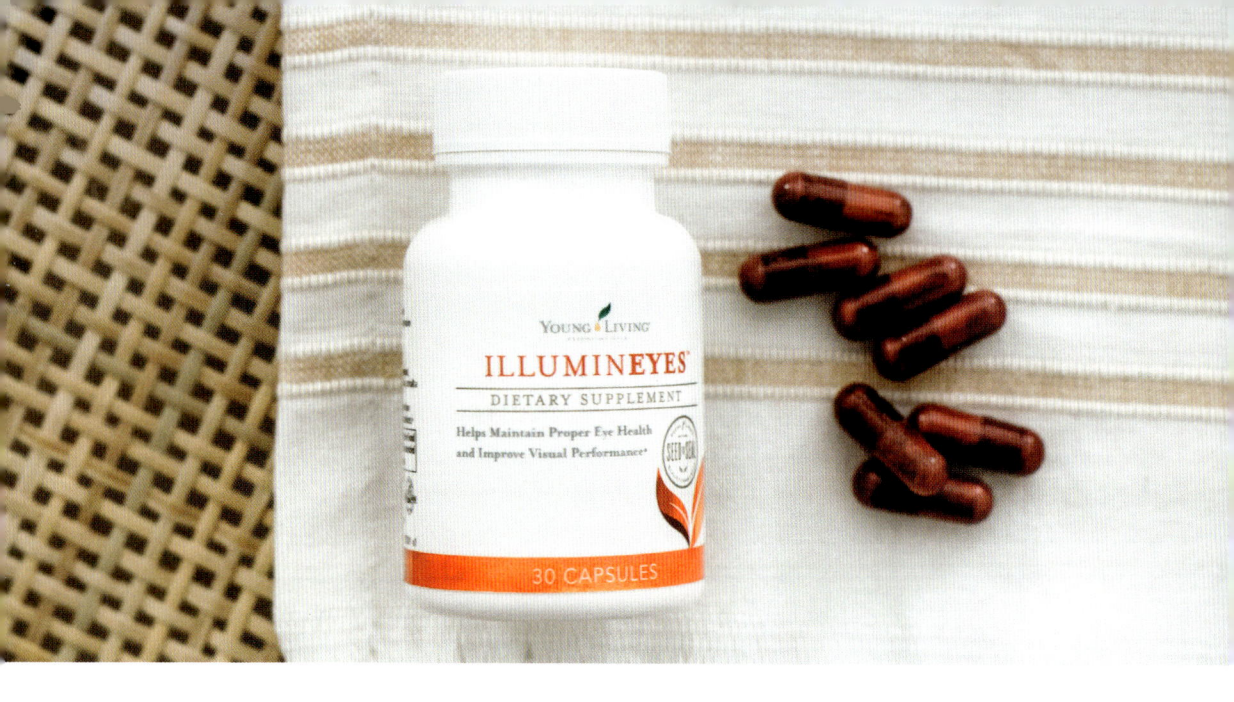

ILLUMINEYES™

IlluminEyes™ is a powerful eye health supplement that includes lutein and zeaxanthin and helps to reduce eye strain. It protects eyes from damaging blue light, maintains long-term eye health, and promotes vibrant skin and hair.

BENEFITS OF ILLUMINEYES™
- Protects eyes from damaging blue light
- Supports vision in low-light settings
- Helps to reduce eye fatigue and eye strain
- Increases macular pigment optical density
- May help to reduce eye health deterioration, which is common with age
- Maintains healthy-looking skin

IlluminEyes™ contains all the great eye health vitamins in the age-related eye disease study (AREDS) formulations you'll find at the pharmacy. Lutein and zeaxanthin are key players in the blend, and vitamins A and C have properties that reduce eye health deterioration, which is commonly related to age.
- **Vitamin A**: Vitamin A is a powerful antioxidant that improves eye health, reduces macular degeneration[164], increases collagen production, treats mild acne, and moisturizes the skin.
- **Vitamin C**: Vitamin C is a potent antioxidant that helps to reduce macular degeneration[164]. It is essential for the growth and repair of tissues, healing wounds, and the repair and maintenance of cartilage, bones, and teeth.

- **Vitamin E**: Vitamin E is a natural antioxidant that helps to reduce macular degeneration[164], minimizes free radical damage within the body, and promotes healthy cell function and overall health.
- **Lutein (from marigold flower):** This well-known antioxidant supports eye health, protects against macular degeneration[165], fights free radical damage from blue light exposure, helps to protect skin health[166], and may be beneficial in diabetes[167].
- **Zeaxanthin (from marigold flower):** This popular antioxidant works alongside lutein to promote eye health, protect against macular degeneration[165], and reduce damage from ultraviolet light exposure.
- **Wolfberry fruit powder:** The wolfberry is one of the best known antioxidant nutrients. It is wonderful for strengthening the immune system, promoting overall wellness, and combating carcinogens.
- **Marigold flower extract:** Marigold lowers inflammation and reduces free radical damage.
- **Acerola cherry extract:** This antioxidant supports eye and skin health and is a source of vitamin C and phytonutrients.

AREDS TRIALS[168]

The National Eye Institute conducted the following two trials on supplementation for eye health and cataract and age-related macular degeneration (AMD)—AREDS and the follow-up AREDS2. The studies found that the participants who took the antioxidants lutein and zeaxanthin with zinc and copper were 25%-30% less likely to develop advanced AMD than those who had originally been assigned a placebo. The formulations that were tested in the trials are now sold as the AREDS and AREDS2 formulas and contain vitamins A, C, and E, copper, zinc, lutein, and zeaxanthin and are considered the "gold standard" in eye health supplements. IlluminEyes™ from Young Living also contains these same ingredients.

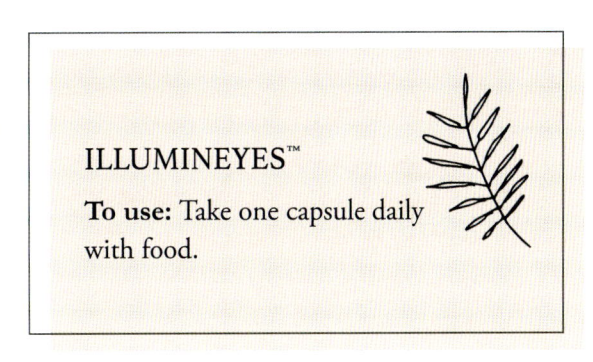

ILLUMINEYES™

To use: Take one capsule daily with food.

Safety notes: Keep out of reach of children. If you are pregnant, nursing, taking medication, or have a medical condition, consult a health professional before use.

K&B™

K&B™ is a kidney and bladder supplement that helps to maintain a healthy fluid balance and urinary and digestive health. K&B™ combines juniper berries, parsley, uva ursi, and essential oils for a tincture that helps to fortify the kidney and bladder against infections and other conditions.

BENEFITS OF K&B™
- Formulated to support normal kidney and bladder health
- Helps to fight against infection and other kidney and bladder conditions
- Combines herbs and essential oils
- Includes juniper berry extract, uva ursi extract, and parsley extract
- Includes the kidney and bladder supportive oils clove, fennel, Roman chamomile, sage, and juniper

The kidneys are two bean-shaped organs that are located just below the rib cage on each side of the spine. The kidneys maintain a healthy balance of water, salts, and minerals, such as sodium, calcium, phosphorus, and potassium, which is essential for nerves, muscles, and other tissues in the body to work normally. In addition, the kidneys make hormones that help to control blood pressure, produce red blood cells, and maintain healthy bones.

The kidneys work constantly to filter the blood by removing waste and extra water to make urine. Urine flows from the kidneys to the bladder, where it is stored until it's excreted. A healthy kidney and bladder system is crucial to overall health, and when this system is out of balance, the effects are often painful. K&B™ works to promote healthy kidney and bladder function with herbs and essential oils that purify and support these organs internally.

- **Juniper berry extract:** Juniper is a natural antiseptic that cleanses the urinary tract. It is high in antioxidants and promotes healthy filtration in the kidneys.
- **Parsley leaf extract**: Parsley leaf is commonly used in herbal medicine to cleanse and purify the urinary tract and is high in antioxidants, which support liver health.
- **Uva ursi leaf extract:** This herb contains flavonoids, tannins, terpenoids, and hydroquinone glycosides that can help to treat urinary tract infections and reduce bacteria that accumulate in the urethra and bladder. It acts as a natural diuretic to promote filtration in the kidneys.
- **Dandelion root extract**: Dandelion root is commonly used in herbal teas and supplements for digestive support and promotes healthy bile flow and liver function.
- **Royal jelly:** Royal jelly is a natural bee product that is fed to queen bees and is rich in amino acids, minerals, and B vitamins. It stimulates the adrenal glands and has antioxidant and anti-inflammatory properties.
- **Geranium essential oil:** Geranium promotes healthy hormone balance, aids circulation, and is a natural diuretic with anti-inflammatory and antimicrobial properties, which makes it a great choice for kidney and bladder support.

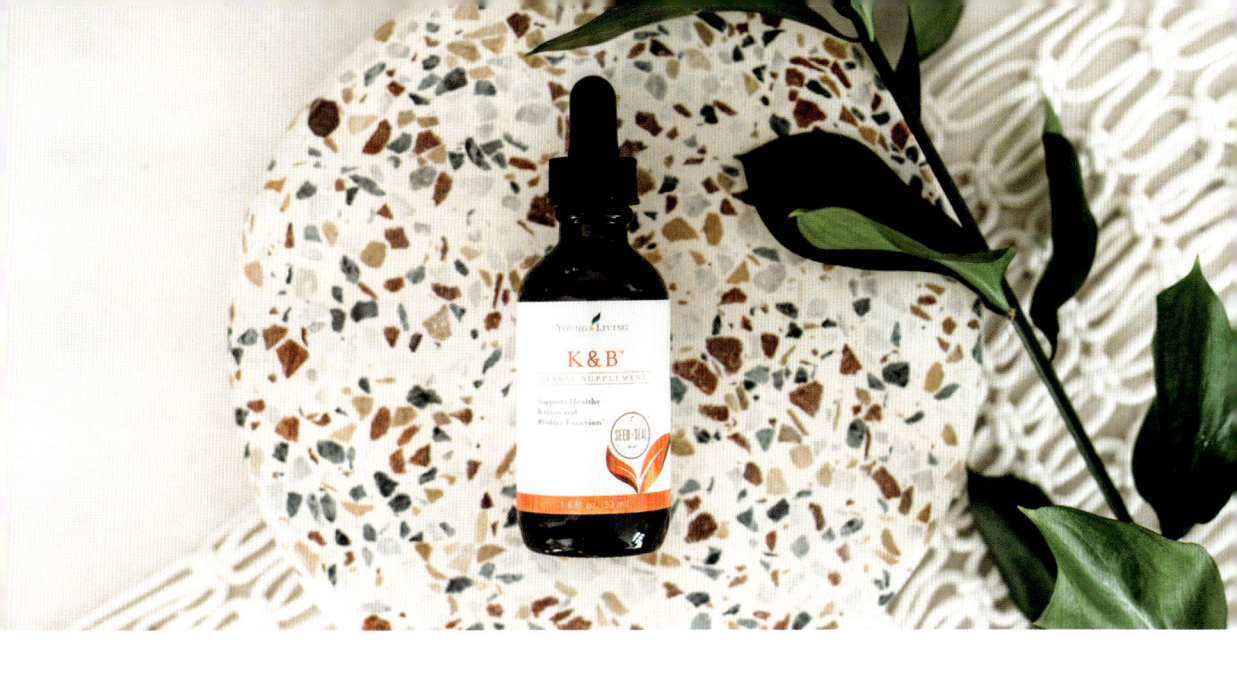

- **Fennel essential oil**: Fennel supports digestion, eases intestinal discomfort, supports pancreas and liver function, provides immune support, and promotes the excretion of toxins.
- **Clove essential oil**: Clove has a range of health benefits, most of which are due to its high antioxidant and anti-inflammatory activity. It has an average ORAC value of over 290,000[19] and can be effective at stopping the growth of some bacteria and fungi[20], including *Candida*[21], at higher doses.
- **Roman chamomile essential oil**: Roman chamomile contains antioxidants that promote healthy bile flow, which is an essential component of detoxification in the liver. It has anti-inflammatory properties that may be beneficial for kidney stones and infections.
- **Sage essential oil**: Sage helps to regulate hormones, promotes healthy digestion, has antioxidant, antiseptic, antiviral, and antifungal properties, stimulates the gallbladder, and supports healthy cholesterol levels[82].
- **Juniper essential oil**: Juniper is an antiseptic oil that purifies and helps to detoxify the kidney and bladder system. It acts as a diuretic to promote the excretion of toxins from the body.

K&B™

To use: Take three half droppers (3 mL) three times daily in distilled water, or as needed. Shake well before use.

Safety notes: Keep in a cool, dry place. Keep out of reach of children. Do not expose to excessive heat or direct sunlight. If pregnant or under a doctor's care, consult your physician or healthcare provider before use.

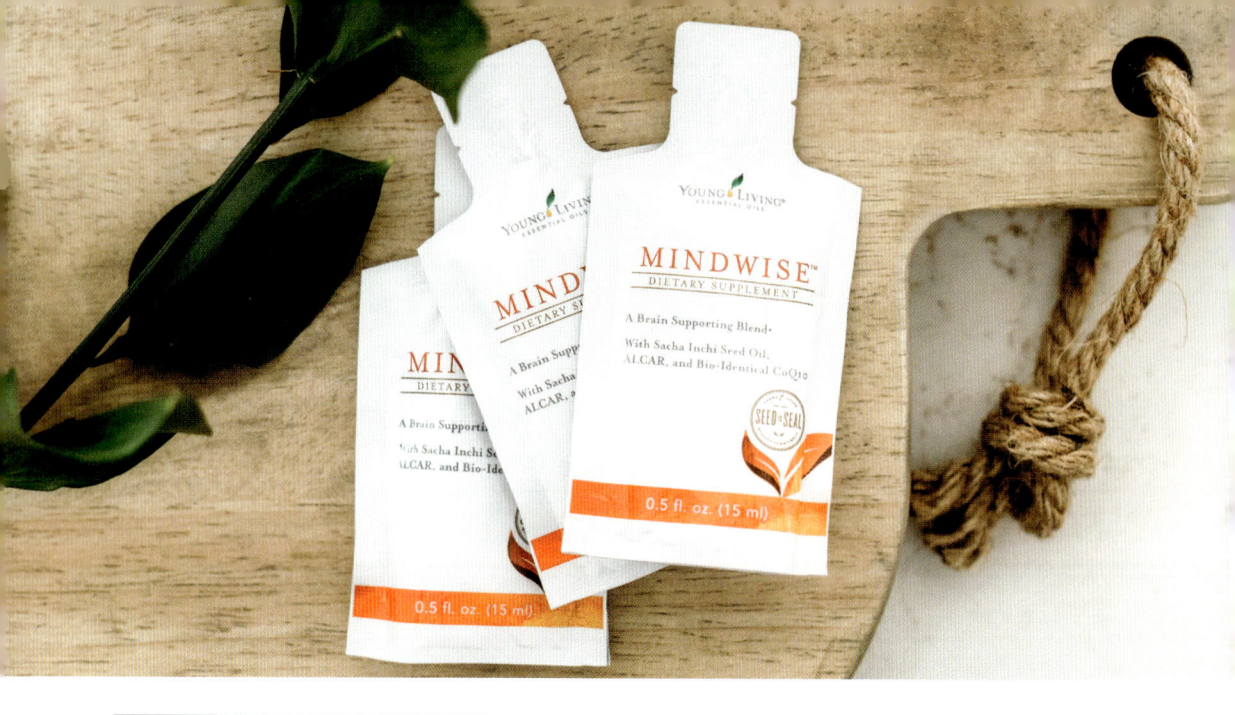

MINDWISE™

MindWise™ uses a combination of fruit juices and extracts, turmeric, and essential oils to create a heart and brain health supplement in liquid form. MindWise™ includes powerhouse ingredients, such as CoQ10, L-alpha glyceryl phosphorylcholine (GPC), and Acetyl-L-Carnitine (ALCAR), all of which are known to improve energy levels and cognitive health.

BENEFITS OF MINDWISE™
- Supports normal brain and heart function
- Contains a high proportion of unsaturated fatty acids and omega-3 fatty acids
- Includes GPC and ALCAR, which improve cognitive function
- Contains bioidentical CoQ10, which supports energy levels
- Includes vitamin D and turmeric, which are known for their health benefits

MindWise™ contains multiple ingredients that are beneficial for overall health, including vitamin D, turmeric root, medium-chain triglycerides (MCTs), and CoQ10. CoQ10 is an important ingredient in this supplement, as it is required within every cell of the body for the cell to function. Although many things can cause low levels of CoQ10, such as chronic diseases, vitamin B deficiency, and statin drugs, as we age, our levels naturally decline. This is when we need even more support from oxidative stress, which is why supplementation is a great choice.

- **Vitamin D:** Vitamin D is an essential vitamin for optimal brain health, hormone levels, bone, teeth, and joint health, and overall well-being. Additionally, it plays a role in mood regulation, immunity, and general wellness.
- **Pomegranate fruit extract:** This is an antioxidant source that supports cardiovascular health and cholesterol levels.

- **Rhododendron leaf extract:** Rhododendron leaf supports healthy blood pressure and cholesterol levels and has antioxidant and anti-inflammatory properties.
- **GPC:** GPC quickly and reliably delivers choline to the brain to create the cognition-boosting neurotransmitter acetylcholine and improves mood and cognitive function[169].
- **ALCAR:** This is a form of the amino acid L-carnitine, which can cross the blood brain barrier. This enables it to improve energy utilization and cognitive function and provide mood support.
- **Coenzyme Q10:** This antioxidant and coenzyme is required by every cell in the body;. It supports energy levels and cardiovascular health, slows the effects of aging, and supports cognitive health.
- **Turmeric root powder:** Turmeric has strong anti-inflammatory properties[2] that match the effectiveness of some anti-inflammatory drugs[3,4]. It is a potent antioxidant that can neutralize free radicals[5] and boosts the activity of the body's own antioxidant enzymes[6].
- **Sacha inchi seed oil:** Sacha inchi seed oil is a rich source of plant-based omega-3 and omega-6 fatty acids, which support healthy cholesterol levels, cognitive health, and heart health.
- **MCTs** (from fractionated coconut oil): MCTs protect heart health, lower LDL ("bad cholesterol) levels, raise HDL ("good" cholesterol) levels[170], and are supportive of brain and gut health. They can also combat harmful bacteria, viruses, fungi, and parasites.
- **Peppermint essential oil:** Peppermint soothes digestion, supports muscles and tendons, helps the body to absorb minerals, and supports the body's response to inflammation.
- **Fennel essential oil:** Fennel supports digestion, the pancreas, and liver, eases intestinal discomfort, provides immune support, and promotes the excretion of toxins.
- **Anise essential oil**: Anise supports overall digestion, acts as a diuretic to remove excess fluid from the body, supports circulation, has anti-inflammatory properties that help to ease intestinal cramping, and improves digestion.

MINDWISE™

To use (bottle):
- Adult initial dose: Take two tbsp. once daily for the first seven to ten days.
- Adult maintenance dose: Take one tbsp. once daily or as needed.
- Child dose (aged 4 to 12): Take one to two tsp. once daily.
- For optimal effect, adults should follow the initial dose schedule for seven to ten days, followed by the maintenance dose. MindWise™ should be taken with a meal. Shake well before use and refrigerate after opening.

To use (MindWise™ sachets):
- Drink one sachet daily. Consume promptly after opening. Should be taken with a meal. Shake well before use.

- **Lemon and lime essential oils:** These citrus oils are high in limonene, a constituent that strengthens the immune system and helps to decongest the lymphatic system. D-limonene alters the signaling pathways within cancer cells in a way that stops cancer cells from multiplying and causes their death[22].

Safety notes: Keep out of reach of children. If you are pregnant, nursing, taking medication, or have a medical condition, consult a health professional before use. Not recommended for children under the age of four. Do not drink directly from the bottle.

OLIVE ESSENTIALS™

Olive Essentials™ supports overall well-being and heart health with a combination of olive leaf oil, hydroxytyrosol, and key essential oils, such as Rosemary Vitality™ and Parsley Vitality™. These ingredients bolster immunity, protect heart health, and promote overall longevity.

BENEFITS OF OLIVE ESSENTIALS™
- Helps to support vascular and heart health
- Supports total body wellness, a healthy immune system, and internal cleansing
- Contains hydroxytyrosol, a powerful antioxidant that is derived from olive fruit and olive leaves
- Provides as much hydroxytyrosol as a liter of extra virgin olive oil in each capsule
- Features the antioxidant-rich, cleansing oils rosemary and parsley

According to an analysis of scientific studies, diets that are high in good-quality extra virgin olive oil are associated with "a lower incidence of atherosclerosis, cardiovascular disease, and certain types of cancer.[171]" The constituents of olive oil have powerful heart protective effects and can help to raise HDL ("good") cholesterol levels and lower LDL ("bad") cholesterol and triglycerides levels[172]. In addition, olive oil helps to reduce age- and disease-related inflammatory changes to the heart and blood vessels[173] and has antioxidant action that fights age-related cognitive decline[174].

Olive Essentials™ contains all the benefits of a Mediterranean diet in a convenient capsule. This formula specifically helps to promote a healthy heart with olive oil, hydroxytyrosol, and essential oils.
- **Hydroxytyrosol** (from olive fruit): This is a powerful antioxidant, whose physical structure allows it to easily enter cells and mitigate and repair cellular damage. It promotes healthy cholesterol levels and heart, brain, and skin health.

- **Olive fruit and extract**: This is a source of powerful antioxidants that have antioxidant, antihypertensive, and anti-inflammatory properties to promote immune, cardiovascular, cognitive, and skin health. It supports aging, promotes emotional balance, and may lower the risk of diabetes[175].
- **Parsley essential oil:** Parsley great source of the antioxidants luteolin, apigenin, lycopene, beta-carotene, and alpha-carotene, which reduce inflammation and free radical damage. It promotes intestinal cleansing, acts as a mild diuretic, supports kidney health[176], and bolsters immunity.
- **Rosemary essential oil**: Rosemary helps to balance the endocrine system, cleanses the liver, reduces free radical damage, and lowers cortisol (stress hormone)[162]. It promotes heart health and helps to maintain healthy blood sugar levels[163].

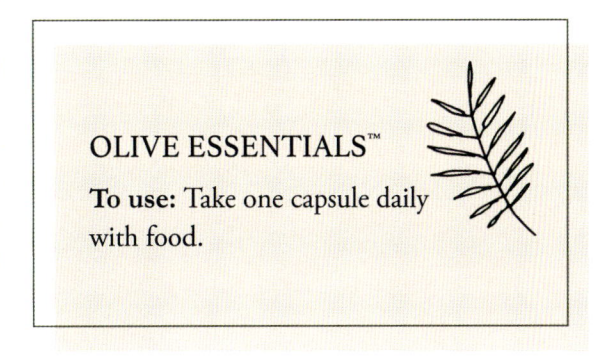

> **OLIVE ESSENTIALS™**
> **To use:** Take one capsule daily with food.

Safety notes: Keep out of reach of children. If you are pregnant, nursing, taking medication, or have a medical condition, consult a healthcare professional before use. Store in a cool, dark place.

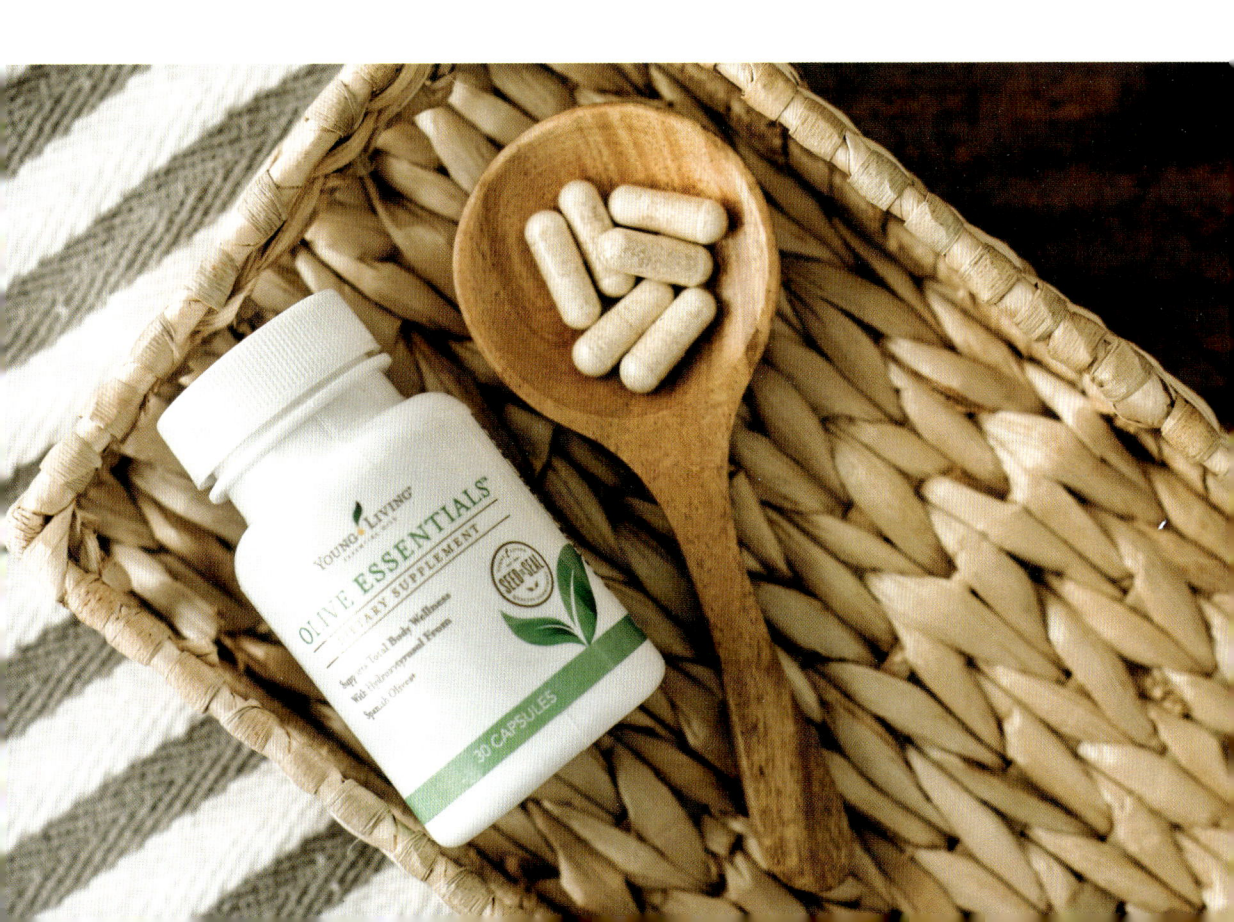

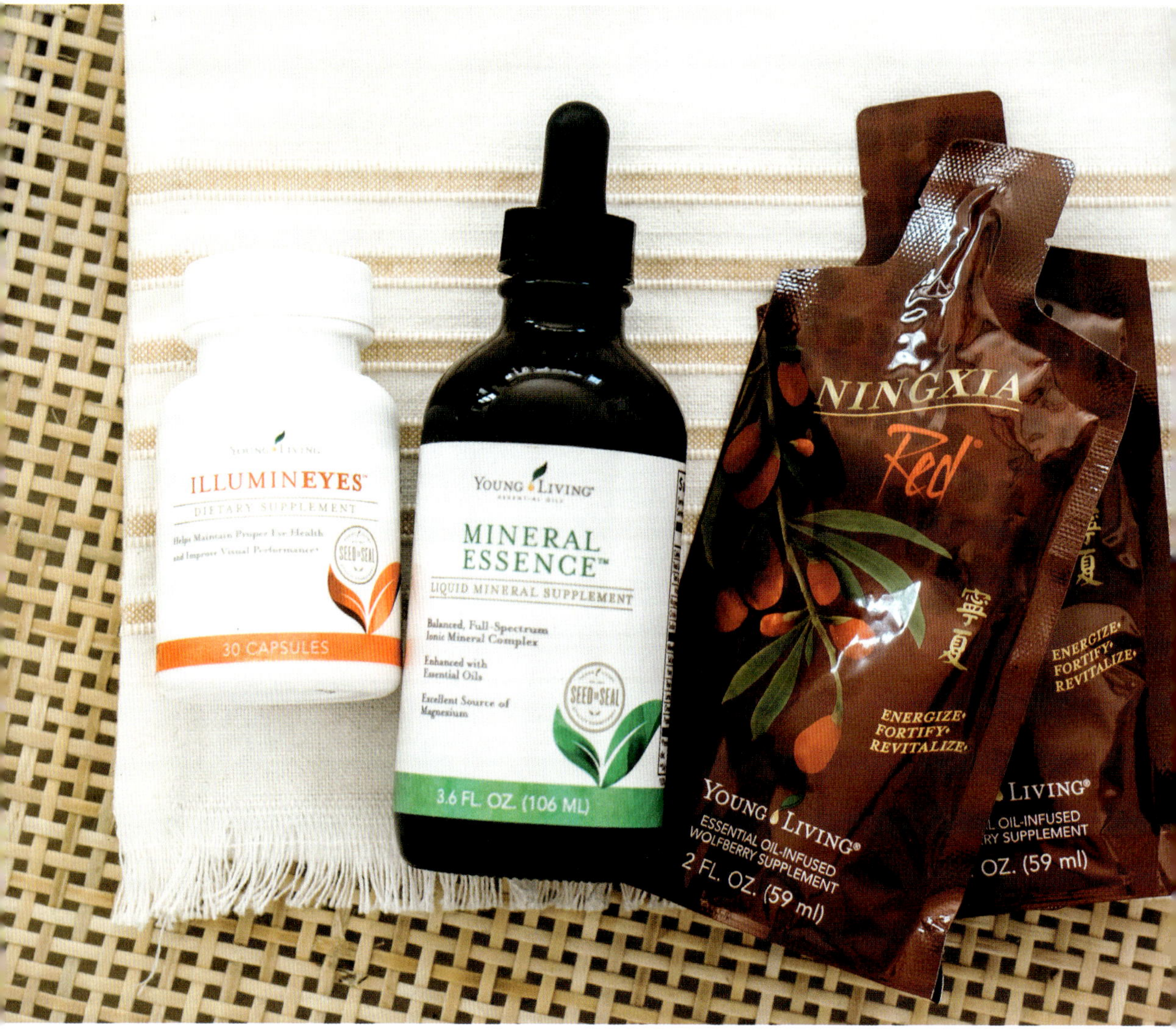
ILLUMINEYES™
DIETARY SUPPLEMENT
30 CAPSULES
YOUNG LIVING
MINERAL ESSENCE™
LIQUID MINERAL SUPPLEMENT
Balanced, Full-Spectrum Ionic Mineral Complex
Enhanced with Essential Oils
Excellent Source of Magnesium
3.6 FL. OZ. (106 ML)
NINGXIA Red®
ENERGIZE• FORTIFY• REVITALIZE•
YOUNG LIVING®
ESSENTIAL OIL-INFUSED WOLFBERRY SUPPLEMENT
2 FL. OZ. (59 ml)

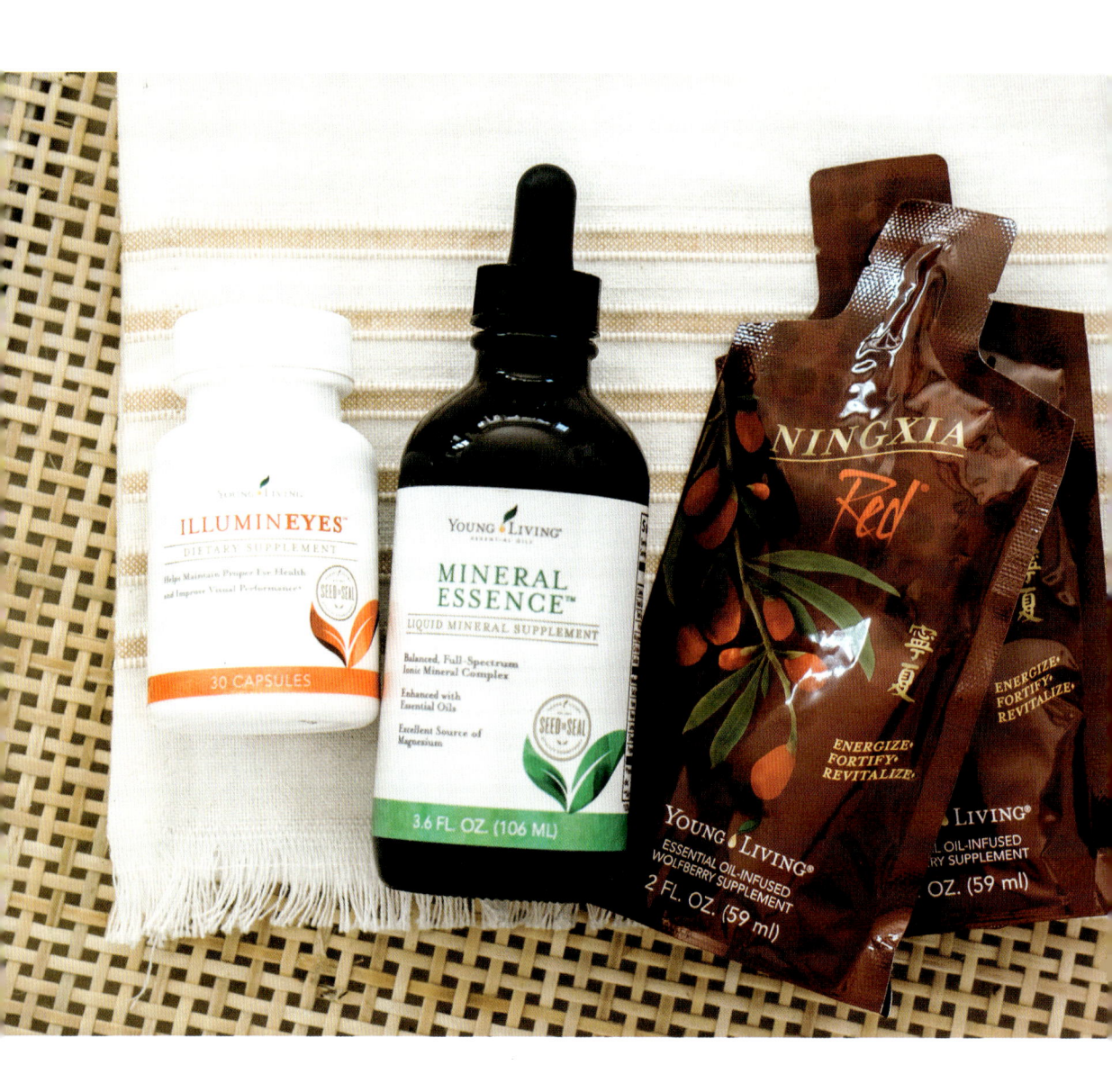

Protocols For Targeted Needs

These areas of health will be ones where you are most likely working with a trusted healthcare provider and may desire to replace conventional treatments with Young Living supplements or herbal alternatives. Although your individual needs may vary, these protocols are a great starting point. As always, open and honest conversations with your care providers are essential. I encourage you to find a provider who listens and respects your health goals.

CARDIOVASCULAR HEALTH
- CardioGize™
- Golden Turmeric™
- Longevity™
- MindWise™
- Mineral Essence™
- NingXia Red®
- OmegaGize3®
- Olive Essentials™
- Super Vitamin D

DIABETES SUPPORT
- Golden Turmeric™
- Life 9®
- IlluminEyes™
- Mineral Essence™
- NingXia Red® (at your discretion)
- Olive Essentials™
- OmegaGize3®
- Super C™
- Super Vitamin D

COGNITIVE SUPPORT
- Golden Turmeric™
- Life 9®
- MindWise™
- Mineral Essence™
- NingXia Red®
- OmegaGize3®
- Super B™
- Super Vitamin D

BEAUTY & SKINCARE
- Golden Turmeric™
- Life 9®
- NingXia Red®
- OmegaGize3®
- Sulfurzyme®
- Super C™
- Options for more targeted support: Progessence Plus™, CBD Beauty Boost™

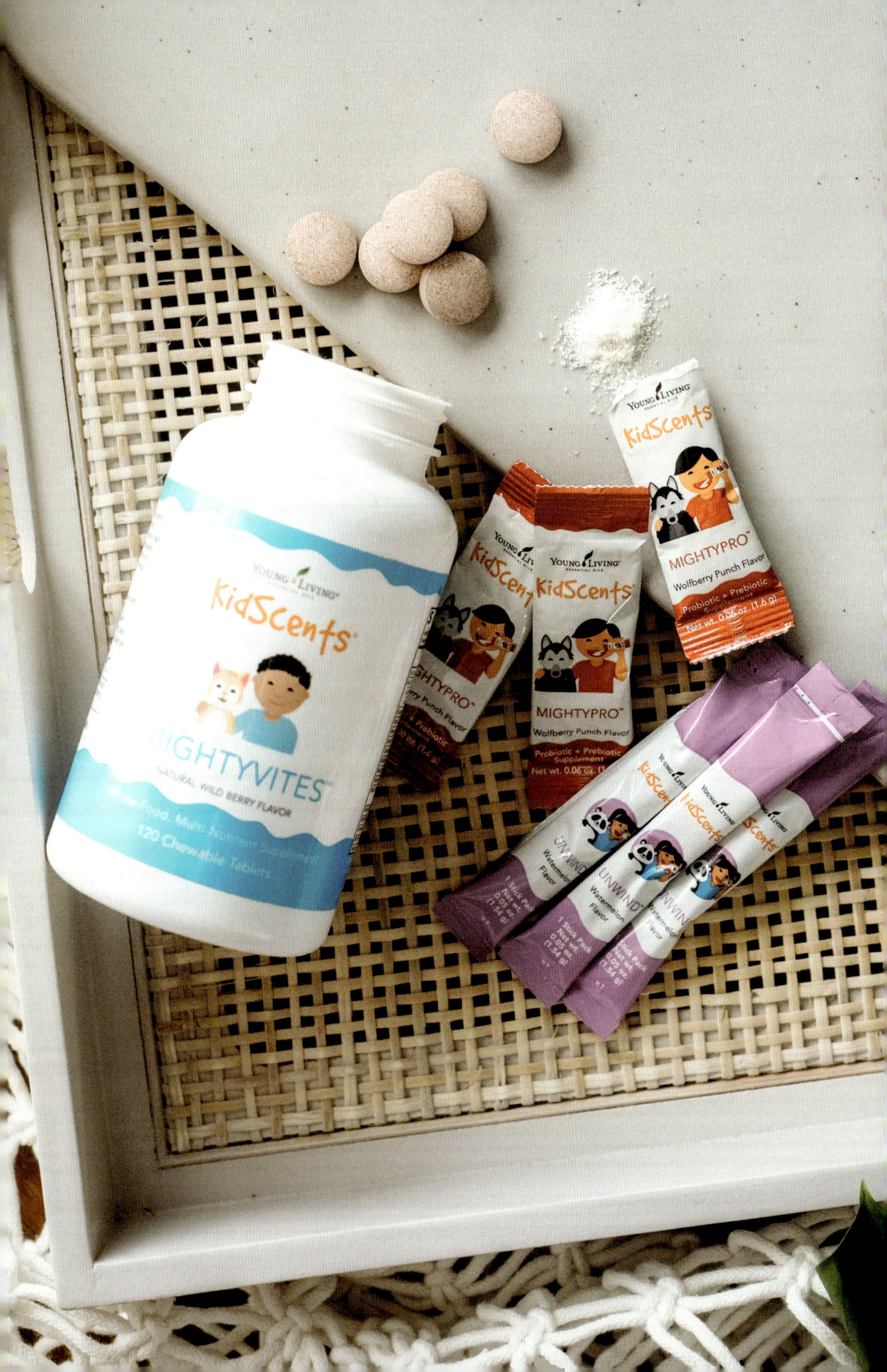
YOUNG LIVING
KidScents
NATURAL WILD BERRY FLAVOR
120 Chewable Tablets
KidScents
MIGHTYPRO
Wolfberry Punch Flavor
Probiotic + Prebiotic Supplement
KidScents
UNWIND
Watermelon Flavor

Part 7: CHILDREN'S SUPPLEMENTS

When it comes to our children's health, there is so much that we can do to promote wellness within our lifestyle and diet. Real, whole foods that are nutrient-dense go a long way when it comes to adequate levels of vitamins and minerals. However, even with a diet that is filled with raw milk, grass-fed proteins, pastured eggs, and organic backyard vegetables*, there are often gaps for our children (and for us as adults). Making sure that our children have essential vitamins, such as vitamins A, B, C, and D, and calcium, zinc, and magnesium is especially important as their bodies and minds grow and develop.

While these supplements were designed with children in mind, they are not just for children. Many adults (myself included) use these supplements because of their dosage forms and ease of use.

Dietary considerations are a very personal decision, and I respect that other families have different views on what is ideal. For more information on the importance of high-quality, nutrient-dense foods, I highly recommend the research of the Weston A. Price Foundation. https://www.westonaprice.org

Supplements discussed:

KIDSCENTS® MIGHTYPRO™
KIDSCENTS® MIGHTYVITES™
KIDSCENTS® MIGHTYZYME™
KIDSCENTS® UNWIND™

CHILDREN'S SUPPLEMENTS AT A GLANCE

	USED FOR	KEY INGREDIENTS	NOTES
MIGHTYPRO™	Pre and probiotic powder	NingXia wolfberry, synergistic blend of probiotics	Can be mixed with water or taken on its own
MIGHTYVITES™	Chewable multivitamin	Full spectrum of vitamins and minerals, including vitamins B, C, D, E, and folate	Can add Super C™ Chewable and Super Vitamin D as desired
MIGHTYZYME™	Chewable digestive enzymes	Food-based plant extracts, folate, enzyme blend	Good for digestive health and nutrient absorption
UNWIND™	Sleep support powder	Magnesium, L-theanine, 5-HTP Griffonia extract	Helps the body to relax into sleep

KIDSCENTS® MIGHTYPRO™

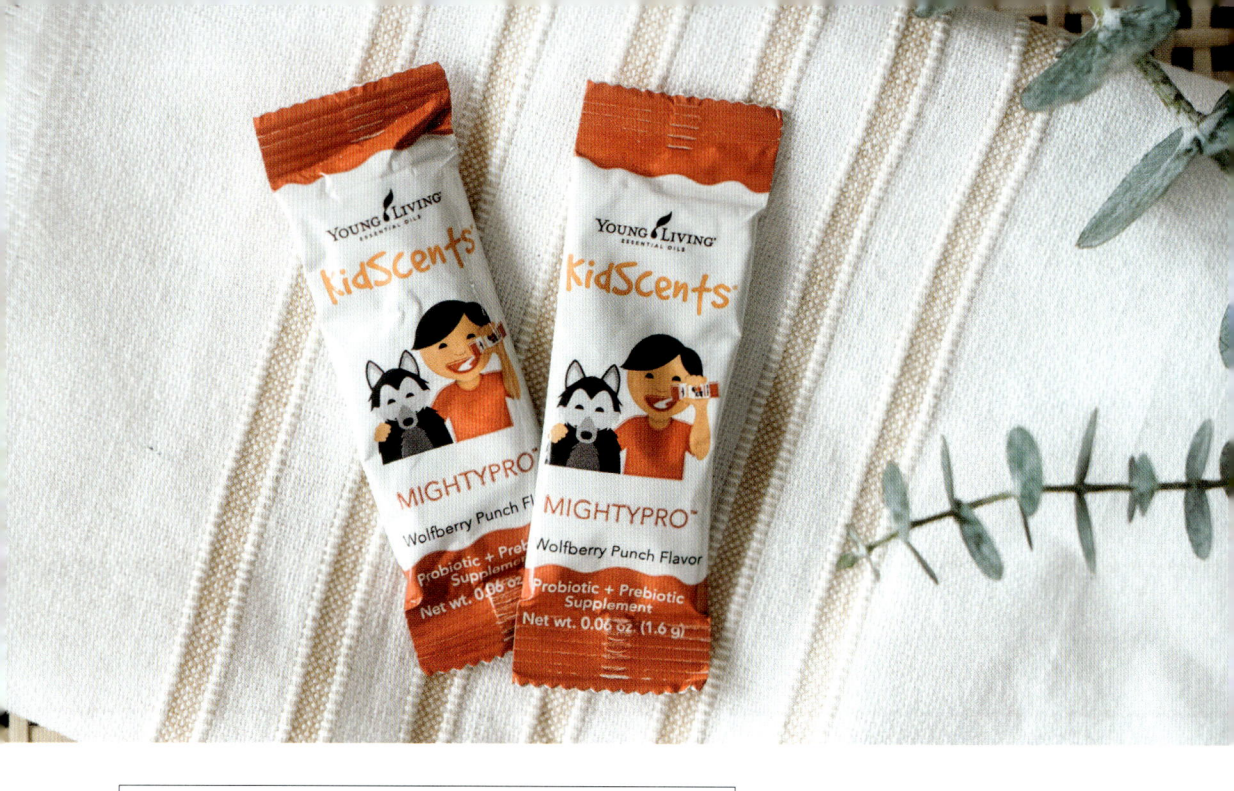

KidScents® MightyPro™ is a great-tasting blend of prebiotics and probiotics that features over 8 billion active, live cultures that are specially formulated to support gastrointestinal, digestive, and immune health in children. Stress, medications, illness, sugar and processed grain consumption, and modern-day chemicals all serve to deplete our natural probiotic stores. Because your immune system starts in your gut, many consider taking a high-quality probiotic to be key to good overall health, both in adults and children.

BENEFITS OF MIGHTYPRO™
- Supports gastrointestinal and immune health in children
- Promotes general health for children
- Promotes healthy bacteria in the gut
- May help with occasional bouts of constipation
- Helps with diarrhea, gas, and bloating
- Promotes overall digestive health
- No added colors, flavors, or artificial sugars

KidScents® MightyPro™ is a unique, synergistic blend of prebiotics (from our beloved NingXia wolfberry, which is a powerhouse herb) and probiotics all in one supplement, and it has been specially formulated for children. MightyPro™ features over 8 billion active, live cultures in combination with NingXia wolfberry fibers, which feed the good bacteria. This combination supports gastrointestinal and immune health and maintains gut health in children, them up and active.

- **NingXia wolfberry:** This is an antioxidant-packed prebiotic that enables the healthy bacteria to multiply from one cell to 35 billion cells in just 12 hours. It boosts immunity, energy levels, and overall wellness and vitality.
- **Fructooligosaccharides:** This is a prebiotic source that feeds the good bacteria in the digestive tract.
- **Lactobacillus paracasei:** This bacterium helps to promote immune system function and overall gut health.
- **Lactobacillus acidophilus**: Lactobacillus acidophilus is the most common probiotic of "friendly" bacteria that live naturally in the body to protect against disease-causing bacteria. It helps to balance the good bacteria in the gut.
- **Lactobacillus plantarum:** This bacterium acts as an antioxidant, may support the body's response to inflammation, and may help to maintain healthy blood sugar levels.
- **Lactobacillus rhamnosus:** This has beneficial properties for the digestive and immune systems, particularly against urinary and intestinal pathogens.
- **Streptococcus thermophilus:** Streptococcus thermophilus stimulates disease-fighting cells, stunts the growth of tumors, and strengthens the immune system.
- **Bifidobacterium infantis:** This is commonly used in fermented foods and supplies the body with good bacteria to overrule unhealthy overgrowth.

MightyPro™ is not just for children! Anyone can use these, especially when traveling with Life 9® is difficult (Life 9® has to be refrigerated after opening).

> **KIDSCENTS® MIGHTYPRO™**
>
> **To use:** For children aged two years and older, empty the contents of one packet into the mouth and allow it to dissolve. Take one packet daily with food to provide optimal conditions for healthy gut bacteria. Can be combined with cold food or drinks. Do not add to warm or hot food or beverages.

Safety notes: Keep out of reach of children. Do not exceed recommended dosage. If you are pregnant, nursing, taking medication, or have a medical condition, consult a health professional before use.

KIDSCENTS® MIGHTYVITES™

KidScents® MightyVites™ includes a full range of vitamins, minerals, antioxidants, and phytonutrients that deliver whole-food support to children's general health and well-being. As it can be difficult to get nutrients into our kids, even with the best dietary habits, taking a well-rounded multivitamin is a great way to promote health and wellness.

BENEFITS OF MIGHTYVITES™
- Provides premium vitamins, minerals, and food-based nutrients to support general health and well-being
- Energizes, builds, and supports your child's wellness
- Combines nutrient-dense, food-based superfruits, plants, and vegetables to deliver a full spectrum of vitamins, minerals, antioxidants, and phytonutrients
- Fortified with Orgen-FA, which is the best available source for naturally derived folate
- Contains no preservatives, synthetic flavors, or colors
- Formulated with wolfberry powder

Research shows that daily multivitamins containing zinc help to facilitate the growth and development of our children[177]. Unfortunately, conventional options are full of ingredients that we do **not** want our kids ingesting, including fillers, parabens, and artificial colors and dyes that have been linked to ADD/ADHD and gut issues. As both a healthcare professional and a mom, I feel good about the ingredients in Young Living's MightyVites™.

- **Vitamin A**: Vitamin A is a powerful antioxidant that is necessary for growth and development, immune system function, and healthy bones[178], skin, and vision.
- **Vitamin C**: Vitamin C is a potent antioxidant that is essential for the growth and repair of tissues, healing wounds, and the repair and maintenance of cartilage, bones, and teeth.
- **Vitamin D:** Vitamin D is an essential vitamin for optimal brain health, hormone levels, bone, teeth and joint health, and overall well-being. Additionally, it plays a role in mood regulation, immunity, and general wellness.
- **Vitamin E**: Vitamin E is a natural antioxidant that minimizes free radical damage within the body and promotes healthy cell function and overall health.
- **Thiamin** (Vitamin B1): B1 is essential for healthy energy levels, carbohydrate metabolism, and nerve function at the cellular level.
- **Riboflavin** (Vitamin B2): B2 assists with the production of cellular energy and helps to regenerate the liver while supporting normal cellular health.
- **Niacin**: Niacin is important for the conversion of carbohydrates into an energy source and supports healthy cholesterol and blood sugar.
- **Pyridoxine** (Vitamin B6): B6 supports a healthy heart and blood vessels.
- **Folate:** Folate is essential for vitamins B6 and B12 to be assimilated into the body. It is superior to folic acid, as the body cannot easily convert folic acid into folate.
- **Methylcobalamin** (Vitamin B12): B12 is essential for red blood cell production, immune function, and nervous system function. It works with vitamin B6 to support heart health.

- **Biotin** (Vitamin B7): B7 helps to convert fats and amino acids into energy, supports healthy hair and nails, and combats yeast and fungus overgrowth.
- **Pantothenic acid** (Vitamin B5): B5 assists with the secretion of hormones and supports the adrenal glands.
- **Zinc**: Zinc is necessary for immune support, cell regeneration, and the proper function of hormones, such as insulin and the growth hormones. It promotes healthy bones, muscles, and teeth.
- **Selenium**: Selenium is an essential trace element that helps the body to produce antioxidant enzymes. It prevents cell damage, helps to protect the body from the poisonous effects of heavy metals, plays a role in immune and reproductive health, and is necessary for normal growth and development[31].
- **Barley grass leaf powder**: Barley grass is a nutrient-rich superfood that is loaded with vitamins and minerals, such as vitamins A, C, E, K, and the B vitamins. It is high in antioxidants and is an excellent source of both soluble and insoluble fiber.
- **Broccoli sprout powder**: Broccoli sprout is high in fiber, antioxidants, nutrients, and vitamins, including vitamin C, which is a potent antioxidant that supports digestive, heart, and immune health.

Safety notes: Keep out of reach of children. Do not exceed recommended dosage. If you are pregnant, nursing, taking medication, or have a medical condition, consult a health professional before use.

KIDSCENTS® MIGHTYVITES™

To use: For children aged 4 to 12, take four chewable tablets daily. Can be taken separately or in a single dose.

These chewable vitamins aren't just for kids. Anyone who requires or desires a chewable vitamin can use these.

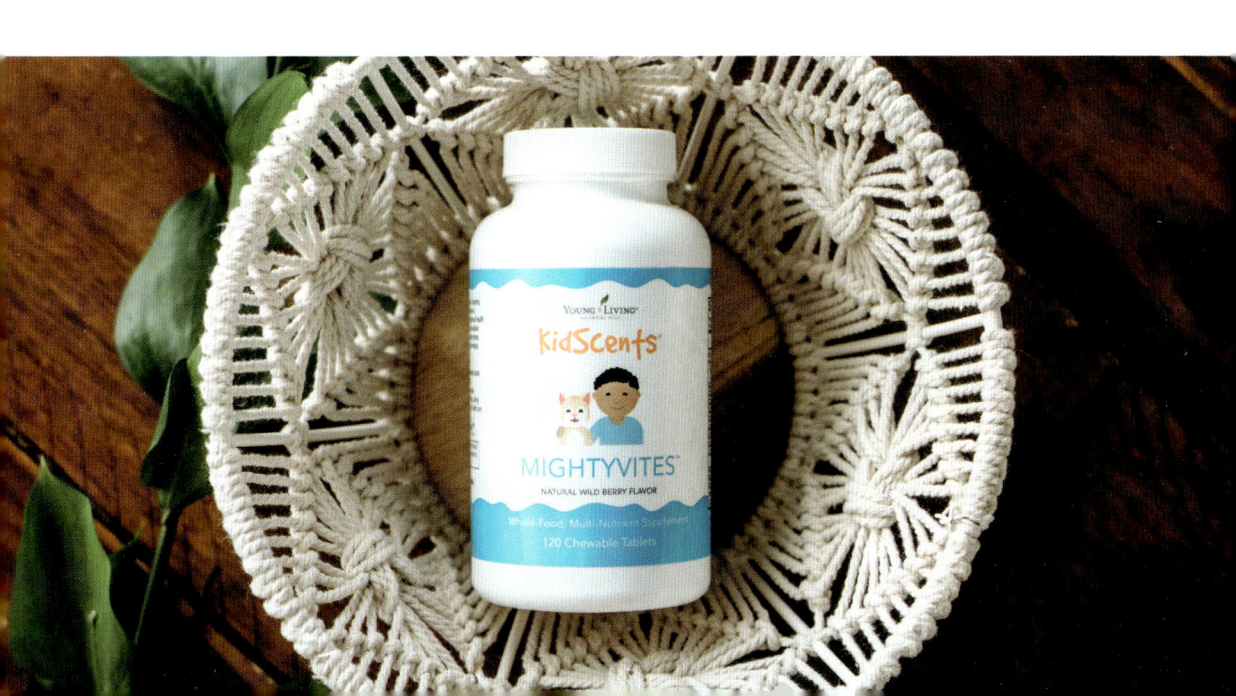

KIDSCENTS® MIGHTYZYME™

KidScents® MightyZyme™ contains enzymes that support and assist the digestive needs of growing bodies and the normal digestion of foods. MightyZyme™ helps with nutrient absorption and helps to relieve occasional symptoms of fullness, pressure, bloating, gas, flatulence, pain, and/or minor cramping that may occur after eating.

Enzymes are crucial to our health and digestion, and in an ideal world, our foods would be rich in natural enzymes. Unfortunately, the average diet and even the soil quality of our produce lead us to be sorely depleted in enzymes at an early age. Without these little workers, we are not assimilating the nutrients that we need, and we all know that growing bodies need those nutrients!

BENEFITS OF MIGHTYZYME™
- Good to relieve feelings of fullness, pressure, bloating, gas, pain, and/or minor cramping that may occur after eating
- Chewable enzyme tablet for children or adults
- Plant-based formula
- Suitable for children aged two and older
- Contains peppermint essential oil to support healthy digestion

Enzymes are protein molecules that are manufactured by all plant and animal cells and are critical for those cells to perform their everyday tasks. Enzymes are essential for our bodies to function. They allow the body's cells to communicate with each other, assist in cell turnover (cell life, growth, and death—an essential natural process), and are responsible for every chemical reaction in our bodies. As enzymes are utilized in and support all systems in the body, there are many areas of health that enzymes can support.
- Gut health and digestion
- Focus and attention
- Mood and disposition
- Energy levels
- Nutrient absorption

KidScents® MightyZyme™ contains enzymes that naturally occur in the body to support the digestive needs of growing bodies. Each ingredient is specifically chosen to support normal digestion and proper nutrient absorption.
- **MightyZyme™ Blend:**
  - **Protease**: These are protein-digesting enzymes that are stable in the varying pH conditions of the digestive tract. They fight off bacteria, yeast, and parasites in the intestines.

- **Amylase**: Amylase is a starch-digesting enzyme that prevents the fermentation of starches in the digestive tract.
- **Peptidase**: Peptidase supports the formation and absorption of amino acids.
- **Bromelain**: Bromelain is a proteolytic enzyme found in pineapples that supports carbohydrate digestion.
- **Cellulase**: Cellulase breaks down cellulose into simpler sugars for digestion.
- **Lipase**: Lipase is a fat-dissolving enzyme that is vital for the absorption of vitamins A, D, and E.
- **Phytase**: This enzyme necessary to break down minerals, such as zinc, magnesium, and potassium, that are found in grains, nuts, seeds, and other foods.

- **Orgen-Kid Blend**: This is a 100% organic, nutrient-dense, food-based superfruit, plant, and vegetable complex that provides natural folate.
  - **Curry leaf extract:** This is an excellent source of antioxidants and bolsters the immune system.
  - **Guava fruit extract:** Guava is high in antioxidants, potassium, and fiber.
  - **Sesbania leaf extract:** Sesbania leaf is high in vitamins C and B9, which support immunity and skin health.
  - **Amla fruit extract:** Amla fruit works synergistically with the other ingredients to promote digestive health.
  - **Holy basil extract**: This herb supports the endocrine, immune, and respiratory systems and helps to reduce stress on the body.
  - **Annatto seed extract:** Annatto seed is antioxidant source that supports healthy digestion.

- **Beetroot juice powder:** Beetroot helps to cleanse and nourish the liver and supports cardiovascular health.
- **Orange and strawberry fruit juice powders:** These fruit powders are real food sources of antioxidants, vitamins, and minerals.
- **Wolfberry fruit powder:** The wolfberry is high in antioxidants that mitigate and repair DNA damage. It acts as a prebiotic to support healthy bacteria in the gut, strengthens the immune system, promotes overall wellness, and combats carcinogens.
- **Barley grass:** Barley grass is a nutrient-rich superfood that is loaded with vitamins and minerals, such as vitamins A, C, E, K, and

---

KIDSCENTS® MIGHTYZYME™

To use:
- **Children aged six or older:** Chew one tablet three times daily before or with meals.
- **Children two to six years:** Chew 1/2 to one tablet (crushed if needed and mixed with yogurt or applesauce).

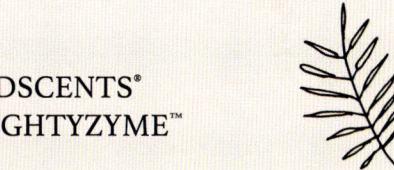

the B vitamins. It is high in antioxidants and is an excellent source of both soluble and insoluble fiber.
- **Broccoli sprout powder**: Broccoli sprout is high in fiber, antioxidants, vitamins, and nutrients, including vitamin C, which is a potent antioxidant that supports digestive, heart, and immune health.

MightyZyme™ isn't just for kids. If you are looking for a chewable enzyme, this is for you too!

Safety notes: Keep out of reach of children. Do not exceed the recommended dosage. If pregnant, nursing, taking medication, or have a medical condition, consult a health professional before use.

KIDSCENTS® UNWIND™

KidScents® Unwind™ is specially formulated for children to promote a calm and relaxed state, reduce restlessness, and improve focus and mental clarity both at home and in the classroom. When we are well rested, we perform better in all areas of life, and our kids are no different. Unwind™ can help them to get a restful night's sleep.

BENEFITS OF UNWIND™
- Contains magnesium and calming essential oils
- Helps with occasional sleeplessness
- Reduces restlessness
- Improves focus and mental clarity at home and in the classroom
- Eases occasional irritability and stress
- Promotes quality, restful sleep

When our children are well rested, it makes a big difference in their health, attention span, and mood. Therefore, prioritizing quality rest goes a long way. KidScents® Unwind™ is there to support you through those times of occasional irritability and/or restlessness that can keep restful sleep at bay. Magnesium, L-theanine, and calming essential oils are combined with other natural ingredients to help your little ones to sleep soundly.
- **L-theanine**: L-theanine acts as a natural stress reliever to promote healthy sleep and supports physical and emotional relaxation[178].
- **Mineral magnesium complex**: This magnesium complex helps to promote muscle relaxation, decrease leg cramps and muscle spasms, and reduce tension to promote restful sleep.
- **5-HTP Griffonia seed extract**: This is a precursor to the neurotransmitter serotonin that enhances relaxation and calms the mind and body. It may increase natural melatonin levels.

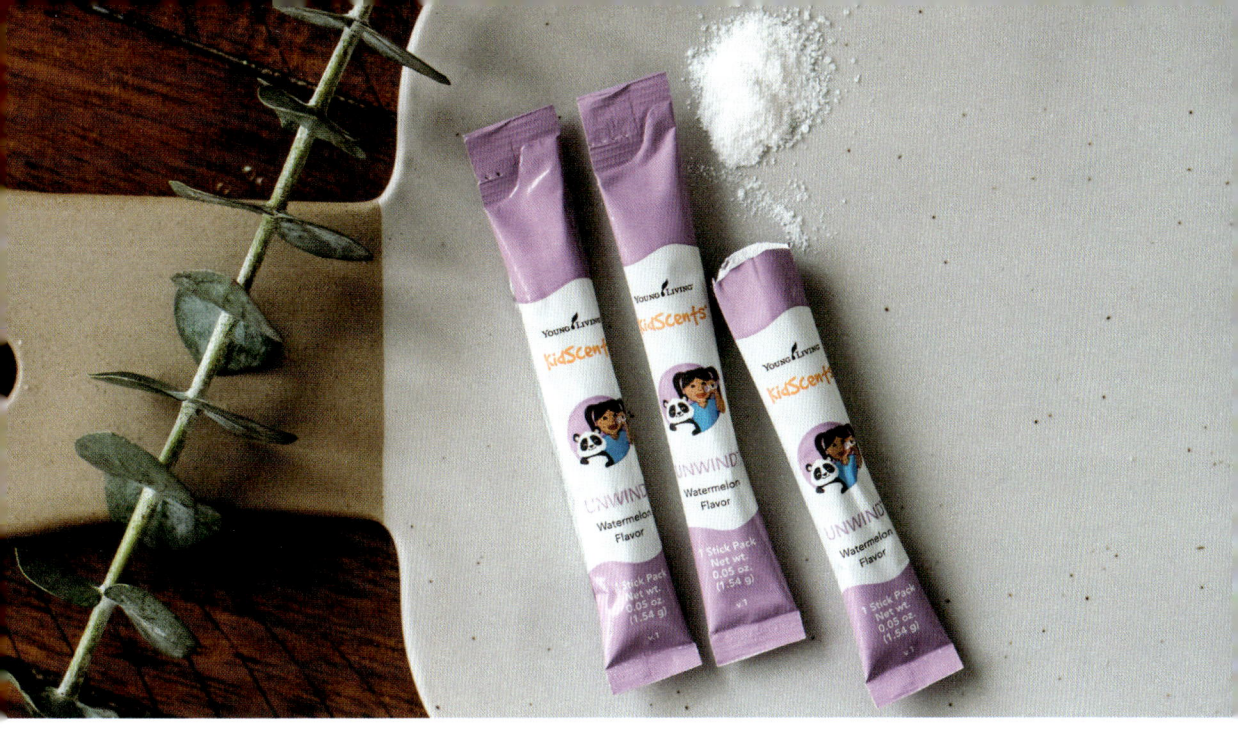

- **Lavender essential oil**: Lavender is well known for its ability to support physical and emotional relaxation and decrease the stress response within the body[115]. It has also shown antidepressant activity in clinical studies[116].
- **Roman chamomile essential oil:** Roman chamomile contains antioxidants that promote overall health and wellness and are calming and soothing to the mind and body.

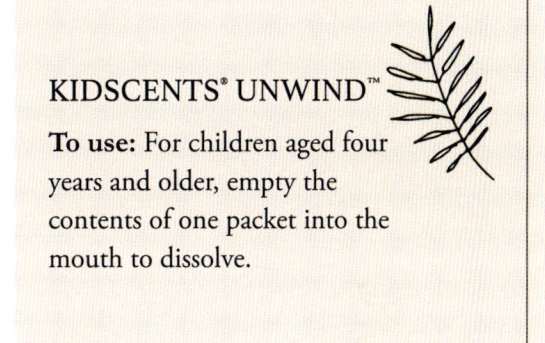

KIDSCENTS® UNWIND™

To use: For children aged four years and older, empty the contents of one packet into the mouth to dissolve.

Create a bedtime routine!

- Fill diffusers with SleepyIze™, Peace & Calming®, or your favorite calming blend.
- Take a KidScents® Unwind™ packet.
- Roll on your favorite bedtime oil—SleepyIze™, Gentle Baby™, Lavender, or Tranquil®.
- Set the tone with white noise, a cool temperature, and a dark space.
- Massage tired legs and feet with Lavender or Relaxation™ Massage Oil.

Safety notes: Keep out of reach of children. If you are pregnant, nursing, taking medication, or have a medical condition, consult a healthcare professional before use. For human consumption only. Not intended for animal use.

Protocols For Children's Health

When it comes to our children's health, we have so much power in our daily habits, and these Young Living supplements are a great foundation for promoting the healthy growth and development of our kids.

CHILDREN'S HEALTH
- KidScents® MightyPro™
- KidScents® MightyVites™
- KidScents® MightyZyme™
- NingXia Red®
- Super C™ Chewable
- Super Vitamin D

In addition, you have the option to add more targeted support as desired at appropriate ages. Some commonly used supplements for children include Pure Protein Complete™ (if needing additional nutritional support), Inner Defense® (for ages 12+ as needed, or you can poke a hole in a capsule and apply it to the spine of a younger child at your discretion), Golden Turmeric™ (as desired for inflammatory needs), Sulfurzyme® (wonderful for active children), Progessence Plus™, and other hormone-supporting supplements (at your discretion and at an appropriate age for hormone balance in young women).

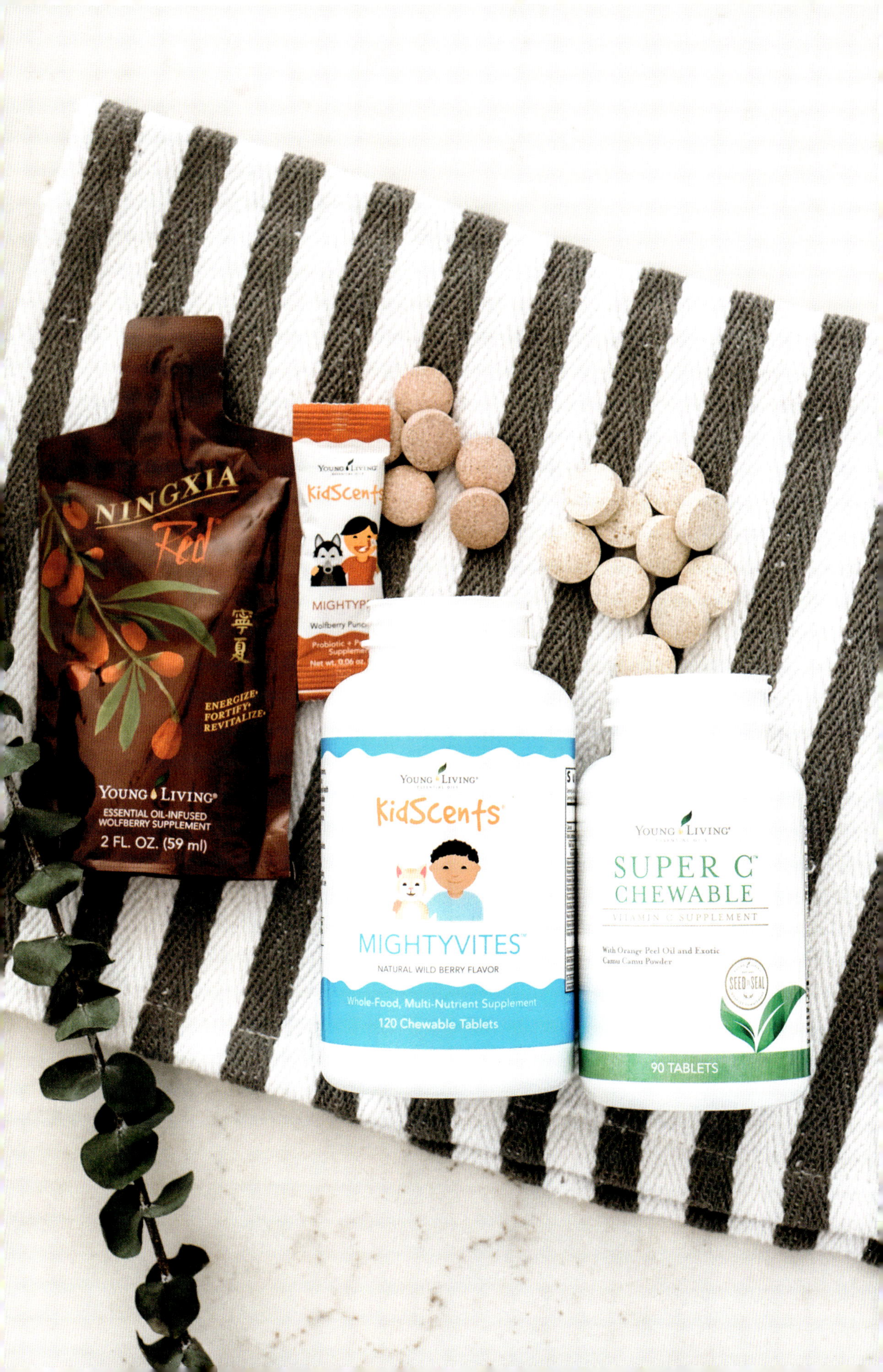
NINGXIA Red
寧夏
ENERGIZE
FORTIFY
REVITALIZE
YOUNG LIVING
ESSENTIAL OIL-INFUSED WOLFBERRY SUPPLEMENT
2 FL. OZ. (59 ml)
YOUNG LIVING
KidScents
YOUNG LIVING
KidScents
MIGHTYVITES
NATURAL WILD BERRY FLAVOR
Whole-Food, Multi-Nutrient Supplement
120 Chewable Tablets
YOUNG LIVING
SUPER C
CHEWABLE
VITAMIN C SUPPLEMENT
With Orange Peel Oil and Exotic Camu Camu Powder
SEED TO SEAL
90 TABLETS

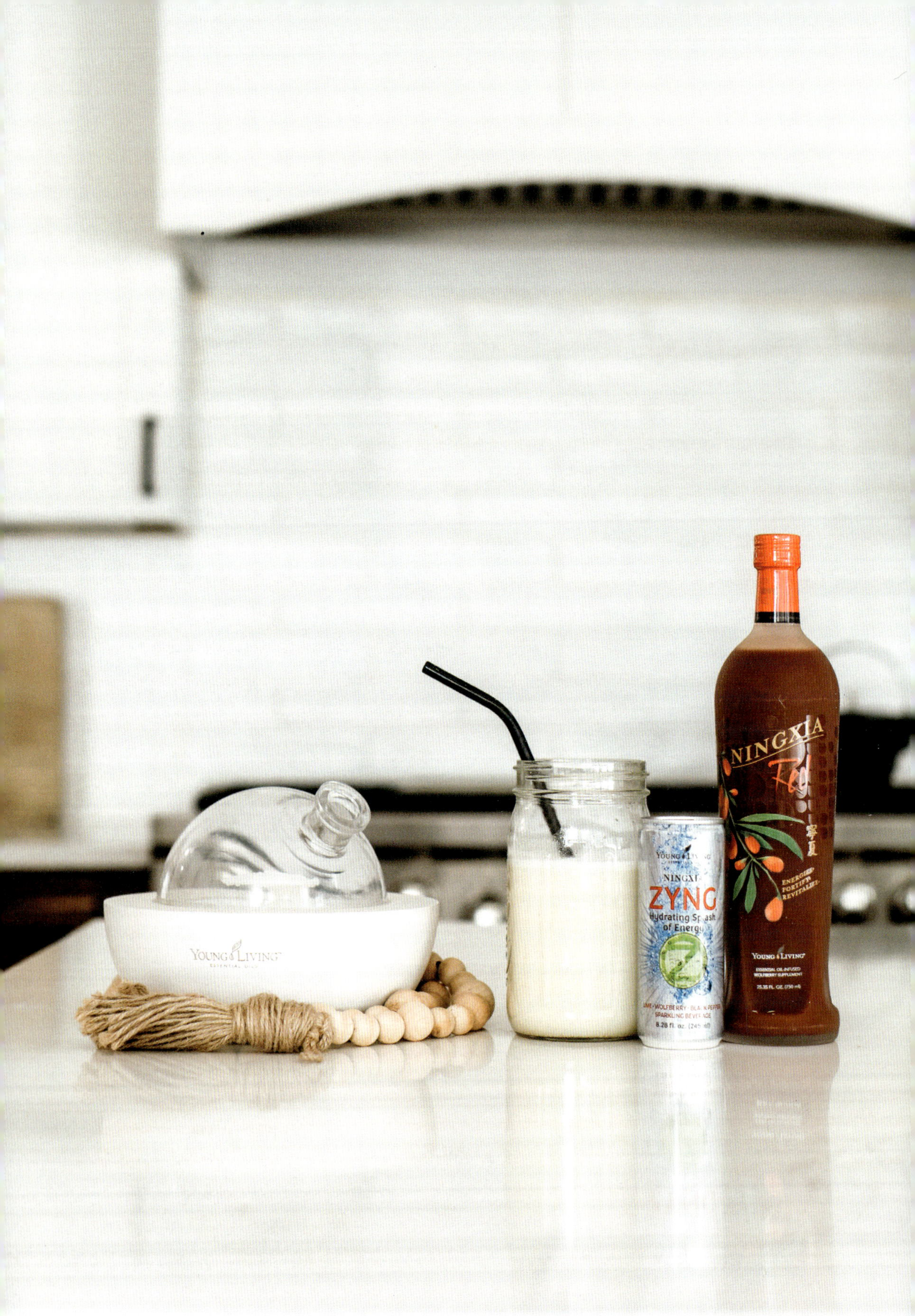
YOUNG LIVING
ZYNG
Hydrating Splash
of Energy
NINGXIA
Red
YOUNG LIVING

Part 8: NUTRITIONAL SUPPLEMENTS

When it comes to our health, nutrition is critical. We could write an entire book on this topic alone! And while there are so many nuances to nutrition and individual needs, there are many things that we can do and products that we can use daily to support our bodies, regardless of our dietary restrictions or needs.

For more information on the importance of nutrient-dense foods and how to add them to your diet, check out the Weston A. Price Foundation. https://www.westonaprice.org

Supplements discussed:

BALANCE COMPLETE™
PURE PROTEIN COMPLETE™
NINGXIA RED®
NINGXIA NITRO™
NINGXIA ZYNG®
SLIQUE® PRODUCT LINE
VITALITY DROPS

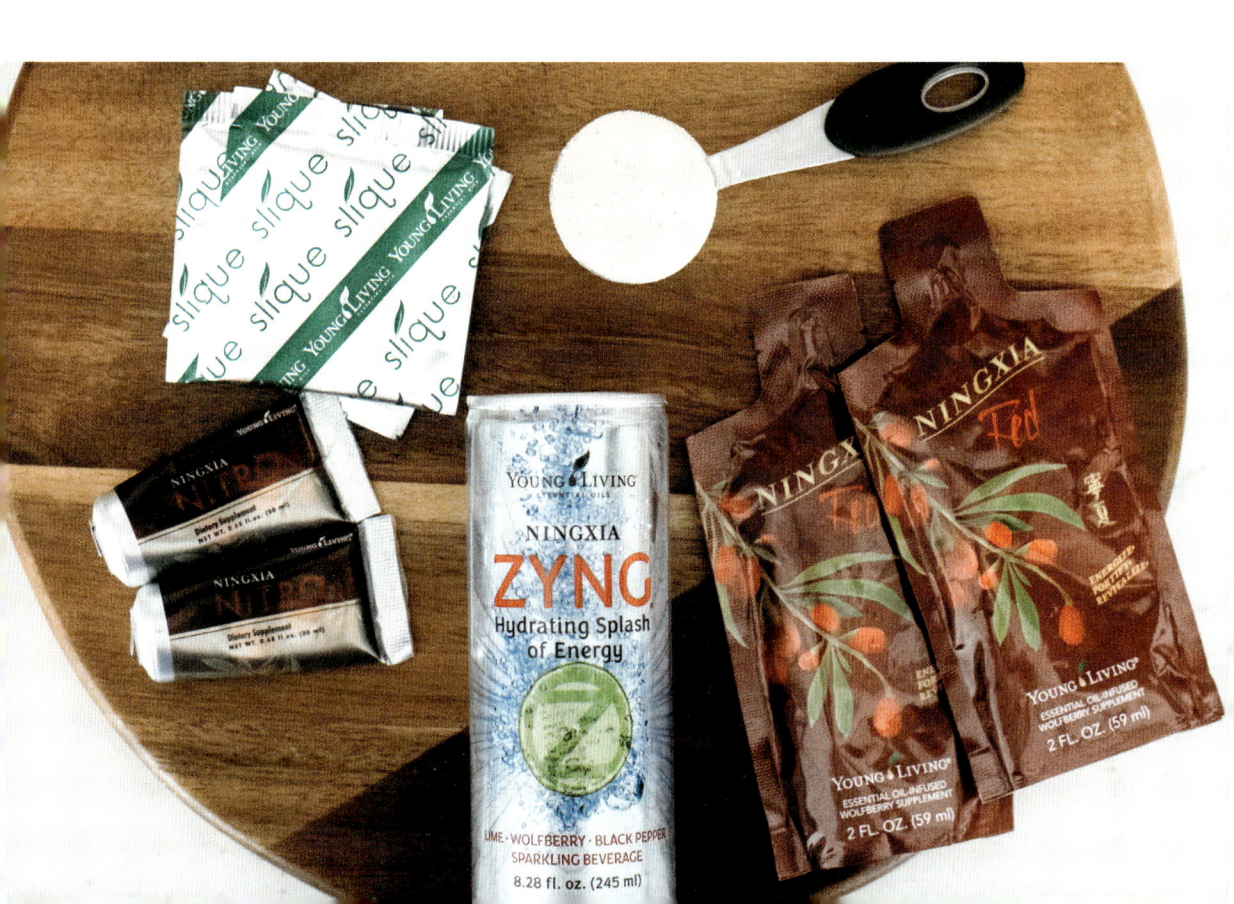

BALANCE COMPLETE™

Balance Complete™ is a nutritive, food-based powder that can be used as a meal replacement, energizer, and cleanser. It contains brown rice bran, barley grass, and extra virgin coconut oil, which makes it high in fiber, protein, and minerals. In addition, Balance Complete™ contains NingXia wolfberry powder, aloe vera, cinnamon powder, and Young Living's premium whey protein blend.

BENEFITS OF BALANCE COMPLETE™
- Healthy meal replacement option
- Effective approach to weight-loss goals and cleansing
- High in protein (12 g of protein per serving)
- Formulated with whey protein to support muscle growth and recovery
- Good source of fiber, which supports digestive health
- Supports a gentle daily cleansing of the digestive system and the absorption of toxins
- Supports a healthy immune system

Balance Complete™ is high in fiber and protein and contains the good fats, enzymes, vitamins, and minerals that are necessary for a nutritionally complete meal replacement. In addition, it supplies an amazing 11 g of fiber and 12 g of protein per serving, absorbs toxins, and satisfies the appetite while balancing the body's essential requirements.

- **NingXia wolfberry fruit powder:** The NingXia wolfberry is one of the most well known antioxidant nutrients. It is wonderful for strengthening the immune system, promoting overall wellness, and combating carcinogens.
- **Rice bran:** Rice bran is rich in essential fatty acids and antioxidants. It is an excellent source of manganese, selenium, and magnesium.
- **Barley grass powder:** This nutrient-rich superfood is loaded with vitamins, minerals, and antioxidants. It works as a cleansing agent to help the body to remove toxins and waste.
- **Enzyme complex (lactase, amylase, bromelain, lipase, and papain):** These enzymes break down lactose, starch, protein, and fat for energy. They are required for the proper absorption of fat-soluble vitamins A, D, and E. Bromelain (proteolytic enzyme

> **BALANCE COMPLETE™**
>
> **To use:** Add two scoops to 8-10 oz. of cold water or milk of choice. Shake, stir, or blend until smooth. For added flavor, add fruit or essential oils. You can also replace your least nutritious meal of the day with Balance Complete™. During Young Living's five-day nutritive cleanse, replace your three daily meals with Balance Complete™ and follow the recommended schedule.

from pineapples) has several health benefits, including immune bolstering and free radical scavenging.
- **Cinnamon powder:** Cinnamon is a super nutrient that strongly supports the immune system. It is an antioxidant and great for helping to promote a healthy weight and blood sugar levels.
- **Calcium, zinc, chromium, selenium, and magnesium:** These minerals are required by the body for various functions. They support all body systems, including the muscles, heart, brain, immunity, and hormone balance.
- **Vitamins A, B, C, and E:** These vitamins are all necessary for our bodies to function properly and stay healthy. They support the immune system and promote healthy eyesight, muscles, bones, teeth, and hair.

Safety notes: Keep out of reach of children. If you are pregnant, nursing, taking medication, or have a medical condition, consult a health professional before use. Contains milk and soy.

NINGXIA RED®

Find more information on NingXia Red® in the "Foundational Supplements" section on page 41.

NingXia Red® is one of Young Living's most popular products, and for good reason. This wolfberry puree is so much more than a delicious addition to your day. NingXia Red® is a nutrient-dense fuel source for our bodies. Much like a car runs better with proper fuel, our bodies perform better when they are supplied with all the nutrients that they need.

BENEFITS OF NINGXIA RED®
- Supports a healthy immune system
- Helps us to be proactive against all the germs coming our way
- A huge source of antioxidants
- Supports brain and joint health
- Supports healthy hormone levels
- Supports healthy blood sugar levels
- Curbs sugar cravings
- Infused with citrus essential oils, which are high in limonene
- Whole-food, nutrient-dense supplement full of vitamins, minerals, amino acids, and polyphenols

NingXia Red® is a powerful antioxidant supplement drink that is made from wolfberry puree, blueberry, plum, cherry, Aronia, and pomegranate juices, grape seed extract, and yuzu, tangerine, lemon, and orange essential oils. The essential oils that are in NingXia Red® act as catalysts to help deliver the antioxidants and nutrients through the cell membranes while assisting in the removal of cellular waste.

NingXia Red® is rich in ellagic acid, polyphenols, flavonoids, vitamins, and minerals. In addition, it has 18 amino acids, 21 trace minerals, beta-carotene, and vitamins B1, B2, B6, and E. It is an excellent whole-food source of nutrients that provides energy and strength to the body without harmful stimulates. In addition, it has an amazing low glycemic index of 11 that does not spike blood sugar levels.

> **NINGXIA RED®**
>
> **To use:** Take 2-4 oz. daily on its own or mixed with water or juice. In addition, NingXia Red® can be added to a smoothie.

NINGXIA NITRO™

NingXia Nitro™ is a delicious wolfberry drink that is infused with essential oils, botanical extracts, D-ribose, Korean ginseng, and green tea extract to increase cognitive alertness, enhance mental fitness, and support overall performance. NingXia Nitro™ is a great pick-me-up to increase energy reserves, sharpen the mind, and increase focus.

BENEFITS OF NINGXIA NITRO™
- Supports alertness
- Promotes cognitive fitness
- Supports physical fitness
- Great source of iodine
- Provides natural energy

With ingredients that have been specifically chosen to kick it up a notch, NingXia Nitro™ is the supplement that you want to reach for when you're starting to feel that afternoon slump, you have a to-do list to tackle, or anytime you want to increase your energy and concentration.
- **NingXia Nitro™ juice**: cherry, kiwi, blueberry, black currant, raspberry, strawberry, and cranberry juices, which are packed full of antioxidants to support our bodies, especially when they are running low on energy.
- **Nitro™ Energy blend**: This blend includes D-ribose, vitamin B3, vitamin B6, folate, vitamin B12, choline, potassium, green tea extract, mulberry leaf extract, Korean ginseng extract, and wolfberry seed oil. All of these are plant-derived vitamins and herbs that help support energy levels naturally.

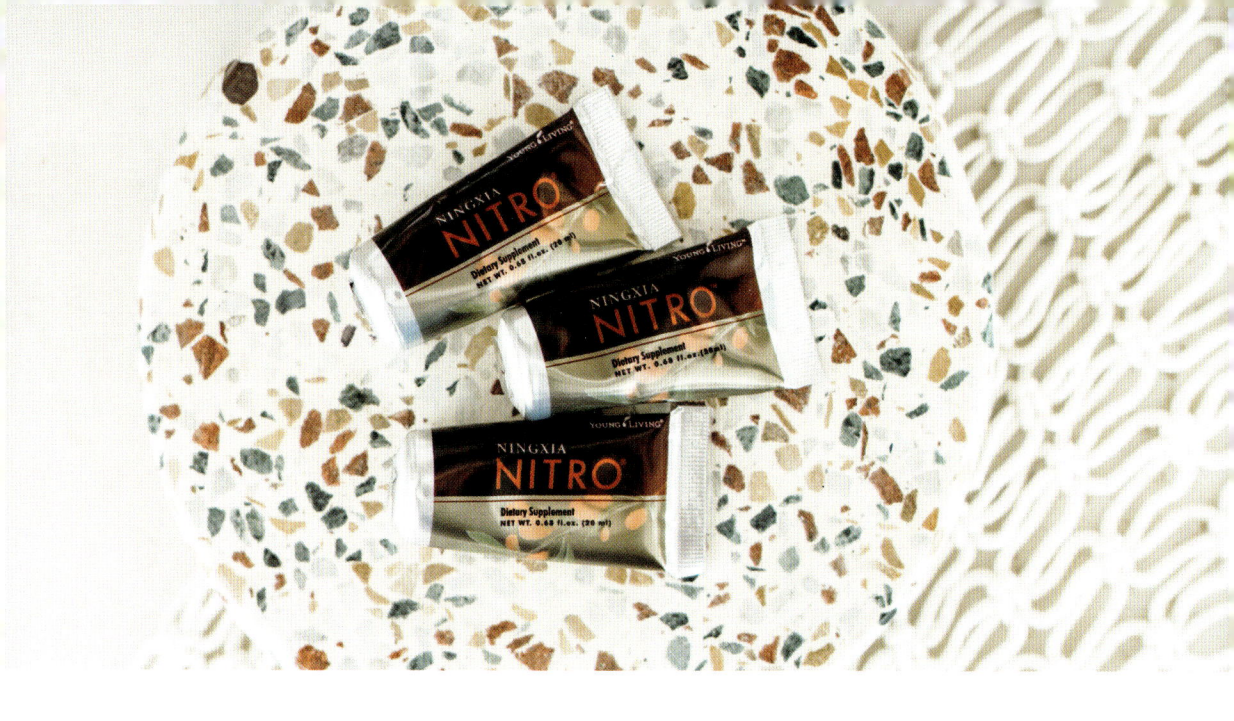

- **D-ribose**: D-ribose is essential to help build ATP in the body. ATP is the body's energy currency and is required for all essential functions, including breathing, pumping blood to the muscles, heart contractions, firing of neurons, and more.
- **Korean ginseng**: This herb supports energy levels and normal cognition and helps to decrease inflammation.
- **Green tea extract**: Green tea is a natural caffeine source (approximately 30 mg of caffeine per tube of Nitro™).
- **B vitamins**: These are critical for the firing of neurons in the brain and support normal cognitive/brain function.
- **Choline**: Choline is an essential micronutrient for all cells and is necessary for numerous bodily processes, including nerve function, cholesterol processing, brain development, muscle mobility, and liver function. It is an essential building block for neurotransmitters, particularly acetylcholine.
- **Nitro™ Alert blend**: This blend includes vanilla, chocolate, yerba mate, spearmint, peppermint, nutmeg, and black pepper. These oils are great for digestion, support the adrenal system (the "fight-or-flight" system, which is often turned on too much, especially in the face of constant stress, blue light exposure, demanding jobs, etc.), and improve energy levels.

Safety notes: Not recommended for children. If you are pregnant, nursing, taking medication, or have a medical condition, consult a health professional before use. Individuals who may be sensitive to caffeine should exercise care when consuming more than two tubes daily.

NINGXIA NITRO™

To use: Consume directly from the tube or mix with 1 oz. of NingXia Red® or 4 oz. of water. Best served chilled.

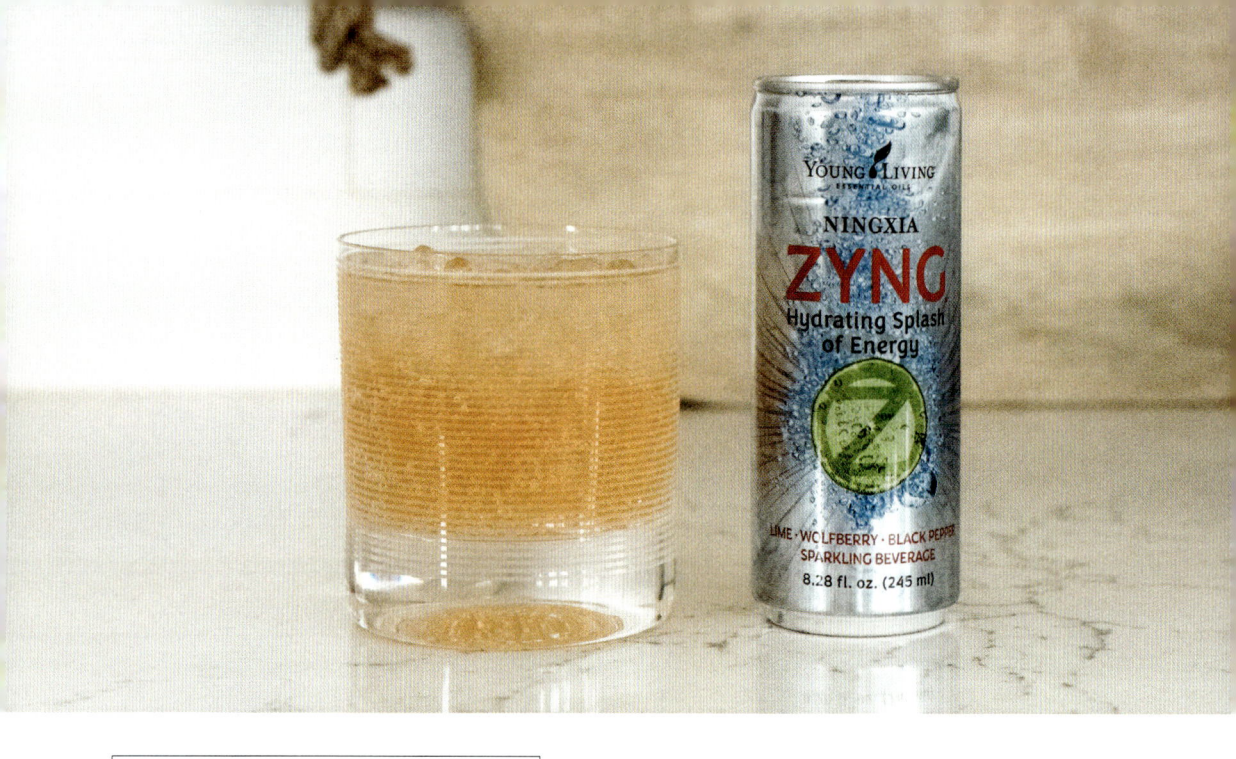

NINGXIA ZYNG®

NingXia Zyng® is a refreshing, lightly carbonated drink that combines NingXia wolfberry puree, pear and blackberry juices, and essential oils with naturally occurring caffeine for an energizing boost.

BENEFITS OF NINGXIA ZYNG®
- Sparkling and refreshing with light carbonation
- Contains B vitamins
- Contains natural lime and black pepper essential oils
- No artificial flavors, colors, sweeteners, or preservatives

NingXia Zyng® combines the nutrient-dense NingXia wolfberry with sparkling water, pear and blackberry juices, a hint of Lime and Black Pepper Vitality™ essential oils, and naturally occurring caffeine from white tea extract. These natural ingredients create a hydrating drink that provides an energy boost without tons of sugar and caffeine, which can be damaging to our health.
- **Wolfberry puree**: The wolfberry is a powerful source of antioxidants and polysaccharides, which bolsters immunity, supports healthy energy levels, and combats carcinogens. It is rich in magnesium, potassium, and vitamin C.
- **Pear and blackberry juices**: These are high in antioxidants, vitamins, and minerals, including vitamin C.
- **White tea leaf extract:** White tea is a natural source of caffeine that is high in antioxidants. It supports the immune system and cognitive function and maintains healthy insulin levels.

- **Niacinamide (vitamin B3), pantothenic acid (vitamin B5), and vitamin B6:** These B vitamins are essential for healthy energy levels, healthy adrenals, and hormone balance.
- **Lime essential oil:** Lime is high in limonene, a constituent that is known to strengthen the immune system and helps to decongest the lymphatic system. D-limonene alters the signaling pathways within cancer cells in a way that stops cancer cells from multiplying and causes their death[22].
- **Black pepper essential oil:** Black pepper is a stimulating and energizing oil that adds a hint of spice and helps to reduce feelings of fatigue.

Unfortunately, conventional energy drinks are filled with ingredients that are harmful to our health. Energy drinks are widely promoted as products that increase energy and enhance mental alertness and physical performance. Next to multivitamins, energy drinks are the most popular dietary supplement that is consumed by American teens and young adults. So, what's wrong with energy drinks?

- *Large amounts of caffeine:* This can cause serious heart and blood vessel problems, such as heart rhythm disturbances and increases in heart rate and blood pressure. It may harm still-developing cardiovascular and nervous systems and can be associated with anxiety, sleep and digestive problems, and dehydration.
- *High amounts of sugar:* A single 16-oz. energy drink may contain 54 g to 62 g of added sugar. This exceeds the maximum amount of added sugar that is recommended for an entire day.

Overall, energy drinks are associated with sugar crashes, energy slumps, and caffeine withdrawal. NingXia Zyng® and NingXia Nitro™ provide a natural, health-supporting option that works even better.

> **NINGXIA XYNG®**
>
> **To use:** Drink one can as desired for a refreshing boost. Best served chilled. Lightly invert the can before opening. Add a tube of NingXia Nitro™ for a sweet twist that supports cognition.

Safety note: Contains naturally occurring caffeine (35 mg).

PURE PROTEIN COMPLETE™

Pure Protein Complete™ combines a blend of five different proteins, amino acids, and ancient peat and apple extracts to create a well-rounded protein powder supplement. This formula supports the muscular system, lean muscle mass, and energy levels and is a great post-workout recovery drink. This delicious protein powder comes in both Vanilla Spice and Chocolate Deluxe flavors and is a great addition to anyone's fitness regimen.

BENEFITS OF PURE PROTEIN COMPLETE™
- An excellent source of protein (25 g)
- Formulated with a variety of amino acids Provides protein metabolism support
- Supports ATP production, the energy currency of the body
- Helps to build lean muscle
- rBGH- and soy-free whey
- Versatile enough for smoothies, baking, and more

The foundation of the Pure Protein Complete™ blend is cow and goat whey, pea protein, egg white protein, and organic hemp seed protein. This specific mix of sources allows for a full range of amino acids, including D-aspartic acid, threonine, l-serine, glutamic acid, glycine, alanine, valine, methionine, isoleucine, leucine, tyrosine, phenylalanine, lysine, histidine, arginine, proline, hydroxyproline, cystine, tryptophan, and cysteine. Additionally, the formula includes a unique enzyme blend, so when paired with these amino acids, this protein supplement supports overall protein utilization in the body. This is of utmost importance when we are focusing on fitness routines and muscle building.

Ancient peat and apple extracts and a powerful B-vitamin blend add to the benefits of this protein powder. This combination of ingredients supports ATP production, which is essential for everything that our bodies do.
- **Potassium, sodium, calcium, zinc, and iron**: These are essential minerals for numerous functions within the body, including muscle health, heart health, energy levels, and immune function.
- **Thiamin (B1), riboflavin (B2), niacin (B3), pyridoxine (B6), methylcobalamin (B12), biotin (B7), and pantothenic acid (B5)**: These B vitamins are required for normal cardiovascular and cognitive health, aid in mood improvement, and help to sustain healthy energy levels.
- **Pure Protein Complete™ proprietary blend**: This is a diverse blend of protein sources that maximizes absorption and allows the body to benefit as much as possible from the formula.
  - **rBGH-free whey protein concentrate**: This is the most bioavailable protein source from grass-fed cows that have not been treated with recombinant bovine growth hormone (rBGH).

- **Pea protein isolate**: Pea protein can help to speed up muscle growth and recovery after a workout.
- **Goat whey protein**: Goat whey is high in natural protein, calcium, potassium, magnesium, and vitamins A and C. It boosts the immune system by encouraging production of white blood cells and antibodies.
- **Egg albumin**: Egg albumin high in proteins, vitamins, and minerals without adding calories.
- **Organic hemp seed protein**: Hemp seed is a complete plant-based protein that is full of vitamins and minerals.
- **Ancient peat and apple extracts**: These extracts support the production of ATP within the body to promote healthy energy levels.
- **Enzyme proprietary complex** (Alpha and Beta amylase, protease, lipase, lactase, cellulase, L. acidophilus, papain, and bromelain): These are enzymes that break down lactose, starch, protein, and fat for energy. They are required for the proper absorption of the fat-soluble vitamins A, D, and E.
  - **Bromelain:** Bromelain is a proteolytic enzyme sourced from pineapples that has many health benefits, including immune bolstering and free radical scavenging.
  - **L. acidophilus:** This is a common probiotic that supports gut and immune health.

WHY MAKE THE SWITCH TO PURE PROTEIN COMPLETE™

Unfortunately, most protein powders contain ingredients that we don't really want to be consuming. Some contain a lot of added sugar (as much as 23 grams per scoop), which can cause an unhealthy spike in blood sugar and insulin levels. Others contain heavy metals and toxins. A study by the Clean Label Project found that many protein powders contain heavy metals (lead, arsenic, cadmium, and mercury), BPA (a chemical that is used to make plastic), pesticides, or other contaminants that are linked to cancer and other health conditions. Some toxins were present in significant quantities. For example, one protein powder contained 25 times the allowed limit of BPA[180].

Because of Young Living's Seed to Seal® standard, we can rest assured that the ingredients that are used are clean, ethically sourced, and good for our bodies and overall health.

> **PURE PROTEIN COMPLETE™**
>
> **To use:** Add two scoops to 8 oz. of cold water or milk of choice, then shake or stir until smooth.

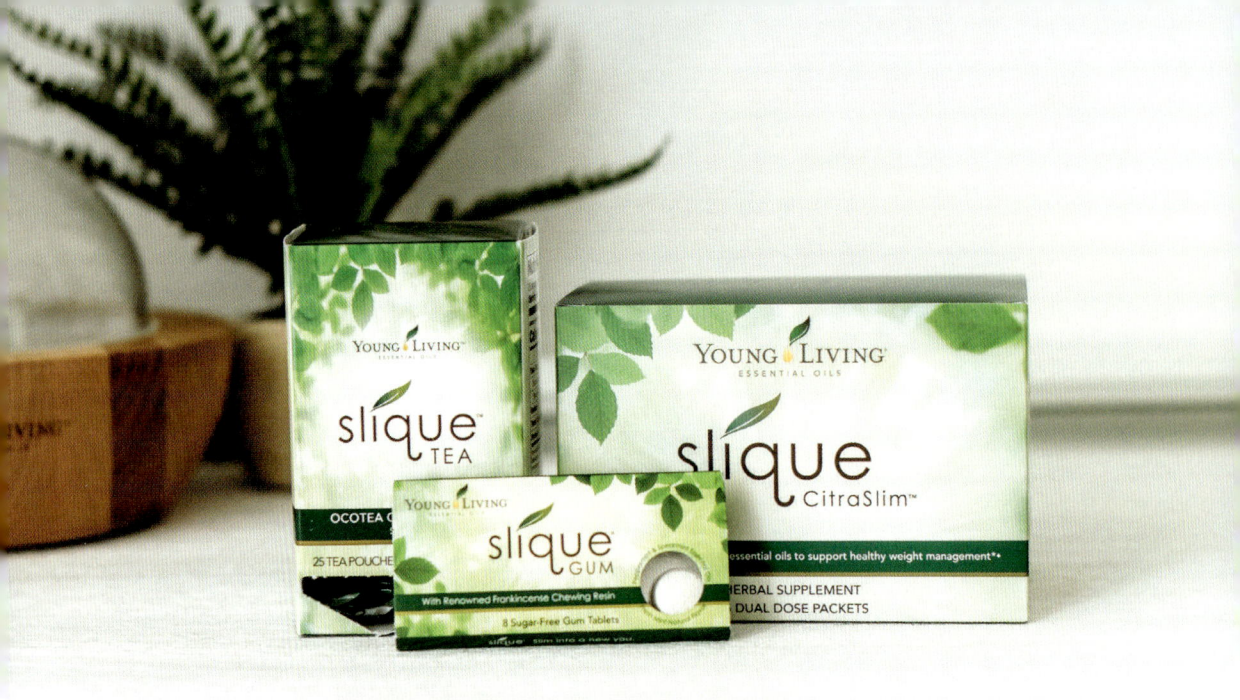

SLIQUE® PRODUCTS

The Slique® line of products is focused on assisting you with your healthy body transformation. For some, that is weight loss, whereas others are focused on increasing metabolism and mobility, and some are looking to increase lean muscle. The goal of the Slique® products is to maximize the results that you can achieve with dietary and exercise programs.

This product line includes:
- **Slique® Shake**: This is a nutrient-rich meal replacement shake.
- **Slique® Bars and Slique® Chocolate Bars**: These bars are a high-fiber snack that helps you stay full longer. It includes baru nuts, cacao nibs, goldenberries, and potato skin extract.
- **Slique® Essence**: This blend combines powerful essential oils with stevia extract and a great citrus flavor to help to satisfy your sweet tooth.
- **Slique® CitraSlim™**: CitraSlim™ is a proprietary citrus extract blend, which some studies suggest may help to support the body in burning excess fat when used in conjunction with a healthy weight-management plan.
- **Slique® Tea**: This herbal tea is formulated with Ocotea, frankincense powder, and other natural ingredients to provide a healthy alternative to sugar-laden beverages.
- **Slique® Gum:** This oil-infused gum has been formulated to help reduce cravings.
- There are also kit options that contain various combinations of the above products.

VITALITY DROPS

Young Living Vitality Drops allow you to hydrate naturally without sugar or artificial colors with the delicious flavor of essential oils. These are a great choice for those wanting extra electrolytes before, during, or after a workout, when someone is dehydrated, or any time you need some extra minerals in your routine.

The Vitality Electrolyte drops contain more than 70 naturally occurring ionic trace minerals, are flavored with essential oils, are lightly sweetened with stevia, and contain no artificial colors.

The drops are available as:
- Vitality Electrolyte Drops Grapefruit Bergamot
- Vitality Electrolyte Drops Lavender Lemonade

VITALITY DROPS+ ENERGY

Vitality Drops+ Energy provide a delicious pick-me-up that you can add to your water to keep your hydration goals on track. This blend combines Brazilian guarana seed extract, green tea, and essential oils to provide optimal levels of natural caffeine to give your hydration a little boost.

The drops are available as:
- Vitality Energy Drops Jade Lemon Berry
- Vitality Energy Drops Spearmint Tangerine

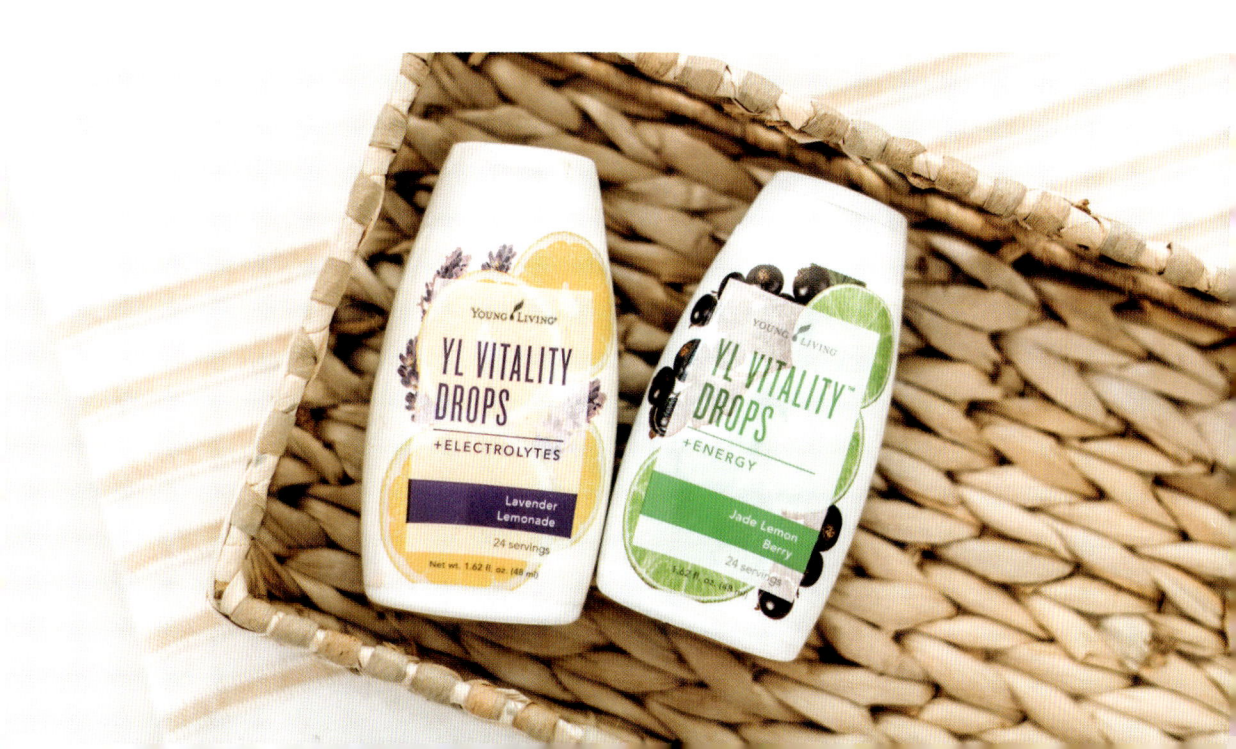

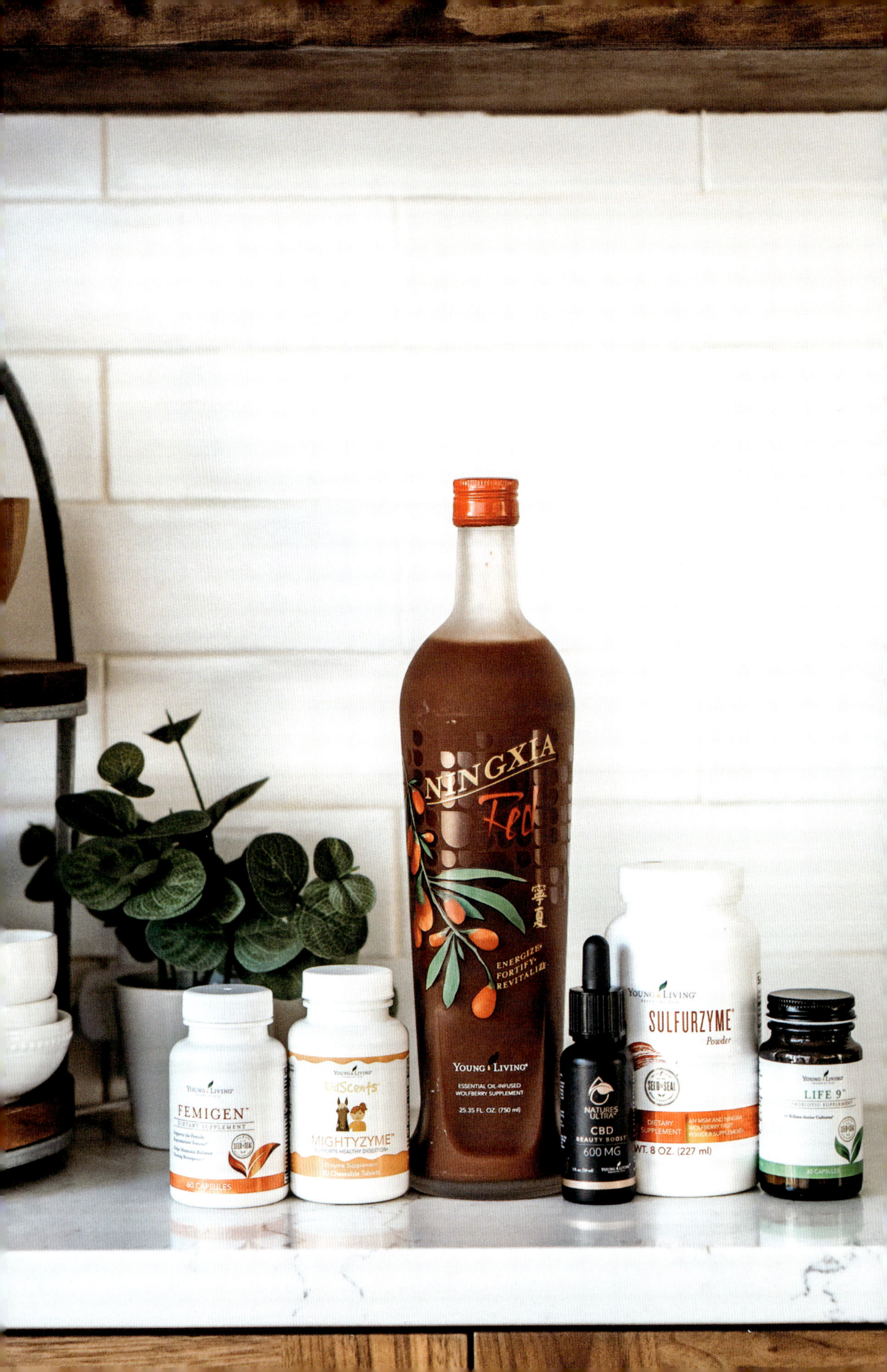
NINGXIA
Red
ENERGIZE
FORTIFY
REVITALIZE
YOUNG LIVING
ESSENTIAL OIL-INFUSED
WOLFBERRY SUPPLEMENT
25.35 FL. OZ. (750 ml)
YOUNG LIVING
FEMIGEN
DIETARY SUPPLEMENT
60 CAPSULES
KidScents
MIGHTYZYME
NATURES ULTRA
CBD
BEAUTY BOOST
600 MG
YOUNG LIVING
SULFURZYME
Powder
DIETARY SUPPLEMENT
WT. 8 OZ. (227 ml)
LIFE 9
30 CAPSULES

CHAPTER 5

PROTOCOL Suggestions

There are so many wonderful options when it comes to Young Living supplements and many ways to use them. Here are a few suggestions for various areas of support and needs to get you started. You can add in other Young Living products and essential oils to support each area as you or your provider see fit. As always, when contemplating a new supplement or health change, speak with a healthcare provider who you trust. For each of these regimens, I would suggest looking at the ingredient amounts in each supplement to determine whether you want to follow the recommended dosage or create a different plan based on your needs. For example, if you know that you need more than 1,000 IU of vitamin D daily, you can alter the protocols or the dosages of the supplements to meet your needs.

AGING SUPPORT
- BLM™ (or AgilEase® if necessary)
- Super Cal Plus™
- Golden Turmeric™
- Longevity™
- Life 9®
- NingXia Red®
- OmegaGize3®
- Sulfurzyme®

BEAUTY & SKINCARE
- Golden Turmeric™
- Life 9®
- NingXia Red®
- OmegaGize3®
- Sulfurzyme®
- Super C™
- Options for more targeted support: Progessence Plus™, CBD Beauty Boost™

CARDIOVASCULAR HEALTH
- CardioGize™
- Golden Turmeric™
- Longevity™
- MindWise™
- Mineral Essence™
- NingXia Red®
- OmegaGize3®
- Olive Essentials™
- Super Vitamin D

CHILDREN'S HEALTH
- KidScents® MightyPro™
- KidScents® MightyVites™
- KidScents® MightyZyme™
- NingXia Red®
- Super C™ Chewable
- Super Vitamin D

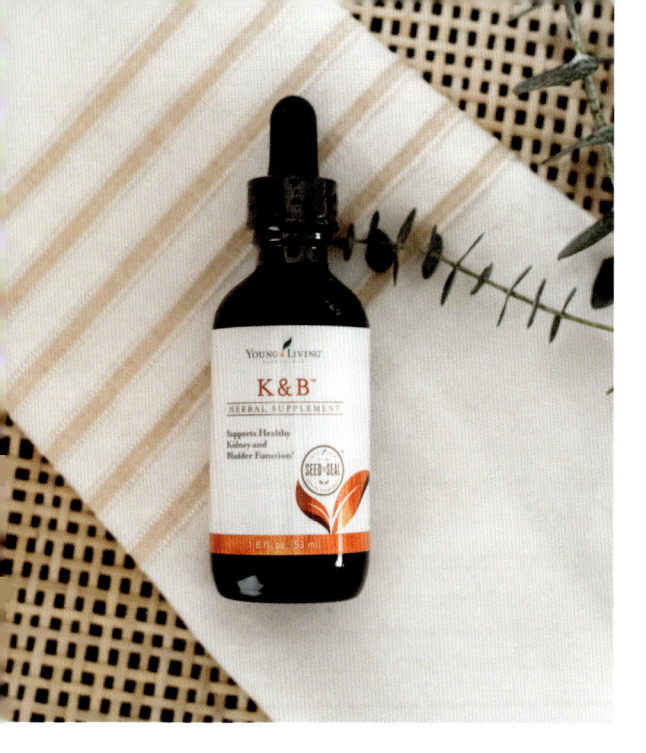

CLEANSING

- Cleansing Trio™ (use annually or as desired for a more in-depth cleanse)
- Detoxzyme™
- Digest & Cleanse™
- ICP™
- NingXia Red®
- Rehemogen™ (use as desired for cleansing)

COGNITIVE SUPPORT

- Golden Turmeric™
- Life 9®
- MindWise™
- Mineral Essence™
- NingXia Red®
- OmegaGize³®
- Super B™
- Super Vitamin D

DIABETES SUPPORT

- Golden Turmeric™
- Life 9®
- IlluminEyes™
- Mineral Essence™
- NingXia Red® (at your discretion)
- Olive Essentials™
- OmegaGize³®
- Super C™
- Super Vitamin D

OVERALL DIGESTIVE HEALTH (FOR MOST ADULTS)

- Digest & Cleanse™
- Essentialzymes-4™ (or Essentialzyme™)
- ICP Daily™
- Life 9®
- Mineral Essence™
- NingXia Red®
- Other options for more support: DiGize™ Vitality™ Essential Oil Blend, Ocotea Vitality™ Essential Oil (great for battling *Candida*)

TARGETED DIGESTIVE HEALTH

- AlkaLime® (especially helpful for those with dietary sensitivities)
- Allerzyme™ (especially helpful for those with dietary or environmental sensitivities)
- ComforTone®
- Digest & Cleanse™
- Essentialzymes-4™ (or Essentialzyme™)
- ICP Daily™
- Life 9®
- Mineral Essence™
- NingXia Red®
- Other options for more support: DiGize™ Vitality™ Essential Oil Blend, Ocotea Vitality™ Essential Oil (great for battling *Candida*)

ENERGY & VITALITY
- Golden Turmeric™
- Longevity™
- MindWise™
- Mineral Essence™
- NingXia Red®
- Super B™

IMMUNE SYSTEM (DAILY SUPPORT)
- Inner Defense® (daily as desired)
- Life 9® (separate from Inner Defense® by at least four hours, ideally eight)
- Mineral Essence™
- MultiGreens™
- NingXia Red®
- Super C™
- Super Vitamin D
- Other options for more support: Thieves® Roll-On, ImmuPower™ Essential Oil Blend

IMMUNE SYSTEM (ACUTE NEEDS)
- ImmuPro™ (take before bed)
- Inner Defense® (up to five times a day)
- Life 9® (separate from Inner Defense® by at least four hours, ideally eight)
- Mineral Essence™
- MultiGreens™
- NingXia Red® (option to increase intake during acute needs)
- Super C™ (up to three times a day)
- Super Vitamin D
- Other options for more support: Thieves® Roll-On, ImmuPower™ Essential Oil Blend, Oregano Essential Oil, Raindrop Massage (or use these oils to make a roller and/or add to an Epsom salt bath)

DAILY LIVER SUPPORT
- Balance Complete™ (use as a gently daily cleanse/meal replacement)
- ICP Daily™
- Life 9®
- Longevity™
- NingXia Red®
- JuvaPower®
- JuvaTone®
- Options for additional support: JuvaFlex™ Vitality™ Essential Oil, Lemon/Lemon Vitality™ Essential Oil, Purification® Essential Oil Blend

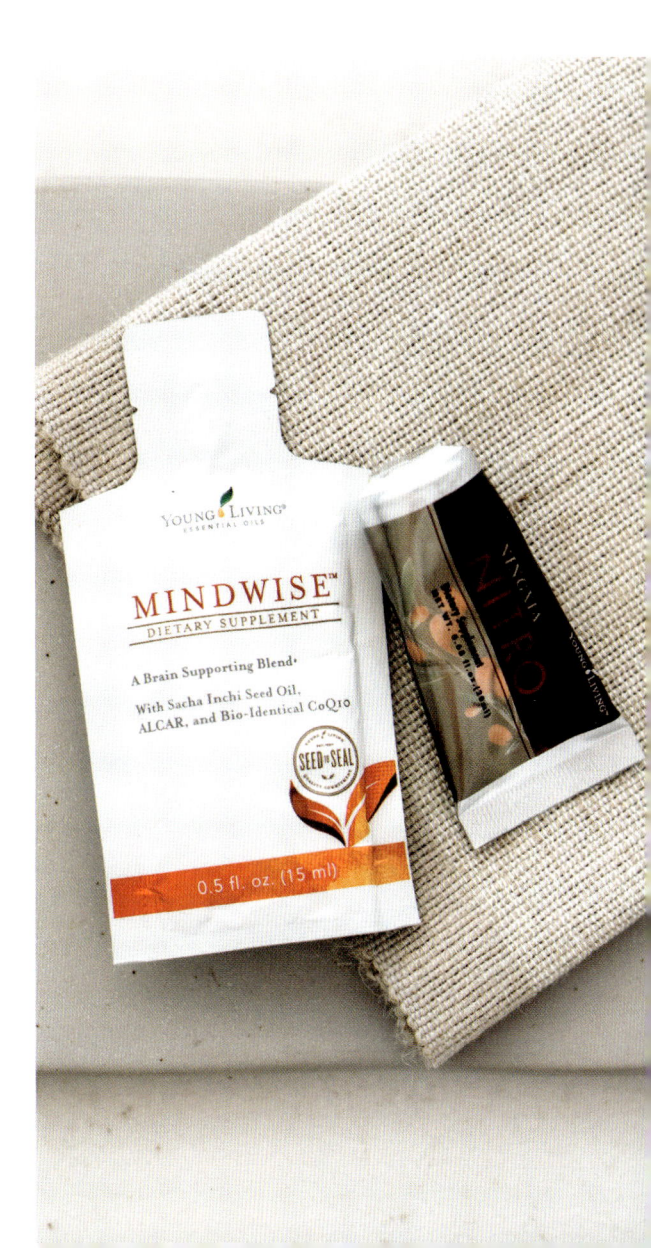

MEN'S HEALTH & HORMONE BALANCE
- Golden Turmeric™
- Life 9*
- Longevity™
- MultiGreens™
- Mineral Essence™
- NingXia Red*
- PowerGize™
- Super B™
- Super Vitamin D
- Options for more targeted support: Prostate Health™, CortiStop* (as needed for stress recovery), Shutran™ Essential Oil Blend, Idaho Blue Spruce Essential Oil, Mister™ Essential Oil Blend

MOOD & EMOTIONS
- Life 9*
- MindWise™
- NingXia Red*
- OmegaGize3*
- Super B™
- Super Vitamin D
- Options for more support: Inner Defense*, Cleansing Trio™, CortiStop*, Progessence Plus™ (women), FemiGen™ (women), EndoFlex™ Vitality™

MUSCLE & BONE HEALTH
- AgilEase* or BLM™
- Golden Turmeric™
- NingXia Red*
- Sulfurzyme*
- Super Cal Plus™
- Super Vitamin D
- Options for more support: AminoWise™, MegaCal™, Pure Protein Complete™

OVERALL WELLNESS (MALE AND FEMALE)
- Golden Turmeric™
- Essentialzymes-4™
- Life 9*
- Longevity™
- Master Formula™
- MultiGreens™
- Mineral Essence™
- NingXia Red*
- OmegaGize3*
- Super B™
- Super C™/Super C™ Chewable
- Super Vitamin D
- Note: can decrease Super B™, C, and D as desired with Master Formula™

PHYSICAL FITNESS & PERFORMANCE
- AgilEase* or BLM™
- AminoWise™
- Golden Turmeric™
- Master Formula™
- NingXia Red*
- PowerGize™
- Pure Protein Complete™
- Sulfurzyme*
- Super B™
- Super Vitamin D

PRE- AND POST-NATAL
- Life 9*
- Master Formula™
- MultiGreens™
- NingXia Red*
- OmegaGize3*
- Super B™
- Super C™ Chewable
- Super Vitamin D

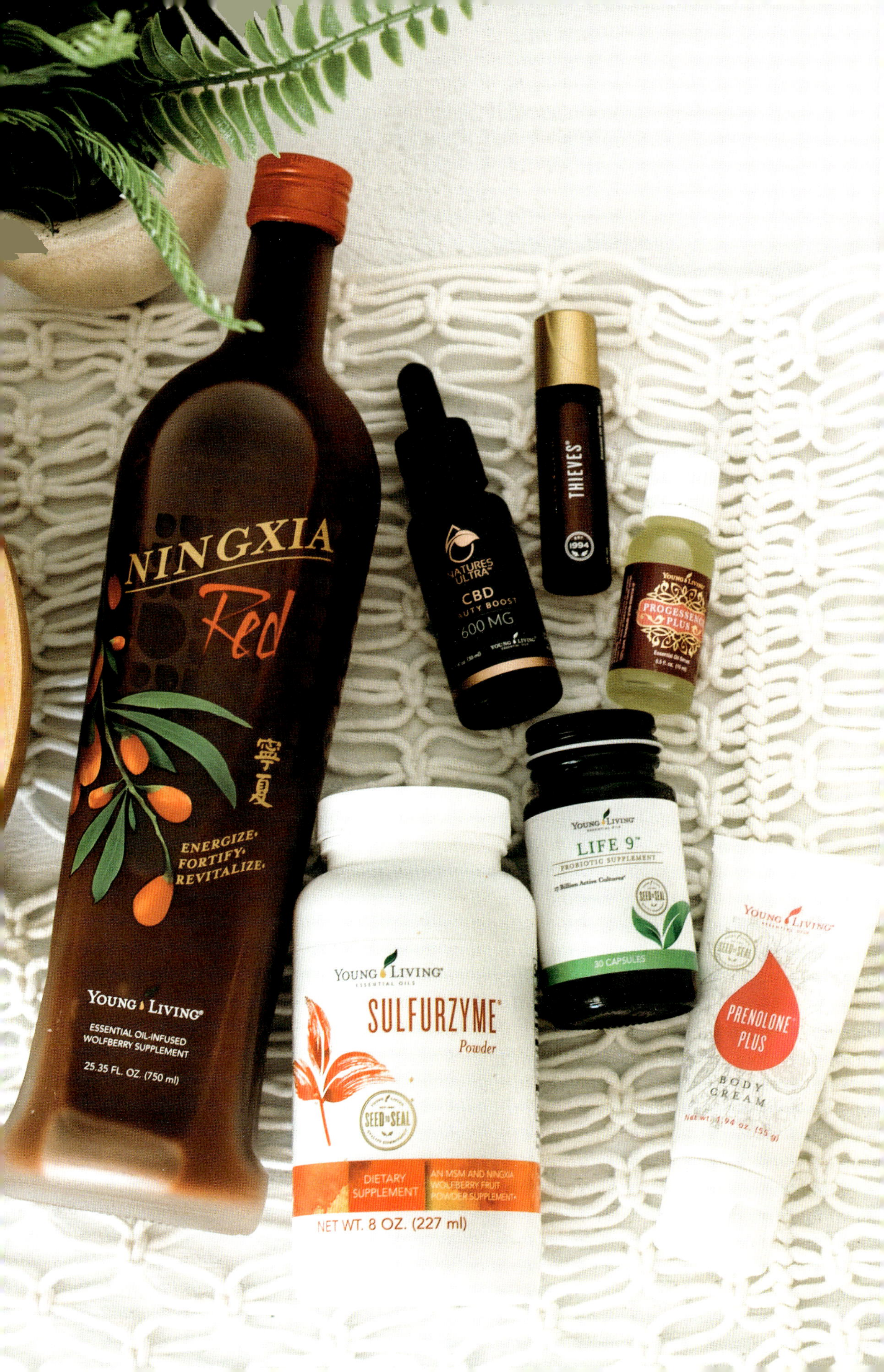
NINGXIA
Red
寧夏
ENERGIZE·
FORTIFY·
REVITALIZE·
YOUNG LIVING
ESSENTIAL OIL-INFUSED
WOLFBERRY SUPPLEMENT
25.35 FL. OZ. (750 ml)
NATURES ULTRA
CBD
600 MG
THIEVES
1994
PROGESSENCE PLUS
YOUNG LIVING
LIFE 9
PROBIOTIC SUPPLEMENT
SEED TO SEAL
30 CAPSULES
YOUNG LIVING
SULFURZYME
Powder
SEED TO SEAL
DIETARY SUPPLEMENT
AN MSM AND NINGXIA WOLFBERRY FRUIT POWDER SUPPLEMENT
NET WT. 8 OZ. (227 ml)
YOUNG LIVING
SEED TO SEAL
PRENOLONE PLUS
BODY CREAM
Net wt. 1.94 oz. (55 g)

STRESS RECOVERY
(ADRENAL SUPPORT)
- CortiStop® (intermittently)
- Golden Turmeric™
- Mineral Essence™
- NingXia Red®
- Super B™
- Super Vitamin D
- Options for more support: EndoFlex™ Vitality™ Essential Oil, Nutmeg Essential Oil

WOMEN'S HEALTH & HORMONE BALANCE
- FemiGen™
- Mineral Essence™
- Progessence Plus™
- NingXia Red®
- Sulfurzyme®
- Super B™
- Super Cal Plus™
- Optional for more targeted support: Thyromin™, Prenolone Plus™, Regenolone™ Moisture Cream

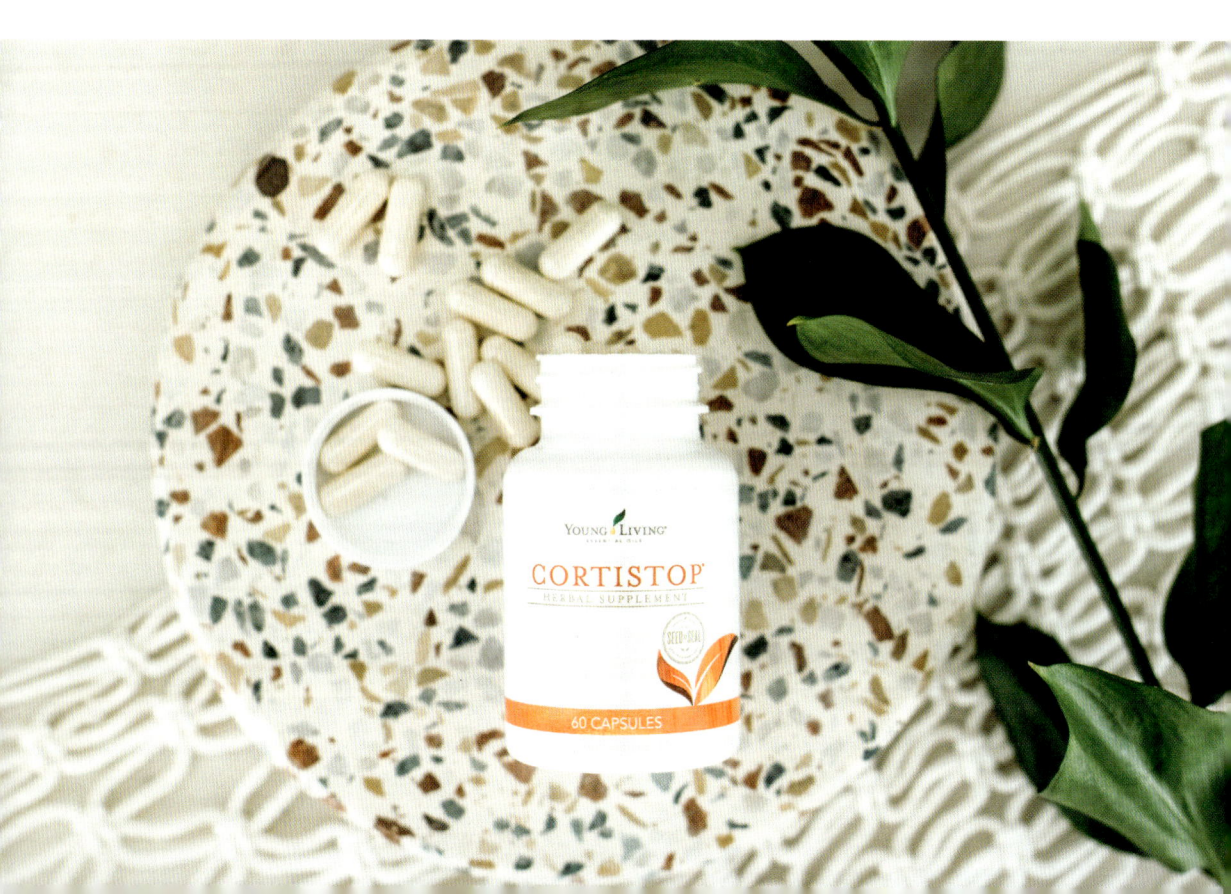

THYROID HEALTH
- Golden Turmeric™
- MultiGreens™
- Mineral Essence™
- NingXia Red®
- Sulfurzyme®
- Thyromin™
- Options for more support: Myrtle Essential Oil, EndoFlex™ Vitality™ Essential Oil

CONVENTIONAL SUPPLEMENTS
& Young Living Alternatives

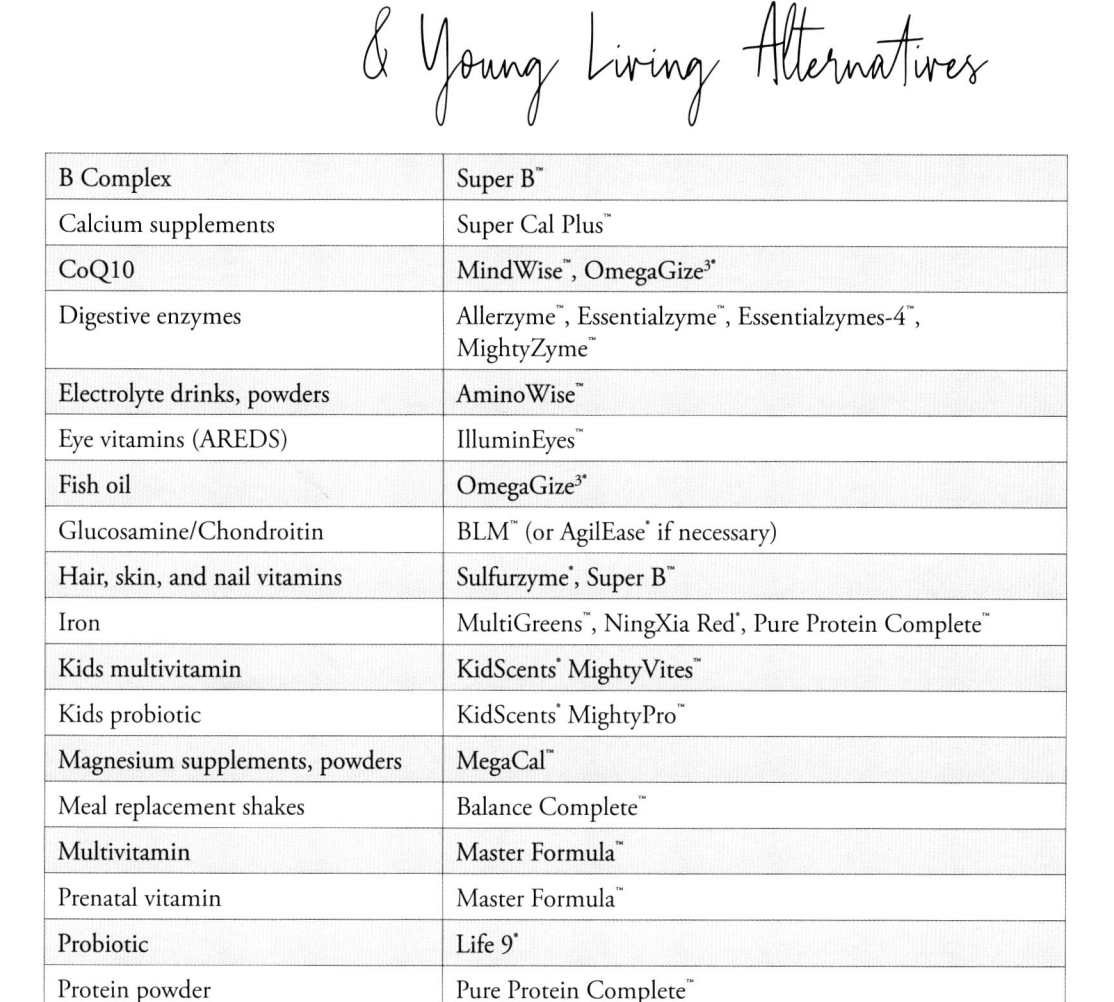

B Complex	Super B™
Calcium supplements	Super Cal Plus™
CoQ10	MindWise™, OmegaGize3™
Digestive enzymes	Allerzyme™, Essentialzyme™, Essentialzymes-4™, MightyZyme™
Electrolyte drinks, powders	AminoWise™
Eye vitamins (AREDS)	IlluminEyes™
Fish oil	OmegaGize3™
Glucosamine/Chondroitin	BLM™ (or AgilEase® if necessary)
Hair, skin, and nail vitamins	Sulfurzyme®, Super B™
Iron	MultiGreens™, NingXia Red®, Pure Protein Complete™
Kids multivitamin	KidScents® MightyVites™
Kids probiotic	KidScents® MightyPro™
Magnesium supplements, powders	MegaCal™
Meal replacement shakes	Balance Complete™
Multivitamin	Master Formula™
Prenatal vitamin	Master Formula™
Probiotic	Life 9®
Protein powder	Pure Protein Complete™
Turmeric supplements	Golden Turmeric™
Vitamin C	Super C™, Super C™ Chewable
Vitamin D	Super Vitamin D
Zinc	Mineral Essence™, Master Formula™, NingXia Red®

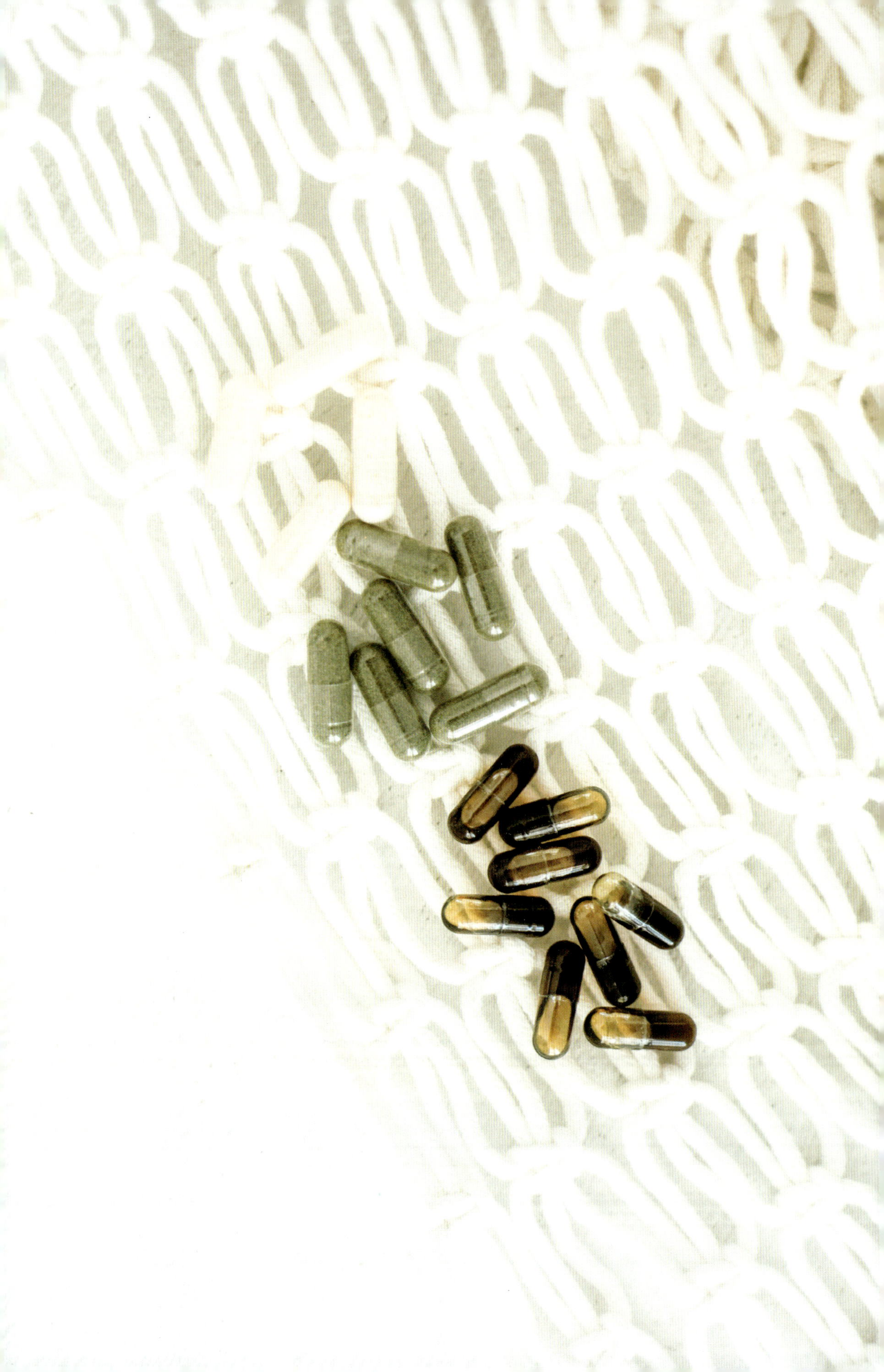

References

1. Pizzino, G., Irrera, N., Cucinotta, M., Pallio, G., Mannino, F., Arcoraci, V., Squadrito, F., Altavilla, D., & Bitto, A. (2017). Oxidative Stress: Harms and Benefits for Human Health. Oxidative medicine and cellular longevity, 2017, 8416763. https://doi.org/10.1155/2017/8416763
2. Jurenka J. S. (2009). Anti-inflammatory properties of curcumin, a major constituent of Curcuma longa: A review of preclinical and clinical research. Alternative medicine review: A journal of clinical therapeutic, 14(2), 141-153.
3. Lal, B., Kapoor, A. K., Asthana, O. P., Agrawal, P. K., Prasad, R., Kumar, P., & Srimal, R. C. (1999). Efficacy of curcumin in the management of chronic anterior uveitis. Phytotherapy research: PTR, 13(4), 318–322. https://doi.org/10.1002/(SICI)1099-1573(199906)13:4<318::AID-PTR445>3.0.CO;2-7
4. Takada, Y., Bhardwaj, A., Potdar, P., & Aggarwal, B. B. (2004). Nonsteroidal anti-inflammatory agents differ in their ability to suppress NF-kappaB activation, inhibition of expression of cyclooxygenase-2 and cyclin D1, and abrogation of tumor cell proliferation. Oncogene, 23(57), 9247-9258. https://doi.org/10.1038/sj.onc.1208169
5. Menon, V. P., & Sudheer, A. R. (2007). Antioxidant and anti-inflammatory properties of curcumin. Advances in experimental medicine and biology, 595, 105-125. https://doi.org/10.1007/978-0-387-46401-5_3
6. Biswas, S. K., McClure, D., Jimenez, L. A., Megson, I. L., & Rahman, I. (2005). Curcumin induces glutathione biosynthesis and inhibits NF-kappaB activation and interleukin-8 release in alveolar epithelial cells: Mechanism of free radical scavenging activity. Antioxidants & redox signaling, 7(1-2), 32-41. https://doi.org/10.1089/ars.2005.7.32
7. Cameron, M., & Chrubasik, S. (2014). Oral herbal therapies for treating osteoarthritis. Cochrane database of systematic reviews, 5, Art. No.: CD002947. DOI: 10.1002/14651858.CD002947.pub2.
8. Mikhaeil, B. R., Maatooq, G. T., Badria, F. A., & Amer, M. M. (2003). Chemistry and immunomodulatory activity of frankincense oil. Zeitschrift fur Naturforschung., Journal of biosciences, 58(3-4), 230-238. https://doi.org/10.1515/znc-2003-3-416
9. Hosseini Sharifabad, M., Esfandiari, E., & Alaei, H. (2004). Effects of frankincense aqueous extract during gestational period on increasing power of learning and memory in adult offsprings. Journal of Isfahan medical school (I.U.M.S), 21(71), 16-20. https://www.sid.ir/en/journal/ViewPaper.aspx?id=48926
10. Chen, Y., Zhou, C., Ge, Z., Liu, Y., Liu, Y., Feng, W., Li, S., Chen, G., & Wei, T. (2013). Composition and potential anticancer activities of essential oils obtained from myrrh and frankincense. Oncology letters, 6(4), 1140–1146. https://doi.org/10.3892/ol.2013.1520
11. Liju, V. B., Jeena, K., & Kuttan, R. (2015). Gastroprotective activity of essential oils from turmeric and ginger. Journal of basic and clinical physiology and pharmacology, 26(1), 95-103. https://doi.org/10.1515/jbcpp-2013-0165
12. Jeena, K., Liju, V. B., & Kuttan, R. (2013). Antioxidant, anti-inflammatory and antinociceptive activities of essential oil from ginger. Indian journal of physiology and pharmacology, 57(1), 51-62.
13. Liu, C. T., Raghu, R., Lin, S. H., Wang, S. Y., Kuo, C. H., Tseng, Y. J., & Sheen, L. Y. (2013). Metabolomics of ginger essential oil against alcoholic fatty liver in mice. Journal of agricultural and food chemistry, 61(46), 11231-11240. https://doi.org/10.1021/jf403523g
14. Maydych, V. (2019). The interplay between stress, inflammation, and emotional attention: Relevance for depression. Frontiers in neuroscience, 13, 384. https://doi.org/10.3389/fnins.2019.00384
15. Steenbergen, L., Sellaro, R., van Hemert, S., Bosch, J. A., & Colzato, L. S. (2015). A randomized controlled trial to test the effect of multispecies probiotics on cognitive reactivity to sad mood. Brain, behavior, and immunity, 48, 258-264. https://doi.org/10.1016/j.bbi.2015.04.003
16. Akkasheh, G., Kashani-Poor, Z., Tajabadi-Ebrahimi, M., Jafari, P., Akbari, H., Taghizadeh, M., Memarzadeh, M. R., Asemi, Z., & Esmaillzadeh, A. (2016). Clinical and metabolic response to probiotic administration in patients with major depressive disorder: A randomized, double-blind, placebo-controlled trial. Nutrition (Burbank, Los Angeles County, Calif.), 32(3), 315-320. https://doi.org/10.1016/j.nut.2015.09.003

17. Lew, L. C., Hor, Y. Y., Yusoff, N., Choi, S. B., Yusoff, M., Roslan, N. S., Ahmad, A., Mohammad, J., Abdullah, M., Zakaria, N., Wahid, N., Sun, Z., Kwok, L. Y., Zhang, H., & Liong, M. T. (2019). Probiotic Lactobacillus plantarum P8 alleviated stress and anxiety while enhancing memory and cognition in stressed adults: A randomised, double-blind, placebo-controlled study. Clinical nutrition (Edinburgh, Scotland), 38(5), 2053–2064. https://doi.org/10.1016/j.clnu.2018.09.010
18. Nisar, M. F., Khadim, M., Rafiq, M., Chen, J., Yang, Y., & Wan, C. C. (2021). Pharmacological properties and health benefits of eugenol: A comprehensive review. Oxidative medicine and cellular longevity, 2497354. https://doi.org/10.1155/2021/2497354
19. Haytowitz, D. & Bhagwat, S.. USDA Database for the Oxygen Radical Absorbance Capacity (ORAC) of Selected Foods, Release 2. May 2010, 11. http://www.orac-info-portal.de/download/ORAC_R2.pdf
20. Schroder, T., Gaskin, S., Ross, K., & Whiley, H. (2017). Antifungal activity of essential oils against fungi isolated from air. International journal of occupational and environmental health, 23(3), 181-186. https://doi.org/10.1080/10773525.2018.1447320
21. Chami, N., Bennis, S., Chami, F., Aboussekhra, A., & Remmal, A. (2005). Study of anticandidal activity of carvacrol and eugenol in vitro and in vivo. Oral microbiology and immunology, 20(2), 106-111. https://doi.org/10.1111/j.1399-302X.2004.00202.x
22. Memorial Sloan Kettering Cancer Center, Integrative Medicine: Herbs. https://www.mskcc.org/cancer-care/integrative-medicine/herbs/d-limonene
23. Sienkiewicz, M., Łysakowska, M., Ciećwierz, J., Denys, P., & Kowalczyk, E. (2011). Antibacterial activity of thyme and lavender essential oils. Medicinal chemistry (Shariqah [United Arab Emirates]), 7(6), 674–689. https://doi.org/10.2174/157340611797928488
24. Zava, D. T., Dollbaum, C. M., & Blen, M. (1998). Estrogen and progestin bioactivity of foods, herbs, and spices. Proceedings of the society for experimental biology and medicine. Society for experimental biology and medicine (New York, N.Y.), 217(3), 369-378. https://doi.org/10.3181/00379727-217-44247
25. Alamgeer, Akhtar, M. S., Jabeen, Q., Khan, H. U., Maheen, S., Haroon-Ur-Rash, Karim, S., Rasool, S., Malik, M. N., Khan, K., Mushtaq, M. N., Latif, F., Tabassum, N., Khan, A. Q., Ahsan, H., & Khan, W. (2014). Pharmacological evaluation of antihypertensive effect of aerial parts of Thymus linearis benth. Acta poloniae pharmaceutica, 71(4), 677-682.
26. Gautam, M., Agrawal, M., Gautam, M., Sharma, P., Gautam, A. S., & Gautam, S. (2012). Role of antioxidants in generalised anxiety disorder and depression. Indian journal of psychiatry, 54(3), 244–247. https://doi.org/10.4103/0019-5545.102424
27. BCM-95® Targets Anxiety and Depression; Positive Results for Natural Dosing of Curcumin for Depression. LANDING, New Jersey, November 22, 2016 via PRNewswire https://tinyurl.com/2p82brpe
28. Lopresti, A., & Drummond, P. (2017). Efficacy of curcumin, and a saffron/curcumin combination for the treatment of major depression: A randomised, double-blind, placebo-controlled study. Journal of affective disorders, 207, 188-196. https://doi.org/10.1016/j.jad.2016.09.047.
29. Akberova, S. I., Musaev Galbinur, P. I., Magomedov, N. M., Babaev, K., Gakhramanov, K., & Stroeva, O. G. (1998). Sravnitel'naia otsenka antioksidantnoĭ aktivnosti paraaminobenzoĭnoĭ kisloty i émoksipina v setchatke [Comparative assessment of antioxidant activity of para-aminobenzoic acid and emoxipin in retina]. Vestnik oftalmologii, 114(6), 39-44.
30. Goyal, S. N., Sharma, C., Mahajan, U. B., Patil, C. R., Agrawal, Y. O., Kumari, S., Arya, D. S., & Ojha, S. (2015). Protective effects of cardamom in isoproterenol-induced myocardial infarction in rats. International journal of molecular sciences, 16(11), 27457-27469. https://doi.org/10.3390/ijms161126040
31. Kieliszek, M., & Błażejak, S. (2016). Current knowledge on the importance of selenium in food for living organisms: A review. Molecules (Basel, Switzerland), 21(5), 609. https://doi.org/10.3390/molecules21050609
32. National Institutes of Health, Health Professional Fact Sheet: Zinc https://ods.od.nih.gov/factsheets/Zinc-HealthProfessional/
33. Komosinska-Vassev, K., Olczyk, P., Kaźmierczak, J., Mencner, L., & Olczyk, K. (2015). Bee pollen: Chemical composition and therapeutic application. Evidence-based complementary and alternative medicine: eCAM, 297425. https://doi.org/10.1155/2015/297425

34. Eraslan, G., Kanbur, M., Silici, S., Liman, B., Altınordulu, S., Sarıca, Z. Evaluation of protective effect of bee pollen against propoxur toxicity in rat, Ecotoxicology and Environmental Safety, Volume 72, Issue 3, 2009, Pages 931-937, ISSN 0147-6513, https://doi.org/10.1016/j.ecoenv.2008.06.008.
35. Denisow, B., & Denisow-Pietrzyk, M. (2016). Biological and therapeutic properties of bee pollen: A review. Journal of the science of food and agriculture, 96(13), 4303-4309. https://doi.org/10.1002/jsfa.7729
36. Rzepecka-Stojko, A., Stojko, J., Jasik, K., & Buszman, E. (2017). Anti-atherogenic activity of polyphenol-rich extract from bee pollen. Nutrients, 9(12), 1369. https://doi.org/10.3390/nu9121369
37. Ke, F., Yadav, P. K., & Ju, L. Z. (2012). Herbal medicine in the treatment of ulcerative colitis. Saudi journal of gastroenterology: Official journal of the Saudi Gastroenterology Association, 18(1), 3-10. https://doi.org/10.4103/1319-3767.91726
38. Araki, Y., Andoh, A., Fujiyama, Y., Kanauchi, O., Takenaka, K., Higuchi, A., & Bamba, T. (2001). Germinated barley foodstuff exhibits different adsorption properties for hydrophilic versus hydrophobic bile acids. Digestion, 64(4), 248-254. https://doi.org/10.1159/000048869
39. Farooq, S. M., Boppana, N. B., Devarajan, A., Sekaran, S. D., Shankar, E. M., Li, C., Gopal, K., Bakar, S. A., Karthik, H. S., & Ebrahim, A. S. (2014). C-phycocyanin confers protection against oxalate-mediated oxidative stress and mitochondrial dysfunctions in MDCK cells. PloS one, 9(4), e93056. https://doi.org/10.1371/journal.pone.0093056
40. Ismail, M. F., Ali, D. A., Fernando, A., Abdraboh, M. E., Gaur, R. L., Ibrahim, W. M., Raj, M. H., & Ouhtit, A. (2009). Chemoprevention of rat liver toxicity and carcinogenesis by Spirulina. International journal of biological sciences, 5(4), 377-387. https://doi.org/10.7150/ijbs.5.377
41. Sayin, I., Cingi, C., Oghan, F., Baykal, B., & Ulusoy, S. (2013). Complementary therapies in allergic rhinitis. ISRN allergy, 938751. https://doi.org/10.1155/2013/938751
42. Cingi, C., Conk-Dalay, M., & Cakli, H. et al. (2018). The effects of spirulina on allergic rhinitis. Eur Arch Otorhinolaryngol, 265, 1219-1223. https://doi.org/10.1007/s00405-008-0642-8
43. Mazokopakis, E. E., Starakis, I. K., Papadomanolaki, M. G., Mavroeidi, N. G., & Ganotakis, E. S. (2014). The hypolipidaemic effects of Spirulina (Arthrospira platensis) supplementation in a Cretan population: A prospective study. Journal of the science of food and agriculture, 94(3), 432-437. https://doi.org/10.1002/jsfa.6261
44. Ismail, M., Hossain, M. F., Tanu, A. R., & Shekhar, H. U. (2015). Effect of spirulina intervention on oxidative stress, antioxidant status, and lipid profile in chronic obstructive pulmonary disease patients. BioMed research international, 486120. https://doi.org/10.1155/2015/486120
45. Torres-Duran, P. V., Ferreira-Hermosillo, A., & Juarez-Oropeza, M. A. (2007). Antihyperlipemic and antihypertensive effects of Spirulina maxima in an open sample of Mexican population: A preliminary report. Lipids in health and disease, 6, 33. https://doi.org/10.1186/1476-511X-6-33
46. Ou, Y., Lin, L., Yang, X., Pan, Q., & Cheng, X. (2013). Antidiabetic potential of phycocyanin: Effects on KKAy mice. Pharmaceutical biology, 51(5), 539–544. https://doi.org/10.3109/13880209.2012.747545
47. Zeisel, S. H., & da Costa, K. A. (2009). Choline: An essential nutrient for public health. Nutrition reviews, 67(11), 615–623. https://doi.org/10.1111/j.1753-4887.2009.00246.x
48. Alexander, P., & Georg, W. (2009). Evidence-based efficacy of adaptogens in fatigue, and molecular mechanisms related to their stress-protective activity. Current Clinical Pharmacology; 4(3). https://dx.doi.org/10.2174/157488409789375311
49. Lee, YJ., Chung, H., Kwak, H., & Yoon S. (2008) The effects of A. senticosus supplementation on serum lipid profiles, biomarkers of oxidative stress, and lymphocyte DNA damage in postmenopausal women. Biochemical and biophysical research communications, 375(1), 44-48.
50. Park, SH., Kim, SK., Shin, IH., Kim, HG., and Choe, JY.. (2009). Effects of AIF on knee osteoarthritis patients: Double-blind, randomized placebo-controlled study. Korean J Physiol Pharmacol. 2009 Feb;13(1), 33–37. https://doi.org/10.4196/kjpp.2009.13.1.33
51. Amraie, E., Farsani, M. K., Sadeghi, L., Khan, T. N., Babadi, V. Y., & Adavi, Z. (2015). The effects of aqueous extract of alfalfa on blood glucose and lipids in alloxan-induced diabetic rats. Interventional Medicine and Applied Science IMAS, 7(3), 124-128. Retrieved Jan 31, 2022, from https://akjournals.com/view/journals/1646/7/3/article-p124.xm

52. Bora, KS., & Sharma, A. (2011). Phytochemical and pharmacological potential of Medicago sativa: A review. Pharmaceutical Biology, 49(2), 211–220. DOI: 10.3109/13880209.2010.504732
53. Kim, M. S., Kim, J. Y., Choi, W. H., & Lee, S. S. (2008). Effects of seaweed supplementation on blood glucose concentration, lipid profile, and antioxidant enzyme activities in patients with type 2 diabetes mellitus. Nutr Res Pract., 2(2), 62-67. https://doi.org/10.4162/nrp.2008.2.2.62
54. Dringen, R. (2000). Metabolism and functions of glutathione in brain. Progress in neurobiology, 62(6), 649-671. https://doi.org/10.1016/s0301-0082(99)00060-x
55. Wenli, S., Shahrajabian, M. H., & Qi, C. (2021). Health benefits of wolfberry (Gou Qi Zi, Fructus barbarum L.) on the basis of ancient Chineseherbalism and Western modern medicine. Avicenna journal of phytomedicine, 11(2), 109-119.
56. Hegarty, B., & Parker, G. (2013). Fish oil as a management component for mood disorders - An evolving signal. Current opinion in psychiatry, 26(1), 33-40. https://doi.org/10.1097/YCO.0b013e32835ab4a7
57. Giles, G. E., Mahoney, C. R., & Kanarek, R. B. (2013). Omega-3 fatty acids influence mood in healthy and depressed individuals. Nutrition reviews, 71(11), 727-741. https://doi.org/10.1111/nure.12066
58. Sanhueza, C., Ryan, L., & Foxcroft, D. R. (2013). Diet and the risk of unipolar depression in adults: Systematic review of cohort studies. Journal of human nutrition and dietetics: The official journal of the British Dietetic Association, 26(1), 56–70. https://doi.org/10.1111/j.1365-277X.2012.01283.x
59. Carr, A. C., & Maggini, S. (2017). Vitamin C and immune function. Nutrients, 9(11), 1211. https://doi.org/10.3390/nu9111211
60. Mahmoud, A. M., Hernández Bautista, R. J., Sandhu, M. A., & Hussein, O. E. (2019). Beneficial effects of citrus flavonoids on cardiovascular and metabolic health. Oxidative medicine and cellular longevity, 5484138. https://doi.org/10.1155/2019/5484138
61. Adams, M. J., Ahuja, K. D., & Geraghty, D. P. (2009). Effect of capsaicin and dihydrocapsaicin on in vitro blood coagulation and platelet aggregation. Thrombosis research, 124(6), 721-723. https://doi.org/10.1016/j.thromres.2009.05.001
62. Institute of Medicine (US) Committee on Military Nutrition Research. Military Strategies for Sustainment of Nutrition and Immune Function in the Field. Washington (DC): National Academies Press (US); 1999. 13, Vitamin E, Vitamin C, and Immune Response: Recent Advances. Available from: https://www.ncbi.nlm.nih.gov/books/NBK230984/
63. Kumar, J., Muntner, P., Kaskel, F. J., Hailpern, S. M., & Melamed, M. L. (2009). Prevalence and associations of 25-hydroxyvitamin D deficiency in US children: NHANES 2001-2004. Pediatrics, 124(3), e362–e370. https://doi.org/10.1542/peds.2009-0051
64. Bounihi, A., Hajjaj, G., Alnamer, R., Cherrah, Y., & Zellou, A. (2013). In vivo potential anti-inflammatory activity of Melissa officinalis l. essential oil. Advances in pharmacological sciences, 2013, 101759. https://doi.org/10.1155/2013/101759
65. Chung, M. J., Cho, S. Y., Bhuiyan, M. J., Kim, K. H., & Lee, S. J. (2010). Anti-diabetic effects of lemon balm (Melissa officinalis) essential oil on glucose- and lipid-regulating enzymes in type 2 diabetic mice. The British journal of nutrition, 104(2), 180-188. https://doi.org/10.1017/S0007114510001765
66. Shenefelt, P.D. Herbal Treatment for Dermatologic Disorders. In: Benzie IFF, Wachtel-Galor S, editors. Herbal Medicine: Biomolecular and Clinical Aspects. 2nd edition. Boca Raton (FL): CRC Press/Taylor & Francis; 2011. Chapter 18. Available from: https://www.ncbi.nlm.nih.gov/books/NBK92761
67. Hăncianu, M., Aprotosoaie, A. C., Gille, E., Poiată, A., Tuchiluș, C., Spac, A., & Stănescu, U. (2008). Chemical composition and in vitro antimicrobial activity of essential oil of Melissa officinalis L. from Romania. Revista medico-chirurgicala a Societatii de Medici si Naturalisti din Iasi, 112(3), 843-847.
68. Cheng, Y. C., Huang, Y. C., & Huang, W. L. (2020). The effect of vitamin D supplement on negative emotions: A systematic review and meta-analysis. Depression and anxiety, 37(6), 549-564. https://doi.org/10.1002/da.23025
69. Jarosz, A. C., & El-Sohemy, A. (2019). Association between Vitamin D status and premenstrual symptoms. Journal of the academy of nutrition and dietetics, 119(1), 115-123. https://doi.org/10.1016/j.jand.2018.06.014
70. Casseb, G., Kaster, M. P., & Rodrigues, A. (2019). Potential role of vitamin D for the management of depression and anxiety. CNS drugs, 33(7), 619-637. https://doi.org/10.1007/s40263-019-00640-4

71. Aloia, J. F., Patel, M., Dimaano, R., Li-Ng, M., Talwar, S. A., Mikhail, M., Pollack, S., & Yeh, J. K. (2008). Vitamin D intake to attain a desired serum 25-hydroxyvitamin D concentration. The American journal of clinical nutrition, 87(6), 1952–1958. https://doi.org/10.1093/ajcn/87.6.1952

72. Lim, D. W., & Kim, Y. T. (2014). Anti-osteoporotic effects of Angelica sinensis (Oliv.) Diels extract on ovariectomized rats and its oral toxicity in rats. Nutrients, 6(10), 4362-4372. https://doi.org/10.3390/nu6104362

73. Circosta, C., Pasquale, R. D., Palumbo, D. R., Samperi, S., & Occhiuto, F. (2006). Estrogenic activity of standardized extract of Angelica sinensis. Phytotherapy research: PTR, 20(8), 665-669. https://doi.org/10.1002/ptr.1928

74. Shen, J., Zhang, J., Deng, M., Liu, Y., Hu, Y., & Zhang, L. (2016). The antidepressant effect of Angelica sinensis extracts on chronic unpredictable mild stress-induced depression is mediated via the upregulation of the BDNF signaling pathway in rats. Evidence-based complementary and alternative medicine: eCAM, 7434692. https://doi.org/10.1155/2016/7434692

75. Mckoy, M.L., Thomas, P.G., Asemota, H., Omoruyi, F. & Simon, O. (2014). Effects of Jamaican bitter yam (Dioscorea polygonoides) and diosgenin on blood and fecal cholesterol in rats. Journal of medicinal food, 17. 10.1089/jmf.2013.0140.

76. Kim, M. S., Lim, H. J., Yang, H. J., Lee, M. S., Shin, B. C., & Ernst, E. (2013). Ginseng for managing menopause symptoms: A systematic review of randomized clinical trials. Journal of ginseng research, 37(1), 30–36. https://doi.org/10.5142/jgr.2013.37.30

77. Arentz, S., Abbott, J. A., Smith, C. A., & Bensoussan, A. (2014). Herbal medicine for the management of polycystic ovary syndrome (PCOS) and associated oligo/amenorrhoea and hyperandrogenism: A review of the laboratory evidence for effects with corroborative clinical findings. BMC complementary and alternative medicine, 14, 511. https://doi.org/10.1186/1472-6882-14-511

78. Nicholson, J. A., Darby, T. D., & Jarboe, C. H. (1972). Viopudial, a hypotensive and smooth muscle antispasmodic from Viburnum opulus. Proceedings of the society for experimental biology and medicine, 140(2), 457-461. doi:10.3181/00379727-140-36479

79. Saltan, G., Süntar, I., Ozbilgin, S., Ilhan, M., Demirel, M.A., Oz, B.E., Keleş, H. & Akkol, E.K. (2016). Viburnum opulus L.: A remedy for the treatment of endometriosis demonstrated by rat model of surgically-induced endometriosis. Journal of Ethnopharmacology, 193, 450-455. https://doi.org/10.1016/j.jep.2016.09.029.

80. Lee, K.B., Cho, E. & Kang, Y.S. (2014). Changes in 5-hydroxytryptamine and cortisol plasma levels in menopausal women after inhalation of clary sage oil. Phytotherapy research, 28(1), 1599-1605 https://doi.org/10.1002/ptr.5163

81. Seol, G.H., Lee, Y.H., Kang, P., You, J.H., Park, M. & Min, S.S. (2013). Randomized controlled trial for Salvia sclarea or Lavandula angustifolia: Differential effects on blood pressure in female patients with urinary incontinence undergoing urodynamic examination. The Journal of Alternative and Complementary Medicine 2013 19(7), 664-670.

82. Sá, C. M., Ramos, A. A., Azevedo, M. F., Lima, C. F., Fernandes-Ferreira, M., & Pereira-Wilson, C. (2009). Sage tea drinking improves lipid profile and antioxidant defences in humans. International journal of molecular sciences, 10(9), 3937-3950. https://doi.org/10.3390/ijms10093937

83. Brown, E. S., Park, J., Marx, C. E., Hynan, L. S., Gardner, C., Davila, D., Nakamura, A., Sunderajan, P., Lo, A., & Holmes, T. (2014). A randomized, double-blind, placebo-controlled trial of pregnenolone for bipolar depression. Neuropsychopharmacology: Official publication of the American College of Neuropsychopharmacology, 39(12), 2867-2873. https://doi.org/10.1038/npp.2014.138

84. Sharma, A.K., Basu, I., & Singh, S. (2018). Efficacy and safety of ashwagandha root extract in subclinical hypothyroid patients: A double-blind, randomized placebo-controlled trial. The Journal of Alternative and Complementary Medicine 2018 24(3), 243-248.

85. Thu, H.E., Mohamed, I.N., Hussain,Z., Jayusman, P.A., Shuid, A.N. (2017). Eurycoma Longifolia as a potential adoptogen of male sexual health: A systematic review on clinical studies. Chinese Journal of Natural Medicines, Volume 15(1), 71-80. ISSN 1875-5364.

86. Chhatre, S., Nesari, T., Somani, G., Kanchan, D., & Sathaye, S. (2014). Phytopharmacological overview of Tribulus terrestris. Pharmacognosy reviews, 8(15), 45-51. https://doi.org/10.4103/0973-7847.125530

87. Salehi, B., Upadhyay, S., Erdogan Orhan, I., Kumar Jugran, A., L D Jayaweera, S., A Dias, D., Sharopov, F., Taheri, Y., Martins, N., Baghalpour, N., Cho, W. C., & Sharifi-Rad, J. (2019). Therapeutic potential of α- and β-pinene: A miracle gift of nature. Biomolecules, 9(11), 738. https://doi.org/10.3390/biom9110738
88. Canning, S., Waterman, M., Orsi, N., Ayres, J., Simpson, N., & Dye, L. (2010). The efficacy of Hypericum perforatum (St John's wort) for the treatment of premenstrual syndrome: A randomized, double-blind, placebo-controlled trial. CNS drugs, 24(3), 207-225. https://doi.org/10.2165/11530120-000000000-00000
89. Grube, B., Walper, A., & Wheatley, D. (1999). St. John's Wort extract: Efficacy for menopausal symptoms of psychological origin. Advances in therapy, 16(4), 177-186.
90. Han, X., Gibson, J., Eggett, D. L., & Parker, T. L. (2017). Bergamot (Citrus bergamia) essential oil inhalation improves positive feelings in the waiting room of a mental health treatment center: A pilot study. Phytotherapy research: PTR, 31(5), 812–816. https://doi.org/10.1002/ptr.5806
91. Hongratanaworakit, T. (2011). Aroma-therapeutic effects of massage blended essential oils on humans. Natural product communications, 6(8), 1199-1204.
92. Suter, A., Saller, R., Riedi, E., & Heinrich, M. (2013). Improving BPH symptoms and sexual dysfunctions with a saw palmetto preparation? Results from a pilot trial. Phytotherapy Research. 27(2), 218–226. https://doi.org/10.1002/ptr.4696
93. Penugonda, K., & Lindshield, B. L. (2013). Fatty acid and phytosterol content of commercial saw palmetto supplements. Nutrients, 5(9), 3617-3633. https://doi.org/10.3390/nu5093617
94. Medjakovic, S., Hobiger, S., Ardjomand-Woelkart, K., Bucar, F., & Jungbauer, A. (2016). Pumpkin seed extract: Cell growth inhibition of hyperplastic and cancer cells, independent of steroid hormone receptors. Fitoterapia, 110, 150–156. ISSN 0367-326X. https://doi.org/10.1016/j.fitote.2016.03.010.
95. Preethi, K. C., Kuttan, G., & Kuttan, R. (2009). Anti-inflammatory activity of flower extract of Calendula officinalis Linn. and its possible mechanism of action. Indian journal of experimental biology, 47(2), 113-120.
96. Ozgoli, G., Selselei, E. A., Mojab, F., & Majd, H. A. (2009). A randomized, placebo-controlled trial of Ginkgo biloba L. in treatment of premenstrual syndrome. Journal of alternative and complementary medicine (New York, N.Y.), 15(8), 845–851. https://doi.org/10.1089/acm.2008.0493
97. Zhu, X. L., Chen, A. F., & Lin, Z. B. (2007). Ganoderma lucidum polysaccharides enhance the function of immunological effector cells in immunosuppressed mice. Journal of ethnopharmacology, 111(2), 219–226. https://doi.org/10.1016/j.jep.2006.11.013
98. Cao, L. Z., & Lin, Z. B. (2002). Regulation on maturation and function of dendritic cells by Ganoderma lucidum polysaccharides. Immunology letters, 83(3), 163-169. https://doi.org/10.1016/s0165-2478(02)00087-1
99. Iwatsuki, K., Akihisa, T., Tokuda, H., Ukiya, M., Oshikubo, M., Kimura, Y., Asano, T., Nomura, A., & Nishino, H. Lucidenic Acids P and Q, Methyl Lucidenate P, and Other Triterpenoids from the Fungus Ganoderma lucidum and Their Inhibitory Effects on Epstein–Barr Virus Activation J. Nat. Prod. 2003, 66, 12, 1582-1585, Publication Date: December 3, 2003. https://doi.org/10.1021/np0302293
100. Wachtel-Galor, S., Szeto, Y. T., Tomlinson, B., & Benzie, I. F. (2004). Ganoderma lucidum ('Lingzhi'); acute and short-term biomarker response to supplementation. International journal of food sciences and nutrition, 55(1), 75-83. https://doi.org/10.1080/09637480310001642510
101. M. Saljoughian. (2009). Adaptogenic or medicinal mushrooms. US Pharmacist: Complementary and Alternative Medicine, 34(4): HS-16-HS-18.
102. Vetvicka, V., & Vetvickova, J. (2014). Immune-enhancing effects of Maitake (Grifola frondosa) and Shiitake (Lentinula edodes) extracts. Annals of translational medicine, 2(2), 14. https://doi.org/10.3978/j.issn.2305-5839.2014.01.05
103. Wisitrassameewong, K., Karunarathna, S. C., Thongklang, N., Zhao, R., Callac, P., Moukha, S., Férandon, C., Chukeatirote, E., & Hyde, K. D. (2012). Agaricus subrufescens: A review. Saudi journal of biological sciences, 19(2), 131-146. https://doi.org/10.1016/j.sjbs.2012.01.003
104. Wang, H., Fu, Z., & Han, C. (2013). The medicinal values of culinary-medicinal royal sun mushroom (Agaricus blazei Murrill). Evidence-based complementary and alternative medicine: eCAM, 842619. https://doi.org/10.1155/2013/842619

105. Peterfalvi, A., Miko, E., Nagy, T., Reger, B., Simon, D., Miseta, A., Czéh, B., & Szereday, L. (2019). Much more than a pleasant scent: A review of essential oils supporting the immune system. Molecules (Basel, Switzerland), 24(24), 4530. https://doi.org/10.3390/molecules24244530
106. Srinivasan, V., Maestroni, G. J., Cardinali, D. P., Esquifino, A. I., Perumal, S. R., & Miller, S. C. (2005). Melatonin, immune function and aging. Immunity & ageing: I & A, 2, 17. https://doi.org/10.1186/1742-4933-2-17
107. D.H. Gilling, M. Kitajima, J.R. Torrey, K.R. Bright. (2014). Antiviral efficacy and mechanisms of action of oregano essential oil and its primary component carvacrol against murine norovirus. Journal of Applied Microbiology. https://doi.org/10.1111/jam.12453
108. Ravishankar, S., Zhu, L., Reyna-Granados, J., Law, B., Joens, L., & Friedman, M. (2010). Carvacrol and cinnamaldehyde inactivate antibiotic-resistant Salmonella enterica in buffer and on celery and oysters. Journal of food protection, 73(2), 234-240. https://doi.org/10.4315/0362-028x-73.2.234
109. Sakkas, H., & Papadopoulou, C. (2017). Antimicrobial activity of basil, oregano, and thyme essential oils. J. Microbiol. Biotechnol. 27, 429-438. https://doi.org/10.4014/jmb.1608.08024
110. Kozics, K., Bučková, M., Puškárová, A., Kalászová, V., Cabicarová, T., & Pangallo, D. (2019). The effect of ten essential oils on several cutaneous drug-resistant microorganisms and their cyto/genotoxic and antioxidant properties. Molecules (Basel, Switzerland), 24(24), 4570. https://doi.org/10.3390/molecules24244570
111. Oliveira, S., Zambrana, J., Iorio, F., Pereira, C., & Antonio, J. (2013). The antimicrobial effects of Citrus limonum and Citrus aurantium essential oils on multi-species biofilms. Brazilian oral research. 10.1590/S1806-83242013005000024.
112. Ben Hsouna, A., Ben Halima, N., Smaoui, S., & Hamdi, N. (2017). Citrus lemon essential oil: Chemical composition, antioxidant and antimicrobial activities with its preservative effect against Listeria monocytogenes inoculated in minced beef meat. Lipids in health and disease, 16(1), 146. https://doi.org/10.1186/s12944-017-0487-5
113. Frassinetti, Stefania & Caltavuturo, L., & Cini, Marianna & Della Croce, Clara & Maserti, Biancaelena. (2011). Antibacterial and antioxidant activity of essential oils from citrus spp. Journal of Essential Oil Research., 23, 27–31. 10.1080/10412905.2011.9700427.
114. Brochot, A., Guilbot, A., Haddioui, L., & Roques, C. (2017). Antibacterial, antifungal, and antiviral effects of three essential oil blends. MicrobiologyOpen, 6(4), e00459. https://doi.org/10.1002/mbo3.459
115. Yogi, W., Tsukada, M., Sato, Y., Izuno, T., Inoue, T., Tsunokawa, Y., Okumo, T., Hisamitsu, T., & Sunagawa, M. (2021). Influences of lavender essential oil inhalation on stress responses during short-duration sleep cycles: A pilot study. Healthcare (Basel, Switzerland), 9(7), 909. https://doi.org/10.3390/healthcare9070909
116. López, V., Nielsen, B., Solas, M., Ramírez, M. J., & Jäger, A. K. (2017). Exploring pharmacological mechanisms of lavender (lavandula angustifolia) essential oil on central nervous system targets. Frontiers in pharmacology, 8, 280. https://doi.org/10.3389/fphar.2017.00280
117. Bruni, O., Ferini-Strambi, L., Giacomoni, E., & Pellegrino, P. (2021). Herbal remedies and their possible effect on the GABAergic system and sleep. Nutrients, 13(2), 530. https://doi.org/10.3390/nu13020530
118. do Vale, T. G., Furtado, E. C., Santos, J. G., Jr, & Viana, G. S. (2002). Central effects of citral, myrcene and limonene, constituents of essential oil chemotypes from Lippia alba (Mill.) n.e. Brown. Phytomedicine: International journal of phytotherapy and phytopharmacology, 9(8), 709-714. https://doi.org/10.1078/094471102321621304
119. Acquaviva, R., Iauk, L., Sorrenti, V., Lanteri, R., Santangelo, R., Licata, A., Licata, F., Vanella, A., Malaguarnera, M., Ragusa, S., & Di Giacomo, C. (2011). Oxidative profile in patients with colon cancer: Effects of Ruta chalepensis L. European Review for Medical and Pharmacological Sciences, 15, 181-191.
120. Carr, A. C., & Maggini, S. (2017). Vitamin C and immune function. Nutrients, 9(11), 1211. https://doi.org/10.3390/nu9111211
121. Doseděl, M., Jirkovský, E., Macáková, K., Krčmová, L. K., Javorská, L., Pourová, J., Mercolini, L., Remião, F., Nováková, L., Mladěnka, P., & On Behalf Of The Oemonom (2021). Vitamin C-sources, physiological role, kinetics, deficiency, use, toxicity, and determination. Nutrients, 13(2), 615. https://doi.org/10.3390/nu13020615

122. Martens, P. J., Gysemans, C., Verstuyf, A., & Mathieu, A. C. (2020). Vitamin D's effect on immune function. Nutrients, 12(5), 1248. https://doi.org/10.3390/nu12051248
123. Lang, P. O., & Aspinall, R. (2017). Vitamin D status and the host resistance to infections: What it is currently (not) understood. Clinical therapeutics, 39(5), 930–945. https://doi.org/10.1016/j.clinthera.2017.04.004
124. Wynn, E., Krieg, M. A., Aeschlimann, J. M., & Burckhardt, P. (2009). Alkaline mineral water lowers bone resorption even in calcium sufficiency: Alkaline mineral water and bone metabolism. Bone, 44(1), 120-124. https://doi.org/10.1016/j.bone.2008.09.007
125. Mozaffarian, D. (2005). Does alpha-linolenic acid intake reduce the risk of coronary heart disease? A review of the evidence. Alternative therapies in health and medicine, 11(3), 24-79.
126. Satyanarayana, S., Sushruta, K., Sarma, G. S., Srinivas, N., & Subba Raju, G. V. (2004). Antioxidant activity of the aqueous extracts of spicy food additives—Evaluation and comparison with ascorbic acid in in-vitro systems. Journal of herbal pharmacotherapy, 4(2), 1-10.
127. Khalil ML. (2006). Biological activity of bee propolis in health and disease. Asian Pacific Journal of Cancer Prevention, 7(1), 22-31.
128. Vimalanathan, S., Schoop, R., Suter, A., & Hudson, J. (2017). Prevention of influenza virus induced bacterial superinfection by standardized Echinacea purpurea, via regulation of surface receptor expression in human bronchial epithelial cells. Virus research, 233, 51-59. https://doi.org/10.1016/j.virusres.2017.03.006
129. Sharma, M., Schoop, R., & Hudson, J. B. (2009). Echinacea as an anti-inflammatory agent: The influence of physiologically relevant parameters. Phytotherapy research: PTR, 23(6), 863-867. https://doi.org/10.1002/ptr.2714
130. Carson, C. F., Hammer, K. A., & Riley, T. V. (2006). Melaleuca alternifolia (tea tree) oil: A review of antimicrobial and other medicinal properties. Clinical microbiology reviews, 19(1), 50-62. https://doi.org/10.1128/CMR.19.1.50-62.2006
131. Minton, B. L. (2008). Red clover shown to improve bone mineral density and lower LDL cholesterol. https://www.naturalnews.com/025089_red_clover_estrogen_isoflavones.html
132. Hertog, M. G., Feskens, E. J., Hollman, P. C., Katan, M. B., & Kromhout, D. (1993). Dietary antioxidant flavonoids and risk of coronary heart disease: The Zutphen Elderly Study. Lancet (London, England), 342(8878), 1007–1011. https://doi.org/10.1016/0140-6736(93)92876-u
133. What are the health benefits of amino acids? How do they work? June 21, 2017 https://tinyurl.com/2yxt8yuw
134. Ispoglou, T., White, H., Preston, T., McElhone, S., McKenna, J., & Hind, K. (2016). Double-blind, placebo-controlled pilot trial of L-Leucine-enriched amino-acid mixtures on body composition and physical performance in men and women aged 65-75 years. European journal of clinical nutrition, 70(2), 182-188. https://doi.org/10.1038/ejcn.2015.91
135. Thomson, J. S., Ali, A., & Rowlands, D. S. (2011). Leucine-protein supplemented recovery feeding enhances subsequent cycling performance in well-trained men. Applied physiology, nutrition, and metabolism = Physiologie appliquee, nutrition et metabolisme, 36(2), 242–253. https://doi.org/10.1139/h10-104
136. Kalogeropoulou, D., Lafave, L., Schweim, K., Gannon, M. C., & Nuttall, F. Q. (2008). Leucine, when ingested with glucose, synergistically stimulates insulin secretion and lowers blood glucose. Metabolism: Clinical and experimental, 57(12), 1747-1752. https://doi.org/10.1016/j.metabol.2008.09.001
137. Sureda, A., Córdova, A., Ferrer, M. D., Pérez, G., Tur, J. A., & Pons, A. (2010). L-citrulline-malate influence over branched chain amino acid utilization during exercise. European journal of applied physiology, 110(2), 341–351. https://doi.org/10.1007/s00421-010-1509-4
138. Bahri, S., Zerrouk, N., Aussel, C., Moinard, C., Crenn, P., Curis, E., Chaumeil, J. C., Cynober, L., & Sfar, S. (2013). Citrulline: From metabolism to therapeutic use. Nutrition (Burbank, Los Angeles County, Calif.), 29(3), 479-484. https://doi.org/10.1016/j.nut.2012.07.002
139. Chu, C. C., Hou, Y. C., Pai, M. H., Chao, C. J., & Yeh, S. L. (2012). Pretreatment with alanyl-glutamine suppresses T-helper-cell-associated cytokine expression and reduces inflammatory responses in mice with acute DSS-induced colitis. The Journal of Nutritional Biochemistry, 23(9), 1092–1099. https://doi.org/10.1016/j.jnutbio.2011.06.002

140. Nakasone, Y., Watabe, K., Watanabe, K., Tomonaga, A., Nagaoka, I., Yamamoto, T., & Yamaguchi, H. (2011). Effect of a glucosamine-based combination supplement containing chondroitin sulfate and antioxidant micronutrients in subjects with symptomatic knee osteoarthritis: A pilot study. Experimental and therapeutic medicine, 2(5), 893-899. https://doi.org/10.3892/etm.2011.298

141. Butawan, M., Benjamin, R. L., & Bloomer, R. J. (2017). Methylsulfonylmethane: Applications and safety of a novel dietary supplement. Nutrients, 9(3), 290. https://doi.org/10.3390/nu9030290

142. Kalman, D. S., Feldman, S., Scheinberg, A. R. et al. (2012). Influence of methylsulfonylmethane on markers of exercise recovery and performance in healthy men: A pilot study. J Int Soc Sports Nutr., 9, 46. https://doi.org/10.1186/1550-2783-9-46

143. Muizzuddin N., Benjamin, R. (2020) Beauty from within: Oral administration of a sulfur-containing supplement methylsulfonylmethane improves signs of skin ageing. International Journal for Vitamin and Nutrition Research, 21:1-10. doi: 10.1024/0300-9831/a000643. Epub ahead of print. PMID: 320835221.

144. International Osteoporosis Foundation Facts & Statistics, https://www.osteoporosis.foundation/facts-statistics

145. Mayo Clinic Patient Care & Health Information https://tinyurl.com/yck5eemn

146. Mühlbauer, R.C., Lozano, A., Palacio, S., Reinli, A., Felix, R. (2003). Common herbs, essential oils, and monoterpenes potently modulate bone metabolism. Bone, 32(4), 372-380, ISSN 8756-3282, https://doi.org/10.1016/S8756-3282(03)00027-9.

147. Hebert, P., Barice, E. J., Park, J., Dyess, S. M., McCaffrey, R., & Hennekens, C. H. (2017). Treatments for inflammatory arthritis: Potential but unproven role of topical copaiba. Integrative medicine (Encinitas, Calif.), 16(2), 40-42.

148. Sunyecz, J. A. (2008). The use of calcium and vitamin D in the management of osteoporosis. Therapeutics and clinical risk management, 4(4), 827–836. https://doi.org/10.2147/tcrm.s3552

149. Ashraf, R., Khan, R. A., Ashraf, I., & Qureshi, A. A. (2013). Effects of Allium sativum (garlic) on systolic and diastolic blood pressure in patients with essential hypertension. Pakistan journal of pharmaceutical sciences, 26(5), 859-863.

150. Ried, K., Frank, O. R., & Stocks, N. P. (2010). Aged garlic extract lowers blood pressure in patients with treated but uncontrolled hypertension: A randomised controlled trial. Maturitas, 67(2), 144-150. https://doi.org/10.1016/j.maturitas.2010.06.001

151. Matsumoto, S., Nakanishi, R., Li, D., Alani, A., Rezaeian, P., Prabhu, S., Abraham, J., Fahmy, M. A., Dailing, C., Flores, F., Hamal, S., Broersen, A., Kitslaar, P.H., & Budoff, M.J. (2016). Aged garlic extract reduces low attenuation plaque in coronary arteries of patients with metabolic syndrome in a prospective randomized double-blind study. The Journal of Nutrition, Volume 146(2), 427S-432S. https://doi.org/10.3945/jn.114.202424

152. Ren, S., Zhang, H., Mu, Y., Sun, M., & Ping Liu. (2013). Pharmacological effects of Astragaloside IV: A literature review. Journal of Traditional Chinese Medicine, 33(3), 413-416. ISSN 0255-2922

153. Wang, K., Cao, P., Shui, W., Yang, Q., Tang, Z., & Zhang, Y. (2015). Angelica sinensis polysaccharide regulates glucose and lipid metabolism disorder in prediabetic and streptozotocin-induced diabetic mice through the elevation of glycogen levels and reduction of inflammatory factors. Food & function, 6(3), 902-909. https://doi.org/10.1039/c4fo00859f

154. Wang, K., Cao, P., Shui, W., Yang, Q., Tanga, Z., Zhang, Y. (2015). Angelica sinensis polysaccharide regulates glucose and lipid metabolism disorder in prediabetic and streptozotocin-induced diabetic mice through the elevation of glycogen levels and reduction of inflammatory factors. Food & function, 3. https://doi.org/10.1039/C4FO00859F

155. Tabassum, N., & Ahmad, F. (2011). Role of natural herbs in the treatment of hypertension. Pharmacognosy reviews, 5(9), 30-40. https://doi.org/10.4103/0973-7847.79097

156. Yano, S., Horiuchi, H., Horie, S., Aimi, N., Sakai, S., Watanab, K. (1991). Ca2+ Channel blocking effects of hirsutine, an indole alkaloid from uncaria genus, in the isolated rat aorta. Planta Med; 57(5), 403–405. DOI: 10.1055/s-2006-960134

157. Orhan, I. E. (2018). Phytochemical and pharmacological activity profile of Crataegus oxyacantha L. (Hawthorn)—A cardiotonic herb. Current medicinal chemistry, 25(37), 4854-4865. https://doi.org/10.2174/0929867323666160919095519

158. Hu, H. J., Luo, X. G., Dong, Q. Q., Mu, A., Shi, G. L., Wang, Q. T., Chen, X. Y., Zhou, H., Zhang, T. C., & Pan, L. W. (2016). Ethanol extract of Zhongtian hawthorn lowers serum cholesterol in mice by inhibiting transcription of 3-hydroxy-3-methylglutaryl-CoA reductase via nuclear factor-kappa B signal pathway. Experimental biology and medicine (Maywood, N.J.), 241(6), 667-674. https://doi.org/10.1177/1535370215627032

159. Verma, S. K., Jain, V., & Katewa, S. S. (2009). Blood pressure lowering, fibrinolysis enhancing and antioxidant activities of cardamom (Elettaria cardamomum). Indian journal of biochemistry & biophysics, 46(6), 503-506.

160. Ibrahim, N. A., El-Seedi, H. R., & Mohammed, M. M. (2007). Phytochemical investigation and hepatoprotective activity of Cupressus sempervirens L. leaves growing in Egypt. Natural product research, 21(10), 857-866. https://doi.org/10.1080/14786410601132477

161. Hancianu, M., Cioanca, O., Mihasan, M., & Hritcu, L. (2013). Neuroprotective effects of inhaled lavender oil on scopolamine-induced dementia via anti-oxidative activities in rats. Phytomedicine: International journal of phytotherapy and phytopharmacology, 20(5), 446-452. https://doi.org/10.1016/j.phymed.2012.12.005

162. Atsumi, T. & Tonosaki, K. (2007). Smelling lavender and rosemary increases free radical scavenging activity and decreases cortisol level in saliva. Psychiatry research, 150(1), 89-96, ISSN 0165-1781, https://doi.org/10.1016/j.psychres.2005.12.012.

163. Hassani, F. V., Shirani, K., & Hosseinzadeh, H. Rosemary (Rosmarinus officinalis) as a potential therapeutic plant in metabolic syndrome: A review. Naunyn-Schmiedeberg's Arch Pharmacol, 389, 931-949. https://doi.org/10.1007/s00210-016-1256-0

164. Age-Related Eye Disease Study Research Group (2001). A randomized, placebo-controlled, clinical trial of high-dose supplementation with vitamins C and E, beta carotene, and zinc for age-related macular degeneration and vision loss: AREDS report no. 8. Archives of ophthalmology (Chicago, Ill.: 1960), 119(10), 1417-1436. https://doi.org/10.1001/archopht.119.10.1417

165. In Brief: Dietary lutein and zeaxanthin may slow macular degeneration. Harvard Health Publishing. December 1, 2007 https://tinyurl.com/2p92kftj

166. Roberts, R.L., Green, J. & Lewis, B. (2009). Lutein and zeaxanthin in eye and skin health. Clinics in dermatology, 27(2), 195–201. ISSN 0738-081X, https://doi.org/10.1016/j.clindermatol.2008.01.011.

167. Arnal, E., Miranda, M., Johnsen-Soriano, S., Alvarez-Nölting, R., Díaz-Llopis, M., Araiz, J., Cervera, E., Bosch-Morell, F., & Romero, F.J. (2009). Beneficial effect of docosahexaenoic acid and lutein on retinal structural, metabolic, and functional abnormalities in diabetic rats. Current eye research, 34(11), 928–938. DOI: 10.3109/02713680903205238

168. National Institutes of Health, National Eye Institute. AREDS/AREDS2 Clinical Trials https://tinyurl.com/4jctstss

169. Parker, A. G., Byars, A., Purpura, M., & Jäger, R. (2015). The effects of alpha-glycerylphosphorylcholine, caffeine or placebo on markers of mood, cognitive function, power, speed, and agility. Journal of the International Society of Sports Nutrition, 12(Suppl 1), P41. https://doi.org/10.1186/1550-2783-12-S1-P41

170. Sung, M. H., Liao, F. H., & Chien, Y. W. (2018). Medium-chain triglycerides lower blood lipids and body weight in streptozotocin-induced type 2 diabetes rats. Nutrients, 10(8), 963. https://doi.org/10.3390/nu10080963

171. João Fernandes, J., Fialho, M., Santos, R., Peixoto-Plácido, C., Madeira, T., Sousa-Santos, N., Virgolino, A., Santos, O., Vaz Carneiro, A. (2020). Is olive oil good for you? A systematic review and meta-analysis on anti-inflammatory benefits from regular dietary intake. Nutrition, 69, 110559. ISSN 0899-9007, https://doi.org/10.1016/j.nut.2019.110559.

172. Cristina Nocella, C., Cammisotto, V., Fianchini, L., D'Amico, A., Novo, M., Castellani, V., Stefanini, L., Violi, F., and Carnevale, R. (2018). Extra virgin olive oil and cardiovascular diseases: Benefits for human health. Endocr Metab Immune Disord Drug Targets.18(1), 4-13.

173. De Santis, S., Cariello, M., Piccinin, E., Sabbà, C., & Moschetta, A. (2019). Extra virgin olive oil: Lesson from nutrigenomics. Nutrients, 11(9), 2085. https://doi.org/10.3390/nu11092085

174. Solfrizzi, V. Panza, F., Torres, F., Mastroianni, F., Del Parigi, A., Venezia, A., Capurso, A. (1999). High monounsaturated fatty acids intake protects against age-related cognitive decline. Neurology, 52(8) 1563. DOI: 10.1212/WNL.52.8.1563

175. Risérus, U., Willett, W. C., & Hu, F. B. (2009). Dietary fats and prevention of type 2 diabetes. Progress in lipid research, 48(1), 44–51. https://doi.org/10.1016/j.plipres.2008.10.002
176. Al-Yousofy, F., Gumaih, H., Ibrahim, H., & Alasbahy, A. (2017). Parsley! Mechanism as antiurolithiasis remedy. American journal of clinical and experimental urology, 5(3), 55-62.
177. Rerksuppaphol, S. & Rerksuppaphol, L. (2016). Effect of zinc plus multivitamin supplementation on growth in school children. Pediatrics international, 58(11), 1193-1199. https://doi.org/10.1111/ped.13011
178. Zhang, X., Zhang, R., Moore, J. B., Wang, Y., Yan, H., Wu, Y., Tan, A., Fu, J., Shen, Z., Qin, G., Li, R., & Chen, G. (2017). The effect of vitamin a on fracture risk: A meta-analysis of cohort studies. International journal of environmental research and public health, 14(9), 1043. https://doi.org/10.3390/ijerph14091043
179. Barrett, J. R., Tracy, D. K., & Giaroli, G. (2013). To sleep or not to sleep: A systematic review of the literature of pharmacological treatments of insomnia in children and adolescents with attention-deficit/hyperactivity disorder. Journal of child and adolescent psychopharmacology, 23(10), 640-647. https://doi.org/10.1089/cap.2013.0059/
180. New Study of Protein Powders from Clean Label Project Finds Elevated Levels of Heavy Metals and BPA in 53 Leading Brands. Published February 27, 2018. https://cleanlabelproject.org/blog-post/new-study-of-protein-powders-from-clean-label-project-finds-elevated-levels-of-heavy-metals-and-bpa-in-53-leading-brands/